Emerging Societies – Coexistence of Childhood Malnutrition and Obesity

Nestlé Nutrition Institute Workshop Series
Pediatric Program, Vol. 63

Emerging Societies – Coexistence of Childhood Malnutrition and Obesity

Editors

Satish C. Kalhan, Cleveland, OH, USA
Andrew M. Prentice, London, UK
Chittaranjan S. Yajnik, Pune, India

KARGER

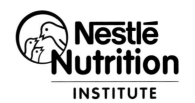

Nestec Ltd., 55 Avenue Nestlé, CH–1800 Vevey (Switzerland)
S. Karger AG, P.O. Box, CH–4009 Basel (Switzerland)   www.karger.com

Printed in Switzerland on acid-free and non-aging paper (ISO 9706) by Reinhardt Druck, Basel
ISBN 978–3–8055–9009–9
e-ISBN 978–3–8055–9010–5
ISSN 1661–6677

Library of Congress Cataloging-in-Publication Data

Nestlé Nutrition Workshop (63rd : 2008 : New Delhi, India)
  Emerging societies : coexistence of childhood malnutrition and obesity /
editors, Satish Kalhan, Andrew M. Prentice, Chittaranjan S. Yajnik.
    p. ; cm. – (Nestlé nutrition workshop series. Pediatric program,
ISSN 1661-6677 ; v. 63)
  Includes bibliographical references and index.
  ISBN 978-3-8055-9009-9 (hard cover : alk. paper)
  1. Malnutrition–Developing countries–Congresses. 2. Obesity–Developing
countries–Congresses. I. Kalhan, Satish. II. Prentice, Andrew. III.
Yajnik, Chittaranjan S. IV. Nestlé Nutrition Institute. V. Title. VI. Title:
Coexistence of childhood malnutrition and obesity. VII. Series: Nestlé
Nutrition workshop series. Paediatric programme ; v. 63.
  [DNLM: 1. Child Nutrition Disorders–epidemiology–Congresses. 2. Child.
3. Comorbidity–Congresses. 4. Developing Countries–Congresses. 5.
Infant Nutrition Disorders–epidemiology–Congresses. 6. Infant. 7.
Malnutrition–complications–Congresses. 8.
Obesity–complications–Congresses. W1 NE228D v.63 2009 / WS 130 N468e
2009]
  RA645.N87N47 2009
  362.196'39091724–dc22
                          2008052592

Basel · Freiburg · Paris · London · New York · Bangalore · Bangkok · Shanghai · Singapore · Tokyo · Sydney

Contents

Contents

Preface

The rapid transition in the developing and emerging societies has manifested as the double burden of disease: the coexistence of as yet unconquered malnutrition and the emerging epidemic of obesity and its related morbidities. A peculiar manifestation of such a double burden in a family is an undernourished child of obese parents, representing two phases of the dual nutritional insult which has led to the current epidemic of chronic non-communicable disease. The interrelationship between these two clinical entities, in spite of a large scientific data, remains to be defined. It perhaps originates in the poor care of pregnant mothers who give rise to a low birthweight baby. Attempts by the parents and the caregivers to feed this baby to 'normalize' its growth may lead to a rapid childhood growth and emergence of obesity and associated morbidities at a relatively young age which leads to higher incidence of type 2 diabetes, hypertension, dyslipidemias and coronary heart disease, the so-called metabolic syndrome. The relationship between intrauterine growth retardation and subsequent obesity, type 2 diabetes and coronary artery disease, described by Barker and colleagues, has now been confirmed in a number of different populations, especially from the developing countries in Asia, Africa and South America. It was in this context that the 63rd Nestlé Workshop was held in New Delhi, India, in order to highlight the coexistence of malnutrition and obesity in different emerging societies, to examine the origin of malnutrition and its links to obesity, to review the possible mechanisms of metabolic injury, and to evaluate the strategies for preventing the projected epidemic of non-communicable disease. Experts in their respective fields from across the world deliberated for 3 days, resulting in the enclosed summary of the state-of-the-art knowledge and the possible areas for future research. We are grateful to all the speakers and participants for a healthy, informative and scientifically exciting dialogue of the various issues. We also appreciate the support of Nestlé Nutrition Institute, in particular Prof. Ferdinand Haschke, Dr. Petra Klassen Wigger, and Elisabeth Chappuis for their support, and from Nestlé India Ltd., Natalie Wagemans and Jeji James for organizing an outstanding workshop. We hope you will find the proceedings both informative and stimulating.

Satish C. Kalhan
Andrew M. Prentice
Chittranjan S. Yajnik

Foreword

Three Nestlé Nutrition Institute Workshops have addressed the topics of obesity and malnutrition; namely the 49th NNW in 2001 on 'Obesity in Childhood and Adolescence', and 'The Malnourished Child' and 'Linear Growth Retardation in Less Developing Countries' in the 1980s. Since then, the problems of malnutrition and obesity and their associated health issues have worsened. The WHO estimates that 22 million children under 5 years of age are overweight at present. In the USA the number of overweight children has doubled since 1980. Despite an overall decrease in the prevalence of stunting in developing countries since 1980, childhood malnutrition remains at a disturbingly high level and as such a major public health problem. The coexistence of these two major public health concerns lead us to organize the 63rd Nestlé Nutrition Institute Workshop entitled 'Emerging Societies – Coexistence of Childhood Malnutrition and Obesity'.

The coexistence of undernutrition (low birthweight, poor growth) alongside overnutrition (mainly obesity) is a phenomenon afflicting many countries as their economies develop and food availability increases. This phenomenon, otherwise known as the 'nutrition transition', is becoming increasingly prevalent in many emerging nations. To date, community-based interventions are the most widely used approaches to counteract malnutrition. However, evidence is growing that interventions targeting the improvement in maternal nutrition and health may deliver the most promising results for improving child nutrition. The nutrition transition now poses the challenge of how to balance short-term benefits versus long-term risks of increased metabolic diseases. India was cited as an example to demonstrate the magnitude of potential long-term consequences, with a 300% increase in the prevalence of diabetes amounting to an estimated 80 million cases by 2025. The contribution not only of nutritional factors, but also genetic background and epigenetic factors, to these outcomes were addressed. In this context, hypotheses such as the thrifty gene hypothesis were discussed as potential mechanisms to explain the increased susceptibility to obesity in emerging nations.

Considerable research still lies ahead in order to address the question of which population segments and at what stage(s) of their lifecycle should be targeted in order to have the most impactful results.

We are deeply indebted to the three chairpersons of this workshop: Prof. *Satish Kalhan* from the Case Western Reserve University in Cleveland; Prof.

Foreword

Andrew Prentice from the London School of Hygiene, and Prof. *Chittaranjan Yajnik* from the King Edward Memorial Hospital in Pune, experts recognized worldwide in their respective fields in nutrition research. Our warm thanks go also to Dr. *Natalia Wagemans* and her team for their excellent logistic support of the workshop and for enabling the participants to enjoy the wonderful Indian culture.

Prof. Ferdinand Haschke, MD, PhD	*Dr. Petra Klassen, PhD*
Chairman	Scientific Advisor
Nestlé Nutrition Institute	Nestlé Nutrition Institute
Vevey, Switzerland	Vevey, Switzerland

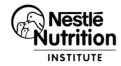

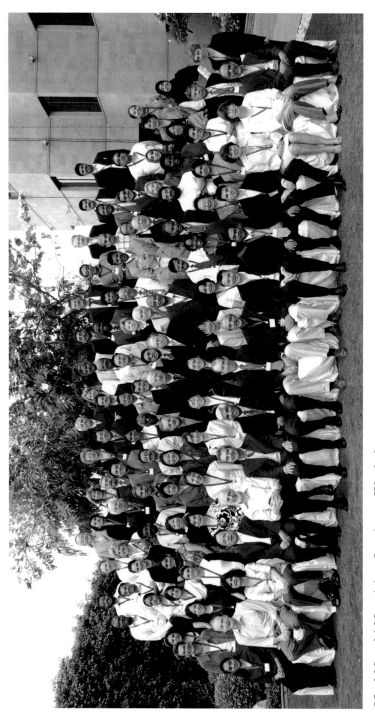

63rd Nestlé Nutrition Institute Workshop
Pediatric Program
New Delhi, March 30–April 3, 2008

Contributors

Chairpersons & Speakers

Dr. Dewan Shamsul Alam

Public Health Sciences Division
ICDDR, B
68 Shaheed Tajuddin Ahmed Sharani
Mohakhali, Dhaka 1212
Bangladesh
E-Mail dsalam@icddrb.org

Prof. Parul Christian

Department of International Health
Program in Human Nutrition
Johns Hopkins Bloomberg School of
Public Health
615 N. Wolfe Street, Rm E2541
Baltimore, MD 21205
USA
E-Mail pchristi@jhsph.edu

Prof. Satish C. Kalhan

Department of Medicine
Cleveland Clinic Lerner College of
Medicine
Case Western Reserve University
Staff, Departments of Pathobiology
and Hepatology, Cleveland Clinic
9500 Euclid Av NE-40
Cleveland, OH 44195
USA
E-Mail sck@case.edu

Prof. Arthur McCullough

Department of Gastroenterology and
Hepatology
Cleveland Clinic Lerner College of
Medicine
9500 Euclid Avenue
Cleveland, OH 44195
USA
E-Mail mcculla@ccf.org

Prof. Staffan Polberger

Neonatal Intensive Care Unit
Department of Paediatrics
University Hospital
SE–221 85 Lund
Sweden
E-Mail Staffan.Polberger@skane.se

Prof. B.M. Popkin

Interdisciplinary Obesity Center
Department of Nutrition
School of Public Health
University of North Carolina
Carolina Population Center
123 West Franklin Street
Chapel Hill, NC 27516-3997
USA
E-Mail popkin@unc.edu

Contributors

Prof. Andrew M. Prentice

MRC International Nutrition Group
London School of Hygiene and
Tropical Medicine
Keppel Street
London WC1E 7HT
UK
E-Mail andrew.prentice@lshtm.ac.uk

Prof. Marc-André Prost

MRC International Nutrition Group
Nutrition & Public Health
Intervention, Research Unit
London School of Hygiene & Tropical
Medicine
Keppel Street
London WC1E 7HT
UK
E-Mail marco@thepep.net

Prof. Eric Ravussin

Pennington Biomedical Research
Center
6400 Perkins Road
Baton Rouge, LA 70808
USA
E-Mail RavussE@pbrc.edu

Prof. K. Srinath Reddy

Public Health Foundation of India
PHD House, Second Floor
4/2, Sirifort Institutional Area
August Kranti Marg, New Delhi
India
E-Mail ksrinath.reddy@phfi.org

Prof. Ana Lydia Sawaya

Department of Physiology
Universidade Federal de São Paulo
Rua Botucatu 862, 2o andar
São Paulo, SP, 04023-060
Brazil
E-Mail alsawaya@unifesp.br

Prof. Prakash Shetty

Institute of Human Nutrition
University of Southampton
Medical School Southampton
Tremona Road
Southampton SO16 6YD
UK
E-Mail prakash.s.shetty@gmail.com

Dr. Vidya Subramanian

Naomi Berrie Diabetes Center
Department of Medicine
Columbia University
1150 St. Nicholas Avenue
New York, NY 10032
USA
E-Mail vs2223@columbia.edu

Prof. Emma Whitelaw

Division of Population Studies and
Human Genetics
Queensland Institute of Medical
Research
300 Herston Road
Herston, Brisbane 4006
Australia
E-Mail Emma.Whitelaw@qimr.edu.au

Prof. Chittaranjan S. Yajnik

King Edward Memorial Hospital
Diabetes Unit
Sardar Moodliar Road
Pune 411011
India
E-Mail diabetes@vsnl.com

Prof. Shi-an Yin

National Institute for Nutrition and
Food Safety
Chinese Center for Disease Control
and Prevention
29 Nan Wei Road, Xuanwu District
Beijing 100050
China
E-Mail shianyin@gmail.com

Moderators

Prof. Kailash Nath Agarwal

D-115, Sector-36
Noida (U.P.) 201301
India
E-Mail adolcare@hotmail.com

Dr. N.K. Arora

The INCLEN Trust
18 Ramanath Building
Yusuf Sarai
New Delhi 110049
India
E-Mail nkarora@inclentrust.org

Prof. Bhaskar Raju

No. 3, 6th Street
Thirunurthy Nagar
Nungambakkam
Chennai 600034
India
E-Mail drdhaskarraju@yahoo.com

Dr. Boindala Sesikaran

National Institute of Nutrition
Jamai Osmania Post
Hydrabad 500007
India
E-Mail dimin_hyd@yahoo.co.in

Invited Attendees

Melissa Wake/Australia
Mahmood Ahmed Chowdhury/Bangladesh
Shafiul Hoque/Bangladesh
Mutaher Ahmed Jaigirdar/Bangladesh
Mohammad Sirajul Islam/Bangladesh
Nelson Ramirez Rodrigquez/Bolivia
Carlos Nogueira De Almeida/Brazil
Roseli Sarni/Brazil
Mehmedali Azemi/Kosovo
Ramush Bejiqi/Kosovo
Hansjosef Bohles/Germany
Zulfikar Ahmed/India
Bikash Bhattacharya/India
Mridula Chatterjee/India
Sukanta Chatterjee/India
Debnath Chaudhuri/India
Dinesh Kumar Chirla/India
Ravindra Chittal/India
Sridhar Ganapathy/India
Anita Jatana/India
Veena Kalra/India
Ishi Khosla/India

Neelam Kler/India
Nitin Chandra Mathur/India
Prashant Mathur/India
John Matthai/India
Anand Pandit/India
Helina Rahman/India
Jaydeb Ray/India
Bela Shah/India
Arvind Shenoi/India
Anupam Sibal/India
Umesh Vaidya/India
Helena Ariaantje Tangkilisan/Indonesia
Mario De Curtris/Italy
Marcello Giovannini/Italy
Valerio Nobili/Italy
Sourideth Seng Chanh/Laos
Myint Myint Zin/Myanmar
Munsur Ahmud Takun/Mauritius
Endrique Romero-Velarde/Mexico
Edgar M. Vasquez/Mexico
Harrie N. Lafeber/Netherlands
Philip Olayeye Abiodun/Nigeria
Abimbola Ajayi/Nigeria

Contributors

Mariam Al Waili/Oman
S. Fancisco Lagrutta/Panama
Demetria Bongga/Philipines
Maria Lourdes Genuino/Philipines
Carla Rego/Portugal
Larisa Shcheplyagina/Russia
Ali Al-Zahrani/Saudi Arabia
Danish Khalid/Saudi Arabia
Martha Herselman/South Africa
H.T. Wickramasinghe/Sri Lanka
Voranuch Chongsrisawat/Thailand

Chongviriyaphan Nalinee/Thailand
Nuthapong Ukarapol/Thailand
Gulden Gokcay/Turkey
Alve Hasanoglu/Turkey
Leyla Tumer/Turkey
Ghazala Balhaj/UAE
Joyce Kakuramatsi Kikafunda/Uganda
Sophie Hawkesworth/UK
Mathilde Savy/UK
Atul Singhal/UK
Brian Wharton/UK

Nestlé Participants

Mr. Abdul Hanan/India
Mr. Jeji James/India
Mr. Christian Van Houtteghem/India
Mr. Leon Wagemans/India
Dr. Natalia Wagemans/India
Mrs. Marjanna Skotnicki-
Hoogland/Netherlands
Mrs. Jhody Digal/Philippines

Mrs. Alice Gravereaux/Switzerland
Prof. Ferdinand Haschke/Switzerland
Dr. Petra Klassen/Switzerland
Dr. Sophie Pecquet/Switzerland
Dr. Yassaman Shahkhalili/Switzerland
Dr. Evelyn Spivey-Krobath/Switzerland
Mrs. Zelda Wilson/UK

Kalhan SC, Prentice AM, Yajnik CS (eds): Emerging Societies – Coexistence of Childhood Malnutrition and Obesity.
Nestlé Nutr Inst Workshop Ser Pediatr Program, vol 63, pp 1–14,
Nestec Ltd., Vevey/S. Karger AG, Basel, © 2009.

Global Changes in Diet and Activity Patterns as Drivers of the Nutrition Transition

Barry M. Popkin

University of North Carolina, Chapel Hill, NC, USA

Abstract

The nutrition transition relates to broad patterns of diet, activity and body composition that have defined our nutritional status in various stages of history. The world is rapidly shifting from a dietary period in which the higher income countries were dominated by patterns of nutrition-related non-communicable diseases (NR-NCDs; while the lower and middle world were dominated by receding famine) to one in which the world is increasingly being dominated by NR-NCDs. Dietary changes appear to be shifting universally toward a diet dominated by higher intakes of caloric sweeteners, animal source foods, and edible oils. Activity patterns at work, leisure, travel, and in the home are equally shifting rapidly toward reduced energy expenditure. Large-scale declines in food prices (e.g., beef prices), increased access to supermarkets, and urbanization of urban and rural areas are key underlying factors.

The Nutrition Transition

The nutrition transition is defined as the shifts in the way we eat and move and subsequent effects on our body composition over the history of man. These broad shifts have occurred and continue to occur around the world in dietary and physical activity patterns. As noted elsewhere, much of the world's attention is focused on the three most recent patterns of the nutrition transition [1, 2]. Until the late 1980s, much of Asia and Africa followed a pattern of diet and activity linked with the 'pattern of receding famine'. Similarly, pockets of the population in Central America and much of South America and the Caribbean were living in a situation where undernutrition and communicable and parasitic diseases dominated. Today, there is a shift in the way we move, eat and drink to a situation where even the poorest countries and in most middle income transitional and all higher income countries, the populations are dominated by the emergence of nutrition-related non-communicable diseases (NR-NCDs). A major health goal today is the move away from this stage of the nutrition transition defined by 'excessive NR-NCDs' toward the 'pattern of behavioral change' where program and policy shifts lead us back toward a healthier lifestyle and reduced adiposity and NR-NCDs. In many ways we want to shift our dietary patterns closer to that of the early hunter-gatherers which focused on plant foods and lean animal source foods.

Around the world, dietary shifts have occurred at various times and rates of change. There are a number of major shifts that are occurring across the lower and middle income world. Within each shift, however, the foods and beverages driving the changes and even the eating behaviors are quite heterogeneous over space.

The Dietary Drivers: More Fats, More Added Caloric Sweeteners, More Animal Source Foods

The Edible Oil Revolution

While a large shift toward increased consumption of edible vegetable oils occurred in the higher income countries in the 1950–1980 period, edible oil has been a major source of dietary change in the lower and middle income countries in the last several decades. The recent shift in the pattern of the nutrition transition in developing countries typically begins with major increases in the domestic production and imports of oilseeds and vegetable oils, rather than meat and milk. Elsewhere, I have written in more depth about the technology behind this shift and the broader nature of these changes in both oil seed extraction technology as well as breeding of new oil seed varieties containing more oil [3]. Principal vegetable oils include soybean, sunflower, rapeseed, palm, and groundnut oil. With the exception of groundnut oil, the global availability of each approximately tripled between 1961 and 1990, and has continued to increase since then though at a slightly reduced global pace.

This dramatic change arose principally from a major increase in the consumption of vegetable fats. The intake of edible oil has increased consistently over the past 15 years. In fact, in some developing countries we have documented an upwards shift in the income elasticity for all groups and a higher one for the poor[4]. In table 1 we present data on the large increase in edible oil intake in China where the major oils are soybean oil and rapeseed oil. The intake for young adults more than doubled to close to 280 kcal of edible oil per day.

Caloric Sweeteners

Sugar is the world's predominant sweetener though its history as the dominant sweetener is only a few centuries old and there are now rapid increases

Table 1. Dietary and physical activity trends of Chinese adults aged 20–45 years

	1989	2006
Food consumption		
Plant oils, g/day	014.8	030.9
All calories per capita from edible oil, %	004.9	012.4
Beef and pork, g/day	052.1	070.6
Poultry, g/day	004.4	009.3
Fish and other aquatic products, g/day	014.4	018.3
Eggs, g/day	009.4	025.1
Dairy, g/day	001.6	011.6
Total animal source foods	102.4	140.5
Physical activity		
Adults in light level occupations, %	024.7	040.0
Households with color TV, %	020.5	095.7
Households with washing machine, %	036.8	072.8
Households with refrigerator, %	013.3	052.7

Source: China Health and Nutrition Survey.

in many other caloric sweeteners. For this article we use the term 'caloric sweetener' instead of added sugar, as there is such a range of non-sugar products used today.

Globally, our research has shown that in 2000, 306 kcals were available for food consumption on a per person per day basis, about a third more than in 1962; caloric sweeteners also accounted for a larger share of both total energy and total carbohydrates consumed [5]. These global figures seem to greatly underestimate the consumption found when one uses detailed food composition data that measure the added sugar in each food item and measure nationally representative dietary intake data for any country. There are only a few countries that have the data to measure added sugar at the individual level and are presented in the examples below.

Figure 1 shows the relationship between the proportion of energy from different food sources and the gross national product for two different levels of urbanization [for a description of the analysis see, 3]. In figure 1a (the less urbanized case) the share of sweeteners increases sharply with income from about 5 to about 15%. In the more urbanized case (fig. 1b), the share is much higher at a lower income (>15%), and hardly increases with income.

We have measured added sugars much more carefully in the US diet. In a recent study we examined added sugars in all foods and beverages and the changes that occurred between 1965 and 2002. In the US there has been a very large increase in both the availability and consumption of high fructose corn syrup and added sugar since 1965 until a slight decline between 2000 and 2004. In the US today the average American consumes 377 kcal/day from added sugar. This represents 16.8% of all calories. Even more important,

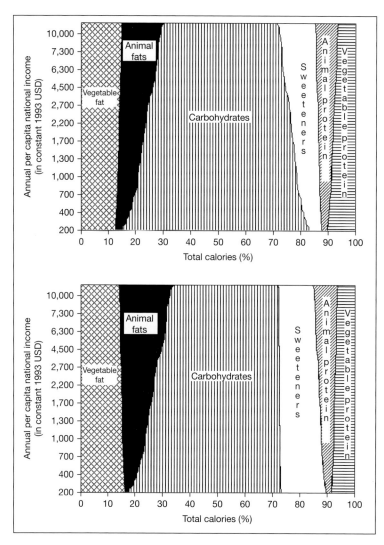

Fig. 1. Relationship between the proportion of energy from each food source and gross national product per capita and urbanization. (*a*) The proportion of the population residing in urban areas is placed at 25% (1990). (*b*) The proportion of the population residing in urban areas is placed at 75% (1990). Sources: Drewnowski and Popkin [3]; food balance data from the FAOUN; gross national product data from the World Bank; regression work by UNC-CH.

among the top 20% of individuals, 896 kcal/person and day of added sugar was consumed [6].

What is most important is the shift in the US in the source of these kilocalories of added caloric sweeteners from foods to beverages. Coke and Pepsi

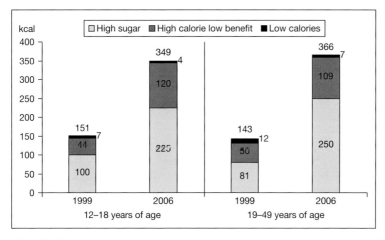

Fig. 2. Beverage consumption trends of Mexican adolescents and adult women, 1999 and 2006. High sugar is composed mainly of soft drinks, sweetened juices, agua frescas and alcohol; high calorie and low benefit is mainly whole milk, and low calories are slightly sweetened coffee and skim milk. Source: Barquera et al. [9] from nationally representative samples of the National Nutrition survey 1999 and 2006.

are global symbols of this shift in how we drink. We have seen a shift in the US since 1965 with a third of our caloric sweeteners coming from beverages to over two thirds. Essentially, in the US over the 1965–2002 period an added 228 cal/day came from caloric beverages and over two thirds of this shift are from sugared drinks [7].

Other countries that have studied aspects of added caloric sweeteners in our diets are Mexico and South Africa [8]. In Mexico, we have completed several analyses of caloric beverage patterns and trends. Mexican adolescents and adults consumed 20.1 and 22.3%, respectively, of their calories from caloric beverages. Whole milk, carbonated and noncarbonated sugared beverages, fruit juice with various sugar and water combinations added, and alcohol represented the four major categories of beverage intake. Unlike the US where soft drinks and other calorically sweetened drinks are dominant, in Mexico sugar added to an array of juice drinks is another major element [9]. A key aspect of Mexico is the more than doubling of intake of caloric beverages between 1999 and 2006 and the potential for far greater increases into the future. Figure 2 shows the trends in caloric beverage intake in Mexico. Another country where juice dominates as the source of caloric beverages is Australia [10].

The shift to beverages as the source of calories is particularly important because they do not sate us and there is an emerging consensus that calories from beverages are a potential source of energy imbalance globally [11]. This is true whether the calories come from high-fat, high-protein or high-carbohydrate beverages.

5

Animal Source Foods

The revolution in animal source foods refers to the increase in demand and production of meat, poultry, fish, and milk in low income developing countries. Delgado [12] has studied this issue extensively in a number of seminal reports and papers. Most of the world's growth in production and consumption of these foods comes from developing countries. Thus, developing countries will produce 63% of meat and 50% of milk in 2020. By 2020, developing countries will consume 107 million metric tons (mmt) more meat and 177 mmt more milk than they did in 1996–1998, dwarfing developed country increases of 19 mmt for meat and 32 mmt for milk. It is a global food activity, transforming the grain markets for animal feed. It also leads to resource degradation, rapid increases in feed grain imports, rapid concentration of production and consumption and social change.

Delgado [12] has shown that the share of the world's meat consumed in developing countries rose from 37 to 48%, and their share of the world's milk rose from 34 to 44%. Pork and poultry accounted for 76% of the large net consumption increase of meat in developing countries from 1982–1984 to 1996–1998.

There are different developing countries that dominate consumption for different animal products. China and Brazil play this role in meat consumption, while India is the key milk consumer. In the mid-1990s, Indian milk consumption amounted to 13% of the world's total and 31% of milk consumption in all developing countries [12]. Table 1 provides data for trends in major components of animal source food intake in China. In China the increase in daily intake per day is over 38 g of animal source foods. Egg and diary intake have been particularly dramatic.

Underlying Eating Behaviors

While there has been extensive research on the economic, sociological, and demographic factors underlying these trends, the shifts in how we eat and how we prepare our food are equally profound, but poorly studied. The critical issues vary in their importance across the globe; however, it is clear that the changes seen in the US, Japan, and Europe are found globally at increasingly earlier stages of each country's economic development. The key issues are:

- We eat more times in a day with snacking events shifting from episodically to 1–3 times/day
- The energy density of snacks has shifted upwards much faster than that for meals. Processed, fried salty snacks, and caloric beverages are the two dominant changes
- Processed foods are replacing unprocessed ones with a large shift toward refined carbohydrates
- Frying and grilling are replacing healthier elements such as boiling and steaming

- Away-from-home consumption and preparation are dominating as the major growth elements and the art of cooking from natural ingredients is losing ground

These trends have been studied extensively in higher income countries; however, few careful studies on these behaviors have occurred in the lower and middle income world [13, 14]. This is in large measure because the collection of nationally representative or large studies of individual dietary intake are infrequent in most low and middle income countries. For instance, India with a population of over a billion does not have a national nutrition monitoring system or any national dietary intake survey system. India does have nationally representative income and expenditure surveys and a rural survey in 9 states that collects limited dietary data. It also has had two nationally representative surveys that collected weight and height data for preschoolers and women of child-bearing age. This is true for many of the world's largest countries. For instance, Brazil and Nigeria, two countries with over 178 and 124 million, respectively, do not have national dietary surveys. China and Mexico, in contrast, do have such nationally representative nutrition surveys that collect dietary data for all individuals.

Physical Activity Dynamics: Changes in the Technology of Work and Movement and Leisure

If individual dietary data are not collected in most low and middle income countries, there is a much greater scarcity of overall measures of physical activity and inactivity. The China Health and Nutrition Survey is one of the very few large scale surveys globally that collects detailed activity data from all age-gender groups. In higher income countries the focus is mainly on the collection of leisure activity and TV viewing, which represent a limited component of overall physical activity. As I show below, there is important variability in activity in all dimensions of life and each has important effects on energy imbalance.

Work at Home
While most of our focus has been on market work and the way this has changed, there are equally large shifts in home production. Time in food preparation has declined over the past half century from about 2 h/day to less than a half hour in the US and variable amounts elsewhere. A vast array of home production technologies from gas and electric stoves to microwaves, cuisinarts, rice cookers, and pressure cookers have reduced the time and effort required in food preparation. The vacuum cleaner, washing machine, and refrigerator have cut time in cleaning and shopping. As Chinese households have obtained these assets, we have found a significant weight gain associated with them [15].

Market Work

Economic work or market work represents one of the areas with the largest shifts in energy expenditures at the population level. The proportion of individuals working in energy expenditure-intensive jobs such as farming, mining, and forestry is way down while manufacturing has increased slightly, but the major shift is toward lower activity service sector jobs. Both lower income and higher income countries have experienced this shift [16]. Equally important has been a major shift in the activity of all occupations. New technology – be it small gas tractors or spraying systems for insecticides for farmers, or computers, faxes for service sector jobs – have led to major declines in activity at the same jobs. For instance, over the 1989–2006 period the proportion of urban Chinese in occupations with light levels of activity has increased from 24.7 to 40% of adults in the 20–45 year age group (table 1) [17].

Transport Shifts from Active to Passive

In most countries the proportion of individuals walking to work or shopping and other activities has declined drastically. In China the shift is from walking and biking to bus, motorcycle, and car use. These shifts again more than double the risk of overweight [18]. There is a great deal of discussion about active transport, namely walking and biking, as a key dimension of activity to promote. However, only in a few high income countries do we have measures of the effects of walking or biking on weight dynamics.

Leisure Is a Major Global Focus for Obesity Control but Is It Earned

We focus far too much attention on attempting to enhance our activity by active leisure pursuits while ignoring all the other dimensions of movement during the day. Part of this is related to the extensive focus on TV viewing. A vast literature has linked TV viewing with increased weight gain; however, most of this has focused on high income countries and there are few studies in higher income countries of other dimensions of activity [19, 20]. In higher income countries there is a focus on promoting walking as a leisure activity. Research at University of North Carolina on women followed for 15 years has shown that walking 2 h/week is linked with 4 kg less weight gain than among those with no walking [21].

There is surprisingly little research in higher income countries of the effect of home production, market work, or even transportation shifts on weight dynamics.

Underlying Environmental Reality

Crime, Pollution and Traffic

Keeping children at home to protect them from crime and the dangers of heavy traffic have been shown to be important in selected studies. For example, in the US, crime has been found to be a key determinant of not just the level of reduced moderate to vigorous physical activity, but also of increased TV viewing time [22–24].

Urban Design

The creation of cities and smaller communities with a focus on low con-nectivity neighborhoods lacking sidewalks and encouraging car use is a com-mon focus. A large number of studies have suggested this is a major issue, but some recent research suggests this might not be such a clear-cut issue [25, 26].

Household Time-Saving Assets and Television Sets

Television and dozens of other time-saving assets represent a major change in the lower and middle income world. The changes in China mirror those throughout Asia. Virtually every household in China has a television set. In fact, by 2006 over 95% of the households had color TV sets. Similarly, the pro-portion of households with washing machines doubled to almost 73% and the proportion with refrigerators increased to more than half of the households (table 1).

Conclusions

Clearly there is great potential that both dietary and physical activity and inactivity patterns are drivers of the growing global shift from a nutrition transition pattern associated with undernutrition to one linked with obesity and other NR-NCDs.

In the dietary area we have limited evidence of trends in eating behavior across the globe; however, there are far less data on overall activity and inac-tivity pattern trends. We have extensive data on total leisure time and TV viewing but little else.

References

1 Popkin B: Nutritional patterns and transitions. Pop Devel Rev 1993;19:138–157.
2 Popkin BM: Global nutrition dynamics: the world is shifting rapidly toward a diet linked with noncommunicable diseases. Am J Clin Nutr 2006;84:289–298.
3 Drewnowski A, Popkin BM: The nutrition transition: new trends in the global diet. Nutr Rev 1997;55:31–43.
4 Du S, Mroz TA, Zhai F, Popkin BM: Rapid income growth adversely affects diet quality in China–particularly for the poor! Soc Sci Med 2004;59:1505–1515.
5 Popkin BM, Nielsen SJ: The sweetening of the world's diet. Obes Res 2003;11:1325–1332.
6 Duffey K, Popkin BM: High-fructose corn syrup: is this what's for dinner? Am J Clin Nutr, in press.
7 Duffey K, Popkin B: Shifts in patterns and consumption of beverages between 1965 and 2002. Obesity 2007;15:2739–2747.

8 Steyn NP, Myburgh NG, Nel JH: Evidence to support a food-based dietary guideline on sugar consumption in South Africa. Bull World Health Organ 2003;81:599–608.
9 Barquera S, Campirano F, Bonvecchio A, et al: Trends and characteristics of caloric beverage consumption in Mexican pre-school and school age children. Cuernevaca,Sanigorski AM, Bell AC, Swinburn BA: Association of key foods and beverages with obesity in Australian school-children. Public Health Nutr 2007;10:152–157.
10 Sanigorski AM, Bell AC, Swinburn BA: Association of key foods and beverages with obesity in Australian schoolchildren. Public Health Nutr 2007;10:152--157.
11 Mourao DM, Bressan J, Campbell WW, Mattes RD: Effects of food form on appetite and energy intake in lean and obese young adults. Int J Obes (Lond) 2007;31:1688–1695.
12 Delgado CL: Rising consumption of meat and milk in developing countries has created a new food revolution. J Nutr 2003;133:3907S–3910S.
13 Wang Z, Zhai F, Du S, Popkin B: Dynamic shifts in Chinese eating behaviors. Asia Pac J Clin Nutr 2008;17:123–130.
14 Adair LS, Popkin BM: Are child eating patterns being transformed globally? Obes Res 2005;13:1281–1299.
15 Monda KL, Adair LS, Zhai F, Popkin BM: Longitudinal relationships between occupational and domestic physical activity patterns and body weight in China. Eur J Clin Nutr 2007 Jul 18, Epub ahead of print. DOI: 10.1038/sj.ejcn.1602849.
16 Popkin BM: Urbanization, lifestyle changes and the nutrition transition. World Dev 1999;27:1905–1916.
17 Bell AC, Ge K, Popkin BM: Weight gain and its predictors in Chinese adults. Int J Obes Relat Metab Disord 2001;25:1079–1086.
18 Bell AC, Ge K, Popkin BM: The road to obesity or the path to prevention: motorized transportation and obesity in China. Obes Res 2002;10:277–283.
19 Food and Nutrition Board: Preventing Childhood Obesity: Health in the Balance. Washington, National Academy Press, 2004.
20 World Health Organization: Obesity: preventing and managing the global epidemic. Report of a WHO consultation. World Health Organ Tech Rep Ser 2000;894:i–xii, 1–253.
21 Gordon-Larsen P, Hou N, Sidney S, et al: Fifteen-year longitudinal trends of walking patterns and their impact on weight change. Am J Clin Nutr, in press.
22 Gordon-Larsen P, McMurray RG, Popkin BM: Determinants of adolescent physical activity and inactivity patterns. Pediatrics 2000;105:E83.
23 Gomez JE, Johnson BA, Selva M, et al: Violent crime and outdoor physical activity among inner-city youth. Prev Med 2004;39:876–881.
24 Owen N, Humpel N, Leslie E, et al: Understanding environmental influences on walking: review and research agenda. Am J Prev Med 2004;27:67–76.
25 Rodriguez DA, Khattak AJ, Evenson KR: Can new urbanism encourage physical activity? Comparing a new urbanist neighborhood with conventional suburbs. J Am Plan Assoc 2006;72:43–54.
26 Frank LD, Schmid TL, Sallis JF, et al: Linking objectively measured physical activity with objectively measured urban form: Findings from SMARTRAQ. Am J Prev Med 2005;28:117–125.

Discussion

Dr. Agarwal: The experiences from China and other countries have been very illuminating. Over 1.3 billion people are overweight, and there is a pattern of nutrition transition in terms of more caloric and fat food and lesser activity, which is really hazardous to health. You gave an example of how things can be improved; in Australia the increase in obesity is 1.3%/year and in Mexico 1.9%. In Mexico the consumption of soft drinks and other caloric beverages was very high, but now there is a shift to using skim milk. So there is a way to improve things. This lecture opens many questions.

Dr. Prentice: I want to go straight to your challenge at the end of your talk. You painted an overwhelming picture of a global juggernaut. How are we going to turn that around? You clearly said that there will be different approaches in different nations and that is well taken. But I wonder if you could start by pointing out some countries in which the obesity rates have at least stabilized or may be decreasing, and trying to show what lessons we might learn from those?

Dr. Popkin: To the best of my knowledge there is only one country in which obesity rates are truly declining in a large segment of the population, and that is among educated women in Brazil, and that is only in two thirds of the Brazilian population, aside from the poor in the northeast. The data show that the rates have increased slowly in Scandinavia, but there is really not a single country where we've managed to turn it around and pull back on the adiposity increases. There are countries that are taking on very aggressive stances right now, for example Mexico. With the Mexican Minister of Health we set up a beverage guidance panel that essentially created a set of guidelines to cut calories from beverages and the country is very aggressively moving on them. Whole milk has already been replaced by 1.5% milk in programs that feed around 20 million people, and will move to 0.5%, close to skim milk, in a year. The same is being done in the schools there. The government is moving now to tax sugar added in beverages and fat added in milk. So Mexico is a country in which caloric beverages are a key part of their huge caloric increases, and it is aggressively taking it on. Today very few countries have the guts and focus of Mexico to try and directly regulate anything on at a national level, other than trying to regulate the mass media.

Dr. Sawaya: As you mentioned very well-educated Brazilian women decreased obesity by avoiding processed food as much as possible and going back to the old traditional staple Brazilian diet which is rice, beans, fruits, legumes. Brazil is also a tropical country where body image and high physical activity are very important. My question is about sweeteners. Were you talking about artificial sweeteners and how important do you think they are?

Dr. Popkin: The sweetener question is a very complex scientific issue today. We actually know very little about the role of sweeteners in our diet, and they are increasing immensely. The receptors that are affected by intense diet sweeteners are exactly the same receptors that are affected by the caloric sugars of all sorts. We understand where the receptors are in the brain and how they act for many other items to which we become both habituated and addicted, but in the case of sweeteners we don't know whether we get habituated to sweeteners and eat more over time or we don't. We have no sense of the long-term effects of exposure to sweeteners and how that changes how we consume. So it is an area that has not really been studied very much. Right now I am actually working on a review of that topic with a colleague of mine because I think it is a major public health concern that has been ignored.

Dr. Arora: While you dealt mostly with food, what is the relative contribution of food or calorie intake versus physical activity on the overall obesity epidemic?

Dr. Popkin: In some ways, the big question is always whether gluttony or sloth is causing the problem. The reality is that the entire world is reducing physical activity, but in a metabolic and energy balance sense we are still in fairly tight regulation. Consider that it only takes 20 cal/day to add 1 kg of weight in a year, so it doesn't take very much dysregulation. We need to realize that we are not extremely far off from energy balance; if we were, the world would be adding many kilograms of weight per year and we are not. Thus very small changes can make a big difference. However, looking at the question of prevention and the question of change, if a person is consuming a soft drink a day, let's say 120 kcal for 225 ml (8 oz), then consider how many kilometers that person must run to burn 120 kcal and you begin to understand the limitations of increased activity. So from that context you can begin to think about all these changes in our diet as we adopted processed foods and shifted from water and breast milk to caloric beverages. It would take a lot of extra activity to prevent the energy imbalance that creates the problem, and from that point of view I think most of us in the nutrition community would recommend dealing more with the diet world. Now the food industry will tell you it is really physical activity, or they did for a long time, but in general most in our nutrition community would say cutting calories is the key. That is, dealing with the food intake side will be more effective than increasing physical activity to deal with whatever dysregulation we are finding.

Dr. D. Chaudhuri: Your studies were done in a sedentary population. What was the average calorie consumption of the population?

Dr. Popkin: First obviously age and gender differences are huge and the changes over time are equally great. So in a country like China, where my colleague and I have worked, and in other countries I have studied in, activity is decreasing and calories are decreasing in general. But relatively speaking, in the US we are now starting to see an increase in caloric intake for reasons I don't understand. This has occurred in the US over the past 30 years. I haven't seen that in any low income country, so it depends on the point in time. On the average for adults in China, we were perhaps talking of 2,400–2,800 cal in the 1980s, today we are talking about closer to 2,200–2,400 cal. Again there is such a huge range, urban, rural, income, region, that it is very hard to deal with average figures anymore, given the vast heterogeneity and energy expenditure as well as the source and the amount of calories.

Dr. Chittal: In most developed countries it has been seen that adult obesity precedes the onset of childhood obesity by perhaps a decade. Why is it that in developing countries like China and India we see a lot of childhood obesity, although it is a less than 1% increase over the last decade, but not much adult obesity?

Dr. Popkin: I am not sure if this is actually correct. My examination of the data from India as well as China, Vietnam, Indonesia, all from nationwide studies, indicates a faster increase in the prevalence of adult than childhood obesity. However, childhood obesity in lower income countries seems to be much more clustered among higher income families whereas poor adults are becoming more obese than rich ones. Thus some samples do find much more in children, but these come from clinics and such. Another issue is that our measurement of childhood obesity is very weak. We are using BMI now, it is not necessarily the best but it is the only option we have, and I don't know what standard you are referring to in India because when I have used the International Obesity Task Force (IOTF) standards for India my point above holds. However, very often people are using weight for height and they are using –1/+1 z score and to compare adults and children, which is almost impossible. The IOTF tried to create a standard that uses a 25 cutoff for adults and a 30 cutoff for BMI and bring it backwards. But as we look at the figures it gets worse and worse as the subjects get younger relative to other measures. So to talk about where there is more, is very complex. In my experience in low income countries, we see later emerging childhood obesity. If it is seen earlier in India, it is probably among the stunted short Indians which is something we found a lot in other parts of the world where we have studied that same issue. I haven't seen other studies that address the point you are raising. In all the other countries I have worked in where there are national standards and we try to use BMI for children and adults, you can't compare the prevalence in children and adults but you can compare the rate of change and it is increasing much more slowly for children.

Dr. Ganapathy: I am a pediatric sleep consultant, so my interest is in the quality of sleep. As you mentioned activity and changes in nutritional trends, don't you feel that we are sleeping less and hence there is more exposure to food? The internet, TV, and lack of sleep lead to a large sleep debt. Therefore during the day people are exhausted and sleepy and their physical activity goes down, which also contributes to obesity [1]. Unfortunately, one third of our population is obese and about 6,000 children die every day because of undernutrition in our country.

Dr. Popkin: First India has the largest absolute number of malnourished and low birthweight children in the world. You brought up several issues. One was the question of sleep deprivation and its effects, and the second was the issue of diet. The complexity with the sleep deprivation issue is we haven't clearly sorted out the causal relationship. How much is adiposity leading to sleep apnea and other problems that cause sleep problems, and how much are sleep, exhaustion and tiredness causing us to eat higher energy processed foods? We have yet to do interventions in the sleep area to try to sort out causality. It is clearly a concern but more important probably in a country like India would be the shift to caloric beverages and processed foods in urban areas. In Latin America and now in Southeast Asia and in the urban rest of the world and in the Middle East, we have moved to the point where first in Latin America over 70% of spending today goes for processed food from supermarkets. In other words people who 20 years ago consumed fresh unprocessed food are today spending 70% of their money on processed food. We don't fully understand what that shift means; how much of it is just refined carbohydrates and other things that come with it, and we don't understand the processing per se other than the components of the food. Clearly there is a huge shift going on and with it is coming a lot of added sugar, added fats and so forth in the food, that we are sure of. But I can't go beyond that and really talk about the major implications of this huge shift in our diet.

Dr. Wharton: You have said the move to animal food is a driver, why? Is it increased fat, or other food displacement or what?

Dr. Popkin: Clearly I was talking about the changes in calories and mixed calories and the increase in energy density, so I am not speaking of fat versus protein. We know in the nutrition world that protein sates and so a high protein diet it can fill and sate you. On the other hand we have another hypothesis and concerns about energy density in the diet and increases, and how that may matter. If you go from a complex carbohydrate diet to an animal food diet, and a diet with a lot more water from fruits and vegetables, to a higher energy-dense diet, there are potential effects. But the causality issue was not my focus. For that we need a set of studies, like those on caloric beverages, on these dietary shift effects on weight in the context of random controlled trials or very well-monitored longitudinal studies. I was not trying to use that to say that therefore consuming more meat causes more adiposity. I was trying to give a sense of the drivers in the change in calories and the change in the composition and the amount of calories. In light of all the research that has been done I would be the last person to say that by giving people a higher protein, higher animal source diet that calories can be lost; calories can be lost with any diet; it is a question of total calorie regulation, and so I wasn't speaking of that. In fact I wish I knew that answer but I don't.

Dr. Yajnik: You talked about all the precipitating factors like diet and physical activity. What could be the susceptibility underlying this? Your slides showed that some of the less developed countries have a very high prevalence of obesity compared to developed countries.

Dr. Popkin: What Dr. Yajnik was talking about was the susceptibility to diet and activity changes in different parts of the world. Essentially what we know is that Caucasians, Europeans of a Caucasian white background, have a very low amount of adiposity around the heart and liver for the same level of BMI compared to almost any other ethnic group in the world, in particular South Asians, and then after that a number of other groups in the world have much higher adiposity. For example Dr. Yajnik shows a wonderful slide of John Ludkin and himself, they both have a BMI of about 21 and John Ludkin has about a third the amount of body fat of Dr. Yajnik, and all of Dr. Yajnik's fatness is around the heart and liver, and the most in the areas that lead the quickest toward diabetes and all the other cardiovascular risk factors that we are so worried about. Aside from Polynesians in parts of Asia, the reality is that at a lower BMI most East Asians, Southeast Asians and South Asians have a greater risk of most of the cardiovascular outcomes that we see. Now in a country like Mexico it is the same, and throughout South America people with a lower BMI are starting to get diabetes and are becoming very insulin-sensitive, and the problems start at a BMI 5–6 points below that seen in the US among White Americans and in England and other places where this has been studied. I think what you are talking about Dr. Yajnik, in terms of sensitivity to diabetes and hypertension, we see much more sensitivity among all groups in the world, aside from Caucasians.

Dr. Rahman: You have mentioned the way people eat in terms of location; sitting in front of a television or something else?

Dr. Shahkhalili: What is the impact of nutrition transition?

Dr. Popkin: These are two different issues. One is the question of movement and sedentarism. You can be sedentary for many reasons. In China children may be sedentary because they are studying, they are not in front of the TV, they are in front of books; in the Philippines and Mexico they are watching TV; sedentarism varies enormously. For adults it again varies across the globe; it just depends on each society. I was asked the question how the shift in the stage of the nutrition transition, where adults are overweight, how does that come back and have an effect on fetal development, and does that play into the long-term intergenerational effects. Clearly adiposity during pregnancy first has an effect on gestational diabetes and a number of other issues. Beyond that on intergenerational transmission, is there a genetic side or is there a behavioral side to that, is there a metabolic transmission, we really don't know. We use adult obesity all the time as an indicator for child obesity but we have not sorted out the causes between behavioral, metabolic and even epigenetic kinds of issues. So I can't answer your question.

Reference

1   Lee-Chiong TL, Carkadon MA, Sateia MJ (eds): Sleep Medicine. Philadelphia, Hanley & Belfus, 2002, chapter 10.

Kalhan SC, Prentice AM, Yajnik CS (eds): Emerging Societies – Coexistence of Childhood Malnutrition and Obesity.
Nestlé Nutr Inst Workshop Ser Pediatr Program, vol 63, pp 15–24,
Nestec Ltd., Vevey/S. Karger AG, Basel, © 2009.

Regional Case Studies – India

K Srinath Reddy

Public Health Foundation of India, New Delhi, India

Abstract

As a proportion of all deaths in India, cardiovascular disease (CVD) will be the largest cause of disability and death, by the year 2020. At the present stage of India's health transition, an estimated 53% of deaths and 44% of disability-adjusted life-years lost are contributed to chronic diseases. India also has the largest number of people with diabetes in the world, with an estimated 19.3 million in 1995 and projected 57.2 million in 2025. The prevalence of hypertension has been reported to range from 20 to 40% in urban adults and 12–17% among rural adults. The number of people with hypertension is expected to increase from 118.2 million in 2000 to 213.5 million in 2025, with nearly equal numbers of men and women. Over the coming decade, until 2015, CVD and diabetes will contribute to a cumulative loss of USD237 billion for the Indian economy. Much of this enormous burden is already evident in urban as well as semi-urban and slum dwellings across India, where increasing lifespan and rapid acquisition of adverse lifestyles related to the demographic transition contribute to the rising prevalence of CVDs and its risk factors such as obesity, hypertension, and type 2 diabetes. The underlying determinants are sociobehavioral factors such as smoking, physical inactivity, improper diet and stress. The changes in diet and physical activity have resulted largely from the epidemiological transition that is underway in most low income countries including India. The main driving forces of these epidemiological shifts are the globalized world, rapid and uneven urbanization, demographic shifts and inter- and intra-country migrations – all of which result in alterations in dietary practices and decreased physical activity. While these changes are global, India has several unique features. The transitions in India are uneven with several states in India still battling the ill effects of undernutrition and infectious diseases, while in other states with better indices of development, chronic diseases including diabetes are emerging as a major area of concern. Regional and urban-rural differences in the occurrence of CVD are the hallmark. All these differences result in a differing prevalence of CVD and its risk factors. Therefore while studying nutrition and physical activity shifts in India, the marked heterogeneity and secular changes in dietary and physical activity practices should be taken into account. This principle should also apply to strategies, policies and nutrition and physical activity guidelines so that they take the regional differences into account.

Chronic diseases account for the greatest share of early death and disability worldwide, especially in low and middle income countries like India [1]. In 2002, the leading chronic diseases – cardiovascular disease (CVD), cancer, chronic respiratory disease, and diabetes – caused 29 million deaths worldwide. At the present stage of India's health transition, chronic diseases contribute to an estimated 53% of deaths and 44% of disability-adjusted life years lost. India also has the largest number of people with diabetes in the world, with an estimated 19.3 million in 1995 and projected 57.2 million in 2025. On the basis of recent surveys, the Indian Council of Medical Research (ICMR) estimates the prevalence of diabetes in adults to be 3.8% in rural areas and 11.8% in urban areas. The prevalence of hypertension has been reported to range between 20 and 40% in urban adults and 12 and 17% among rural adults. The number of people with hypertension is expected to increase from 118.2 million in 2000 to 213.5 million in 2025, with nearly equal numbers of men and women. Over the coming decade, until 2015, CVD and diabetes are likely to contribute to a cumulative loss of USD 237 billion for the Indian economy [2]. Much of this enormous burden is already evident in urban as well as semi-urban and slum dwellings across India, where increasing lifespan and rapid acquisition of adverse lifestyles related to demographic transition are contributing to the rising prevalence of CVDs and its risk factors such as obesity, hypertension, and type 2 diabetes. The underlying determinants lie in socio-behavioral factors such as smoking, physical inactivity, improper diet and stress [3]. Tobacco is the leading avoidable cause of death worldwide, and its rising consumption in developing countries warrants early and effective public health responses. In India alone, the tobacco-attributable toll will rise from 1.4% in 1990 to 13.3% in 2020.

India has experienced a major surge in life expectancy (41.2 years in 1951–1961 to 64 years in 2005). This was principally due to a decline in deaths occurring in infancy, childhood, and adolescence and was related to more effective public health responses to perinatal, infectious, and nutritional deficiency disorders and to improved economic indicators such as per capita income and social indicators such as female literacy in some areas. These demographic shifts have augmented the ranks of middle-aged and older adults. The concomitant decline in infectious and nutritional disorders (competing causes of death) further enhances the proportional burden due to CVD and other chronic lifestyle-related diseases. This shift, representing a decline in deaths from infectious diseases to an increase in those due to chronic diseases, is often referred to as the modern epidemiological transition [4].

Childhood obesity is emerging as a major health problem in India, especially in children from urban higher socioeconomic areas; for example, about 30% of children were overweight in an affluent Delhi school [5]. Thus, identifying potential risk factors for childhood obesity and formulating early interventions is crucial in the management of the obesity epidemic. The adverse health effects of obesity in children justify the need to look for potential risk

Table 1. Risk factors for non-communicable diseases in the South East Asia Region (SEAR) according to the World Health Report [10]

Risk factor	Optimum	SEAR
Mean fruit and vegetable intake, g/day	600	236.2
Mean SBP, mm Hg	115	128.8
Mean cholesterol, mmol/l	3.8	5.0
No physical activity, %	0	16.6
Overweight – mean BMI	21	20.5
Tobacco consumption, %	No	22
Alcohol consumption, %	0	13.6
Urban air pollution, µg/m^3	7.5	25.6

factors and provide suitable interventions. Factors contributing to childhood obesity, such as parental obesity, eating behaviors, TV viewing and lack of physical activity have been studied in Western settings [6, 7]. A cross-sectional survey of urban Delhi and its rural environs revealed that a higher prevalence of coronary heart disease (CHD) in the urban sample was associated with higher levels of body mass index, blood pressure, fasting blood lipids (total cholesterol, ratio of cholesterol to HDL cholesterol, triglycerides), and diabetes.

Unhealthy diets and physical inactivity are two of the main risk factors for raised blood pressure, raised blood glucose, abnormal blood lipids, overweight/obesity, and for the major chronic diseases such as CVDs, cancer, and diabetes [8]. Globally it is estimated that approximately 2.7 million deaths are attributable to low fruit and vegetable intake while 1.9 million deaths are attributable to physical inactivity. A large majority of these deaths occur in low and middle income countries. The changes in diet and physical activity have resulted largely from the epidemiological transition that is underway in most low income countries including India. The main driving forces of these epidemiological shifts are a globalized world, rapid and uneven urbanization, demographic shifts and inter- and intra-country migrations – all of which result in alterations in dietary practices (a shift from high fiber, vegetable and fruit-rich diets to diets rich in saturated fats, trans fats and high salt-containing processed foods) and a decrease in physical activity (due to availability of mass-transport systems and mechanization of daily activities).

While these changes are global, India has several unique features. The transitions in India are uneven with several states in India still battling the ill effects of undernutrition and infectious diseases, while in states with better indices of development, chronic diseases including diabetes are emerging as a major area of concern. The mean fruit and vegetable intake in the South East Asia Region is only 40% of the optimal rate and nearly 17% of the total population is physically inactive (table 1).

What Are the Key Dietary Dimensions?

While nutritional status has improved worldwide over the past 50 years, new nutrition-related problems have also emerged. In India, the nutrition transition is associated with a shift in dietary patterns to more 'Western' diets rich in saturated fat, refined foods and sugar and low in fiber, and leads to an increase in non-communicable diseases (NCDs). As reviewed by Drewnowski and Popkin [10], the global availability of cheap vegetable oils and fats has resulted in greatly increased fat consumption among low-income countries. The transition now occurs at lower levels of the gross national product than previously and is further accelerated by rapid urbanization. The Asian countries, with a diet that is traditionally high in carbohydrates and low in fat, have shown an overall decline in the proportion of energy from complex carbohydrates along with the increase in the proportion of fat. The globalization of food production and marketing is also contributing to the increasing consumption of energy-dense foods poor in dietary fiber and several micronutrients. Water and milk appear to be replaced by calorically sweetened beverages. The World Health Report [9] introduced the term 'risk transition' to describe the changes in consumption of tobacco, alcohol, nutrition and other lifestyles that promote the development of NCDs. This transition does not necessarily affect an entire population but rather segments of it, based on, for instance, the environment (e.g. rural vs. urban) or socioeconomic circumstances.

The ICMR, recognizing the importance of a database on the diet and nutritional status of the community, sponsored multicentric studies to assess the growth and development of Indian children [11] and studies on the nutritional problems of preschool children [12]. These investigations indicated the presence of extensive growth retardation among Indian children as compared to American children and exploded the myth of protein deficiency in Indian diets. Studies by Rao et al. [13] demonstrated for the first time that, in communities which depend mainly on cereals and millets in the diets of preschool children, the primary bottleneck is an energy or food deficit. These and other [14] studies helped to formulate the scientific basis for the supplementary feeding programs in operation in the country.

The major data source for the diet and nutritional status of the Indian population is National Nutrition Monitoring Bureau (NNMB), established by the ICMR in 1972. In the recent past, the Food and Nutrition Board, Department of Women and Child Development, Government of India, also initiated surveys to collect information at the district level on the diet and nutrition profile of the communities in different states of the country. By and large, the National Institute of Nutrition has played a vital role in organizing these studies and surveys. The existence of diverse dietary profiles in India, linked to religion, ethnicity and geographical region, makes assessments on the 'national' dietary profiles difficult. This problem is compounded by the methodological issues related to dietary assessments, which have been extensively reviewed.

Table 2. Change in average calorie consumption by states – urban (kcal/capita/day)

	1972–1973	1983	1993–1994	1999–2000
Andhra Pradesh	2,143	2,009	1,992	2,052
Assam	2,135	2,043	2,108	2,174
Bihar	2,157	2,131	2,185	2,171
Gujarat	2,172	2,000	2,027	2,058
Haryana	2,404	2,242	2,149	2,172
Karnataka	1,925	2,124	2,025	2,045
Kerala	1,723	2,049	1,966	1,995
Madhya Pradesh	2,229	2,137	2,082	2,132
Maharashtra	1,971	2,028	1,989	2,039
Orissa	2,275	2,218	2,251	2,295
Punjab	2,703	2,100	2,059	2,197
Rajasthan	2,357	2,255	2,184	2,335
Tamil Nadu	1,841	2,140	1,922	2,030
Uttar Pradesh	2,151	2,043	2,114	2,131
West Bengal	2,080	2,045	2,131	2,134

Source: Chandrashekhar and Ghosh [15].

Despite these problems, however, periodic data from the National Nutrition Monitoring Bureau and other sources such as the National Family Health Survey (NFHS) indicate that there are clear differences in diet between urban and rural areas within a region. These data have been reviewed earlier, and suggest that the visible fat in poor rural diets is mainly vegetable-based and that the differences in the dietary fat intake between rural and urban populations are largely due to differences in the intakes of visible fats. Urbanization may also be associated with a change in the dietary n-6/n-3 ratio because of increases in the consumption of cheap commercial vegetable oil (n-6 fatty acids). Regional differences and urban-rural differences in the occurrence of CVD is the hallmark. There is marked heterogeneity in the total energy intake in both rural and urban areas (tables 2, 3).

According to the NFHS-3 data, overweight and obesity are more than three times higher in urban than rural areas. Both undernutrition and overweight and obesity are higher among women. Malnutrition levels are lowest in Delhi, Punjab, and several of the small northeastern states. Malnutrition levels are higher among young girls. Almost half of the girls in age 15–19 years are undernourished.

In addition to the rural-urban differences in dietary patterns, there are also important changes that occur with improvements in socioeconomic status. These include:

- An increased intake of legumes, vegetables, milk and, in case of non-vegetarians, foods of animal origin

19

Table 3. Change in average calorie consumption by states – rural (kcal/capita/day)

	1972–1973	1983	1993–1994	1999–2000
Andhra Pradesh	2,103	2,204	2,052	2,021
Assam	2,074	2,055	1,983	1,915
Bihar	2,225	2,159	2,115	2,121
Gujarat	2,142	2,113	1,994	1,986
Haryana	3,215	2,554	2,491	2,455
Karnataka	2,202	2,250	2,073	2,028
Kerala	1,559	1,884	1,955	1,982
Madhya Pradesh	2,423	2,323	2,154	2,062
Maharashtra	1,895	2,144	1,935	2,012
Orissa	1,995	2,103	2,199	2,119
Punjab	3,493	2,577	2,418	2,381
Rajasthan	2,730	2,433	2,470	2,425
Tamil Nadu	1,955	1,861	1,884	1,826
Uttar Pradesh	2,575	2,399	2,307	2,327
West Bengal	1,821	2,027	2,211	2,085

Source: Chandrashekhar and Ghosh [15].

- Substitution of coarse grain by the more prestigious and often highly polished cereals such as rice. There is also a reduction in the overall cereal intake, although this continues to be high by Western standards
- Progressive increases in the intake of edible fat
- Increased intake of sugar and sweets
- Increase in energy intake leading to obesity

What Are the Key Physical Activity Shifts?

Rastogi et al. [16] highlighted the adverse health consequences of physical inactivity and the importance of leisure-time exercise in the prevention of CHD risk among Indians. Earlier studies in India using simple, self-reported categorizations of physical activity status had documented the disparate physical activity patterns in urban and rural populations. A large number of studies, predominantly in developed countries, have linked the risk of a lack of discretionary leisure time activity to the development of NCDs such as diabetes and CHD [17]. In developing countries, however, lower levels of mechanization at home, at work and in transport make the documentation of physical activity within these domains particularly important. For instance, in urban areas in India, about a third of the people who exercise approximately 30 min 5 days a week are sedentary in terms of their composite physical activity levels when all physical activity domains are taken into account. In contrast, individuals in rural areas with little discretionary leisure time activity may be heavily active owing to the nature of their manual occupations. Yet again, simple categorizations of physical activity status on the basis of occupation can lead to erroneous physical activity in the 'non-occupational' domains of physical activity [18]. In India, associations between CHD and physical inactivity have been explored using rudimentary questionnaires. These studies have demonstrated the protective effect of physical activity in preventing CHD, although the extent of this effect in rural and urban areas is variable, in part owing to the fairly basic assessment of physical activity. In assessing physical activity patterns, these studies have used key questions to document occupational and leisure time activity. Data from healthy, educated, urban, employed Indians, using more comprehensive physical activity questionnaires, indicate that 61% of males and 51% of females are either sedentary or mildly active [19]. Physical activity patterns in rural Indians have not been evaluated to any large extent. However, small studies in agricultural workers indicate that they have high levels of physical activity and that this may be true both during the harvest season and during the lean season [20].

The Prospective Urban Rural Epidemiology study showed that there are variable differences in dietary intakes, physical activity patterns and prevalence of chronic diseases among urban and rural populations. There is some evidence of a positive behavioral shift in a higher socioeconomic status urban population to adopting a more physically active lifestyle. In rural areas with a high penetration of urban influences, a degenerative phase of nutrition transition is well underway [21].

Recommended Priority Interventions

An overall measure to be taken for reducing the disease burden in the Indian subcontinent is to develop comprehensive national and local plans/policies which encourage and promote healthy eating and active living. These plans should involve healthcare providers, work sites, schools, media, industries carrying out food production processing, and preparation, in addition to the policymakers. The collective goal should be directed towards attainment of a healthy living by all. Specific interventions depending on local, physical and cultural conditions should be based on careful analysis of existing dietary and activity patterns and their determinants; however, the following interventions as described by Willett et al. [22] can be considered:

Physical Activity
- Developing transportation policies and a physical environment to promote walking and riding bicycles. This intervention includes constructing sidewalks and protected bicycle paths and lanes that are attractive, safe, well-lit, and functional with regard to destinations

21

- Adopting policies that promote livable, walker-friendly communities that include parks and are centered around access to public transportation
- Encouraging the use of public transportation and discourage overdependence on private automobiles
- Promoting the use of stairs by inclusion of accessible and attractive stairways at workplaces, residential complexes, shoppingmalls, etc.

Healthy Diets
- Developing comprehensive school programs that integrate nutrition into core curricula and healthy nutrition into school food services. Regional or national standards to promote healthy eating should be developed for school food services. Programs should also aim at limiting television watching, in part by promoting attractive alternatives
- Working with the agriculture sector and food industries to replace unhealthy fats with healthy fats, including adequate amounts of n-3 fatty acids. This goal can be achieved through a combination of education, regulation, and incentives
- Clear labeling of energy content for all packaged foods, including fast food
- Using tax policies to encourage the consumption of healthier foods. For example, carbonated drinks could be fully taxed and not subsidized in the same way as healthier foods
- Emphasizing the production and consumption of healthy food products in agriculture support and extension programs
- Ensuring that health providers regularly weigh both children and adult patients, track their weights over time, and provide counseling regarding diet and activity if they are already overweight or if unhealthy weight gain is occurring during adulthood. Those activities should be integrated with programs that address undernutrition. Healthcare providers should be encouraged to set a good example by not smoking, by exercising regularly, and by eating healthy diets
- Promoting healthy foods at worksite food services. Worksites can also promote physical activity by providing financial incentives to use public transportation or ride bicycles (and by not subsidizing automobiles by providing free parking). Providing areas for exercise during work breaks and showers may be useful
- Setting standards that restrict the promotion of foods high in sugar, refined starch and saturated and trans fats for children on television and elsewhere
- Setting national standards for the amount of sodium in processed foods

National Campaigns
- Investing in developing locally appropriate health messages related to diet, physical activity, and weight control. This effort is best done in cooperation with government agencies, nongovernmental organizations, and professional organizations so that consistent messages can be used on television and radio, at healthcare settings, schools and worksites, and elsewhere. This effort should use the best social-marketing techniques available, with messages continuously evaluated for effectiveness
- Developing a sustainable surveillance system that monitors weight and height, physical activity, and key dietary variables

Implementation of the recommended policies to promote health and well-being is often not straightforward because of opposition by powerful and well-funded political and economic forces, such as those involved in the tobacco, automobile, food, and oil industries. The solutions will depend on a country's specific political landscape. However, experiences in many countries indicate that alliances of public interest groups, professional organizations, and motivated individuals can overcome such powerful interests. Strategies should start with sound science and can use a mix of mass media, lobbying efforts, and lawsuits. Protection of children can be a powerful lever because of almost universal concern about their welfare and the recognition that they cannot be responsible for the long-term consequences of their diet and lifestyle choices.

All these differences result in a differing prevalence of CVD and its risk factors. For example even among industrial workers and their families who are economically better off than the general community, there are wide-ranging differences in CVD risk factors. In industries located predominantly in urban areas, CVD risk factor levels are high compared to those in peri-urban areas [23]. However local dietary practices may alter the prevalence. For example, the tea garden workers of Assam receive extra salt as compensation for the putative loss of sodium due to their outdoor work. This has resulted in high prevalence of high blood pressure though other CVD risk factors are similar to other industrial populations which are predominantly located in peri-urban areas. Therefore while studying nutrition and physical activity shifts in India, the marked heterogeneity and secular changes in dietary and physical activity practices should be taken into account. This principle should also apply to strategies, policies and nutrition and physical activity guidelines so that they take into account the regional differences.

To summarize, we should aim at telescoping this transition to propagate 'appropriate' rather than 'under' or 'over' nutrition; adopting a life-course approach (with a special focus on children and adolescents), and promoting healthy diets and physical activity by using policy and education as complementary interventions to impact on populations and individuals.

References

1 Lopez AD, Mathers CD, Ezzati M, et al: Global and regional burden of risk factors, 2001:systematic analysis of population health data. Lancet 2006;367:1747–1757.
2 World Health Organization: Country Cooperation Strategy 2006–2011 India. Geneva, WHO, 2006, pp 3–14.
3 Reddy KS, Shah B, Varghese C, Ramadoss A: Responding to the threat of chronic diseases in India. Lancet 2005;366:1744–1749.
4 Reddy KS, Yusuf S: Emerging epidemic of cardiovascular disease in developing countries. Circulation 1998;97:596–601.
5 Kapil U, Singh P, Pathak P, et al: Prevalence of obesity amongst affluent adolescent school children in Delhi. Indian Pediatr 2002;39:449–452.
6 Burke V, Beilin LJ, Simmer K, et al: Predictors of body mass index and associations with cardiovascular risk factors in Australian children: a prospective cohort study. Int J Obes 2005;29:15–23.
7 Jago R, Baranowski T, Baranowski JC, et al: BMI from 3–6 y of age is predicted by TV viewing and physical activity, not diet. Int J Obes 2005;29:557–564.
8 World Health Organization: Prevention and Control of Non-Communicable Diseases: Implementation of the Global Strategy. Geneva, WHO, 2007.

9 World Health Report: Reducing Risks, Promoting Healthy Life. Geneva, WHO, 2002.
10 Drewnowski A, Popkin BM: The nutrition transition: new trends in the global diet. Nutr Rev 1997;55:31–43.
11 Indian Council of Medical Research: Growth and Physical Development of Indian Infant and Children. Tech Report Ser No. 18. New Delhi, Indian Council of Medical Research, 1972.
12 Indian Council of Medical Research: Studies on Preschool Children. ICMR Tech Rep Ser No. 26. New Delhi, Indian Council of Medical Research, 1974.
13 Rao BSN, Rao KV, Naidu AN: Calorie protein adequacy of the dietaries of preschool children in India. J Nutr Diet 1969;6:238–244.
14 Gopalan G, Swaminathan VK, Kumari VK, et al: Effect of calorie supplementation on growth of undernourished children. Am J Clin Nutr 1973;26:563–566.
15 Chandrashekhar CP, Ghosh J: http://www.thehindubusinessline.com/2003/02/11/stories/2003021100210900.htm
16 Rastogi T, Reddy KS, Vaz M, et al: Diet and risk of ischemic heart disease in India. Am J Clin Nutr 2004;79:582–592.
17 Warburton DE, Nicol CW, Bredin SS: Health benefits of physical activity: The evidence. CMAJ 2006;174:801–809.
18 Vaz M, Bharathi AV: How sedentary are people in 'sedentary' occupations? The physical activity of teachers in urban South India. Occup Med (Lond) 2004;54:369–372.
19 Vaz M, Bharathi AV: Attitudes to and characteristics of physical activity patterns in urban, educated, middle-class Indians. Indian J Med 2000;52:301–306.
20 Durnin JV, Drummond S, Satyanarayana K: A collaborative EEC study on seasonality and marginal nutrition: the Glasgow Hyderabad (S. India) study. Eur J Clin Nutr 1990;44:19–29.
21 Vaz M, Yusuf S, Bharathi AV, et al: The nutrition transition in India. S Afr J Clin Nutr 2005;18:198–201.
22 Willett WC, Koplan JP, Nugent R, et al: Prevention of chronic disease by means of diet and lifestyle changes; in Jamison DT, Breman JG, Measham AR, et al (eds): Disease Control Priorities in Developing Countries, ed 2. New York, Oxford University Press, 2006, pp 833–850.
23 Reddy KS, Prabhakaran D, Jeemon P, et al: Educational status and cardiovascular risk profile in Indians. Proc Natl Acad Sci USA 2007;104:16263–16268.
24 Reddy KS, Prabhakaran D, Chaturvedi V, et al: Cardiovascular risk profile across India: results from the CVD Surveillance in Industrial Populations Study. Indian Heart J 2005;57:543–557.

For discussion, see p. 41.

Kalhan SC, Prentice AM, Yajnik CS (eds): Emerging Societies – Coexistence of Childhood Malnutrition and Obesity.
Nestlé Nutr Inst Workshop Ser Pediatr Program, vol 63, pp 25–32,
Nestec Ltd., Vevey/S. Karger AG, Basel, © 2009.

Regional Case Studies – China

Shi-an Yin

National Institute for Nutrition and Food Safety, Chinese Center for Disease Control and
Prevention, Beijing, China

Abstract

Over the last 30 years, the nutritional status of Chinese children has greatly improved due to economic development and improved incomes. In this review, the status of childhood malnutrition and obesity in China is evaluated based on the National Nutrition and Health Survey of 2002 (NNHS2002) and the survey on National Student Health and Physical Fitness in China of 2005. Compared with the NNHS1992 survey, the body weights and heights of preschool children in urban and rural areas have significantly improved, and the prevalence of malnutrition (underweight and stunting) has been significantly reduced. However, micronutrient deficiencies, including calcium, zinc, vitamin A, vitamins B_1 and B_2, are still common in preschool and school children. These data show that the growth and development of Chinese children are under our expectations. On the other hand, the national averaged prevalences of overweight and obesity in the children under 6 years of age are 3.4 or 2.0% as estimated by the Chinese or WHO standards, respectively. We are now facing double challenges: to prevent malnutrition and the increase in overweight and obesity in children.

Over the last 30 years (1979–2008), the nutritional status of Chinese children has greatly improved due to economic development and income increases. At present, typical malnutrition (for example, severe protein-energy malnutrition, vitamin A or thiamine deficiencies) is not common. However, marginal micronutrient deficiencies (iron, vitamin A, iodine, calcium, zinc and vitamin B_1 deficiencies) are common in children in urban cities and rural areas [1–3]. Nutritional deficiencies, including anemia, rickets, vitamin A and zinc, are still serious problems affected the growth and development of children in poor areas. At the same time, the prevalence of overweight and obesity in children is significantly increased year by year in the cities, especially in large cities. Reviewing the results of the National Student Health and Physical Fitness of China survey in 2005, the rates of overweight and obesity were 13.2 and 11.4%, respectively, for boys aged 7–12 years in cities, indicating increases of 1.4 and 2.7%, respectively, compared to the survey conducted in 2000. That is, there has been a significant increase in overweight and obesity in children and adolescents within 5 years [4].

Economic Development and Chronic Non-Communicable Diseases

Economic Development Change from 1979 to 2008 in China

For three decades since 1979, following the reform and opening-up of China, the Chinese have gone through a stage of transition from adequate food and clothing to a well-off society. The goal of quadrupling China's gross national product by 2000 was reached at the end of 1997. Per capita disposable income achieved the breakthrough goal of 10,000 Chinese yuan (= USD 1,220) in 2005. Personal income per capita has significant increased in urban and rural areas and reached USD 1,740 in 2006. The increase in China's economy was 11.4% in 2007 (the fastest pace in 13 years).

Prevalence of Chronic Non-Communicable Diseases Significantly Increases with the Change in Living Pattern at the National Level

It has been reported that the ratio of the number of chronic disease deaths to the total number of deaths has risen from 73.8% in 1991 to 80.9% at the national level in 2000; deaths were 85.3 and 76.5% in urban and rural areas of China, respectively. Over the last 10 years, mortality rates for cancers, cerebrovascular diseases, diabetes and coronary heart disease have shown an upward trend. For example, in China, hypertension has been the number one killer. The prevalence of hypertension in people over the age of 18 is 18.8%. It is estimated that about 160 million people have hypertension; an increase of more than 70 million patients from 1991 to 2002. Another serious threat to health and survival is the increased incidence of diabetes. Based on the data of 2002, the prevalence of diabetes in people over 18 years of age in China was 6.1, 3.7 and 1.8% in large cities, small- and medium-sized cities, and rural areas, respectively. Compared with the rate in 1996, the prevalence in the large cities rose by 40% in only 6 years [1].

Growth Status of Chinese Children

Based on the National Nutritional and Health Survey in 2002, the body weights and heights of preschool children in urban and rural areas improved significantly compared to the results in 1992 (tables 1, 2) [3]. The heights and weights of preschool children in urban and rural areas improved significantly with the increase in household income [3].

Table 1. Changing trend in height (cm) of Chinese children from 1992 to 2002

Age years	Urban boys			girls			Rural boys			girls		
	1992	2002	gain	1992	2002	gain	1992	2002	gain	1992	2002	gain
2[a]	087.6	090.1	2.5	088.2	089.0	0.8	085.5	087.6	2.1	084.7	086.2	1.5
3	095.4	099.7	4.3	094.5	098.8	4.3	092.0	095.1	3.1	091.0	094.2	3.2
4	102.4	106.0	3.6	099.9	105.0	5.1	098.5	101.8	3.3	097.4	101.0	3.6
5	108.2	112.2	4.0	106.6	111.5	4.9	104.9	108.2	3.3	103.8	107.4	3.6
6–7	113.5	118.4	4.9	112.6	117.0	4.4	110.2	113.1	2.9	109.6	112.9	3.3

[a] Measured length for children less than 3 years.

Table 2. Changing trend in body weight (kg) of Chinese children from 1992 to 2002

Age years	Urban boys			girls			Rural boys			girls		
	1992	2002	gain	1992	2002	gain	1992	2002	gain	1992	2002	gain
2	12.8	13.5	0.7	12.7	12.7	0	12.2	12.8	0.6	11.7	11.9	0.2
3	14.7	16.0	1.3	14.5	15.4	0.9	13.8	14.3	0.5	13.2	13.8	0.6
4	16.8	17.8	1.0	15.9	17.0	1.1	15.4	16.0	0.6	15.0	15.5	0.5
5	18.6	19.7	1.1	17.7	19.0	1.3	17.1	17.7	0.6	16.6	17.1	0.5
6–7	20.7	22.2	1.5	20.0	21.1	1.1	19.1	19.4	0.3	18.4	18.7	0.3

Prevalence of Malnutrition in Chinese Children under 7 Years of Age in China

The remarkable nutritional improvement of children in the 1990s is the consequence of the rapid socioeconomic development of China [5, 6]. For example, the prevalence of underweight in urban and rural areas was reduced from 10.1 and 20.0% in 1992 to 3.1 and 9.3%, respectively, in 2002, and the prevalence of stunting in urban and rural areas was reduced from 19.1 and 35.0% in 1992 to 4.9 and 17.3%, respectively in 2002 (tables 3, 4) in the same period.

Prevalence of Overweight and Obesity in Chinese Children and Adolescents

- The national averaged prevalence of overweight and obesity in Chinese children and adolescents is shown in figure 1. The rates of overweight and obesity for the children under 6 years were 3.4 or 2.0% as estimated using the Chinese or WHO standards, respectively, and the prevalence of overweight and obesity for 7–17 years was 4.5% (4.2% by WHO) and 2.1% (1.8% by WHO), respectively, in 2002. Using the Chinese standard, the prevalence of overweight and obesity in children and adolescents in cities and rural areas is presented in figure 2 [1, 7].

Micronutrient Status of Chinese Children in China

The data from the National Nutrition and Health Survey in 2002 showed that the growth and development of Chinese children is far from ideal. Micronutrient deficiencies, including calcium, zinc, vitamin A, vitamins B_1 and B_2, are quite common in preschool and school children. Iron deficiency and iron deficiency anemia are still a serous problem based on the National Nutrition and Health Survey in 2002. This survey showed that the prevalence of anemia in children (6–9 years) was 13–14% in cities [3], indicating that these children are at a high risk of having anemia. The characteristics of anemia in China are that the apparent iron intake is adequate, however, iron deficiency and iron deficiency anemia are the most common nutritional deficiency problems, particularly among young children due to the poor absorption of iron from plant food, and thus the amount of absorbable iron is not enough to meet the iron requirements.

With regard to vitamin A deficiency, the mean vitamin A level in the serum of 10,784 children in five districts of Shenyang City in China was 1.20 ± 0.44 µmol/l [8], and 33.1 and 10.5% of children have serum retinol levels of 0.7–1.05 and 0.35–0.69 µmol/l, respectively, showing that the vitamin A levels of

Table 3. Comparison of underweight prevalence of children under 5 years of age from 1992 to 2002 (%)

Age, years	National			Urban			Rural		
	1992	2002	change	1992	2002	change	1992	2002	change
0	9.7	2.6	−73.2	8.7	1.7	−80.5	10.0	2.9	−71.0
1	19.3	8.4	−56.5	9.8	4.6	−53.1	21.8	9.6	−56.0
2	19.2	9.8	−49.0	10.6	5.1	−51.9	21.0	1.2	−46.7
3	20.7	9.4	−54.6	8.5	2.4	−71.8	23.8	1.7	−50.8
4–5	18.1	9.6	−47.0	12.4	3.4	−72.6	19.5	1.5	−41.0
Total	18.0	7.8	−56.7	10.1	3.1	−69.3	20.0	09.3	−53.5

Table 4. Comparison of stunting prevalence of children under 5 years old from 1992 to 2002 (%)

Age, years	National			Urban			Rural		
	1992	2002	change	1992	2002	change	1992	2002	change
0	14.4	8.0	−44.4	10.7	3.9	−63.6	15.2	9.2	−39.5
1	33.8	18.0	−46.7	19.9	8.6	−56.8	37.3	20.9	−44.0
2	30.3	15.1	−50.2	17.2	8.0	−53.5	33.0	7.3	−47.6
3	36.6	15.2	−58.5	19.0	3.3	−82.6	41.0	9.0	−53.7
4–5	37.4	16.1	−57.0	24.8	4.9	−80.2	40.6	9.6	−51.7
Total	31.9	14.3	−55.2	19.1	4.9	−74.5	35.0	7.3	−50.6

Yin

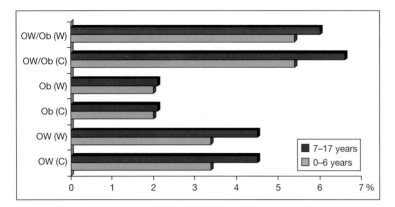

Fig. 1. The prevalence of overweight and obesity in children and adolescents (%). OW = Overweight; Ob = obesity; C = using Chinese standard; W = using WHO standard.

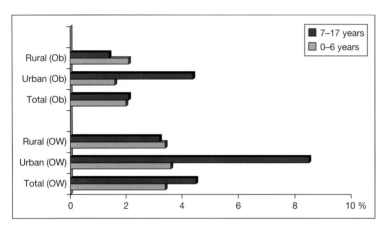

Fig. 2. The prevalence of overweight and obesity in children and adolescents estimated by Chinese standard in different areas (%). OW = Overweight; Ob = obesity.

children aged 3 years old are relatively low. The incidence of marginal vitamin A deficiency (about 40% in children aged 3–12 years) is relatively high. The insufficiency of vitamin A in the diet is the direct cause of vitamin A deficiency [3]. It is well known that vitamin A deficiency may affect the physical development of children. Furthermore, a factor contributing to vitamin A deficiency among Chinese children is that their diets contain even smaller quantities of plant carotenoids than those of adults because plant provitamin A carotenoids account for about 70% of dietary vitamin A in the Chinese population [2]. Thus, preschool children are at high risk of vitamin A deficiency due to their rapid growth (which further increases their vitamin A requirements), their inadequate complementary feeding, and their general aversion to eating green leafy vegetables.

In addition, other micronutrient deficiencies have been observed. As the consumption of milk and its products is relatively low, the lack of calcium in the traditional Chinese diet is very common, making the calcium intake of children less than 40% of the Chinese recommended nutritional intake (RNI; equal to US recommended daily allowance) based on the National Nutrition and Health Survey in 2002 [2]. The zinc intake of children reached 80% of the Chinese RNI; vitamin B_2 intake reached about 60% of the Chinese RNI, and vitamin B_1 was 65–71% of the Chinese RNI [2].

Conclusions

Following the economic development and increase in household income, the nutritional status of Chinese children has greatly improved in the past 30 years. However, the prevalence of non-communicable diseases has significantly increased with the change in living pattern at the national level.

With the increase in household income, the body weights and heights of preschool children in urban and rural areas have significantly improved in the last 10 years.

The prevalence of malnutrition (underweight and stunting) in urban and rural areas has markedly decreased, and can be ascribed to the remarkable nutritional improvement of children in the 1990s as a consequence of the rapid socioeconomic development of China.

The rapid increase in overweight and obesity in children and adolescents in relation to the changes in dietary pattern and physical activities should be a warning.

With regard to treating and solving the double challenges (malnutrition and overweight and obesity), we should not only make strategies on how to eliminate micronutrient deficiencies but also on how to prevent overweight and obesity in children and adolescents.

Acknowledgements

The author would like to thank Dr. Guangwen Tang for assistance in preparing the manuscript.

References

1 Wang LD: General Report on the Nutritional and Health Status of Chinese Population – 2002 National Nutrition and Health Survey. Beijing, People's Medical Publishing House, 2005.
2 Zhai FY, Yang XG: The Status of Dietary and Nutrient Intakes of Chinese Population – 2002 National Nutrition and Health Survey. Beijing, People's Medical Publishing House, 2006.

Yin

3 Yang XG, Zhai FY: The body mass and nutrition status of Chinese population – 2002 National Nutrition and Health Survey. Beijing, People's Medical Publishing House, 2006.
4 Ji CY, Sun JL: Analyses of the epidemiological status of overweight and obesity in Chinese students and the prevalence. J Peking Univ(Health Sci) 2004;36:194–197.
5 Chang S, Fu Z, He W, Chen C: Current situation and trend of child growth in China. J Hyg Res 2000;29:270–274.
6 Chen CM, He W, Fu ZY, et al: Ten-Year Tracking Nutritional Status in China. Beijing, People's Medical Publishing House, 2004.
7 Ma GS, Li YP, Wu YF, et al: The prevalence of body overweight and obesity and its changes among Chinese people during 1992 to 2002. Chin J Prev Med 2005;39:311–315.
8 Yang R, Chen C, Chen L, et al: Investigate the serum vitamin A levels of children aged 0–6 years in Zhejiang Province. Chin J Child Health Care 2001;8:160–161.

For discussion, see p. 41.

Kalhan SC, Prentice AM, Yajnik CS (eds): Emerging Societies – Coexistence of Childhood Malnutrition
and Obesity.
Nestlé Nutr Inst Workshop Ser Pediatr Program, vol 63, pp 33–46,
Nestec Ltd., Vevey/S. Karger AG, Basel, © 2009.

Regional Case Studies – Africa

Andrew M. Prentice

MRC International Nutrition Group, London School of Hygiene and Tropical Medicine,
London, UK, and MRC Keneba, Keneba, The Gambia

Abstract

Africa is the final continent to be affected by the nutrition transition and, as elsewhere, is characterized by the paradoxical coexistence of malnutrition and obesity.
Several features of the obesity epidemic in Africa mirror those in other emerging
nations: it penetrates the richer nations and urban areas first with a strong urban–
rural gradient; initially it affects the wealthy, but later there is a demographic switch as
obesity becomes a condition more associated with poverty, and it shares many of the
same drivers related to the increasing affordability of highly refined oils and carbohydrates, and a move away from subsistence farm work and towards sedentary lifestyles.
Africa also has some characteristics of the obesity epidemic that stand out from other
regions such as: (1) excepting some areas of the Pacific, Africa is probably the only
region in which obesity (especially among women) is viewed culturally as a positive
and desirable trait, leading to major gender differences in obesity rates in many countries; (2) most of Africa has very low rates of obesity in children, and to date African
obesity is mostly an adult syndrome; (3) Africans seem genetically prone to higher
rates of diabetes and hypertension in association with obesity than Caucasians, but
seem to be relatively protected from dislipidemias; (4) the case-specific deaths and
disabilities from diabetes and hypertension in Africa are very high due to the paucity
of health services and the strain that the 'double burden' of disease places on health
systems.

Introduction

The paradoxical coexistence of malnutrition and obesity in Africa is made
vividly apparent by a visit to almost any major hospital in urban Africa where
children's wards are struggling with infectious diseases and the rehabilitation
of severely malnourished children, whilst neighboring adult wards are dealing
with amputations of diabetic feet and other consequences of obesity-related

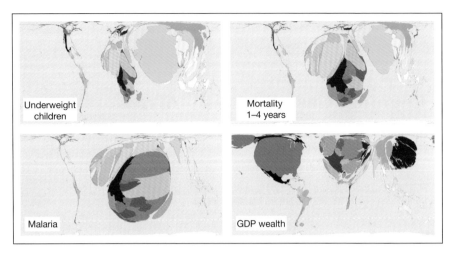

Fig. 1. Africa – the continent left behind by development. Countries have been resized according to the size of the problem being illustrated. Reproduced with permission from www.worldmapper.org

comorbidities. Here we summarize some of the available evidence and seek to contrast the African situation with the case studies from India and China of the preceding chapters [1, 2].

The Epidemiology of Underweight and Overweight in Africa

In sub-Saharan Africa, progress towards meeting one of the key indicators of the first Millennium Development Goals – the proportion of underweight children – is slow and in several countries is in reverse. Current projections indicate that Africa will not meet its target by 2015 [3]. Africa is still the home of the most acute nutritional emergencies with unacceptably high levels of severe acute malnutrition. These are largely in regions of conflict and in countries failed by their political leaders. Figure 1 shows clearly how Africa dominates the world for many infectious diseases (here illustrated by malaria) and under 5-year mortality, comes second to South East Asia in terms of the proportion of underweight children, and is barely visible in terms of gross domestic product wealth. Distressingly Africa also dominates the global picture of countries in serious economic decline.

Proportions of the adult population with a body mass index (BMI) of <18.5 (set as the definition of chronic energy deficiency) are substantial, but less than in many South Asian countries [1, 2, 4], and are a lesser concern. Adult height is also greater than in many Asian countries. In mothers the larger adult stature than in the Indian subcontinent is accompanied by

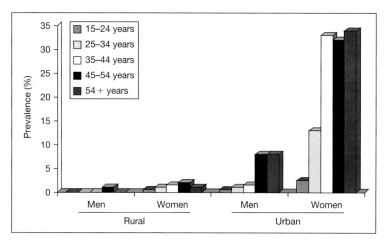

Fig. 2. Rural-urban, gender and age trends in obesity in The Gambia. Redrawn from van der Sande et al. [10].

larger mean birthweights and a lower proportion of low birthweight babies [5].

Yet obesity rates in Africa are escalating fast [6, 7]. The increase is especially rapid in urban areas, though the trends are by no means confined to Africa's cities. There are several features of the obesity epidemic in Africa that mirror those in other emerging nations: it penetrates the richer nations first (in Africa these tend to be in North Africa); it penetrates urban areas first with a strong urban–rural gradient, but this diminishes with time; initially it affects the wealthy, but later there is a demographic switch and obesity becomes a condition more associated with poverty (as in Western nations) [5, 8], and it shares many of the same drivers related to the increasing affordability of highly refined oils and carbohydrates, and a move away from subsistence farm work and towards sedentary lifestyles [9]. Because the obesity epidemic is advancing so rapidly (making national statistics out of date even before they are published) and because data collection systems in Africa are poorly developed, we will not attempt to provide a survey of the latest transcontinental trends. Selected data can be found elsewhere [7]. Here we concentrate instead on outlining features of the obesity epidemic that differ between Africa and other regions and have to rely on 'micro-data' from a few individual studies to illustrate such features.

Figure 2 shows data from a nationally representative survey in The Gambia [10] to illustrate the rural–urban and gender gradients that are frequently reported in Africa. It shows that obesity is virtually unknown in rural areas in both sexes and across all ages. Not surprisingly this is associated with a lower prevalence of obesity-related disease risk factors, though hypertension con-

Prentice

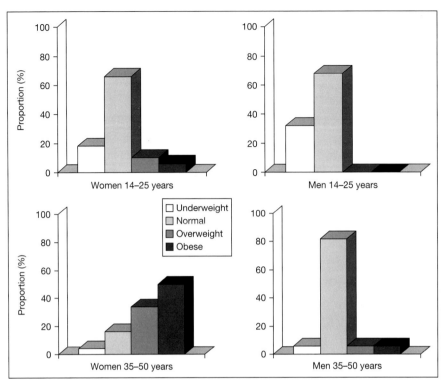

Fig. 3. BMI distribution in young and middle-aged Gambian men and women. Redrawn from Siervo et al. [12].

stitutes a significant problem in rural Africa [10, 11]. In urban areas the average prevalence of obesity (BMI >30) exceeded 30% in women aged 35 years and above. In men, however, there was virtually no obesity until 45 years and even then the rates were a fraction of those in women. Figure 3 illustrates the results from a smaller survey from which the BMI distribution can be plotted for men and women in two age bands (14–25 and 35–50 years) [12]. The gender differences are even more striking as is the development of obesity with middle age in women.

A recently published meta-analysis of 13 studies in West Africa confirms the urban–rural gradient with an odds ratio in urban areas of 2.7 (95% CI 1.7–4.6) [6]. In the same publication a meta-analysis of 26 studies also confirmed the strong sex differences in prevalence with an odds ratio of 4.8 (95% CI 3.3–7.0) in rural areas and 3.6 (95% CI 2.5–4.0) in urban areas [6].

Interestingly a study from urban Benin suggests that although obesity and abdominal obesity rates are much higher in women that in men this does not translate to higher rates of hypertension, hypertriglyceridemia or diabetes [8].

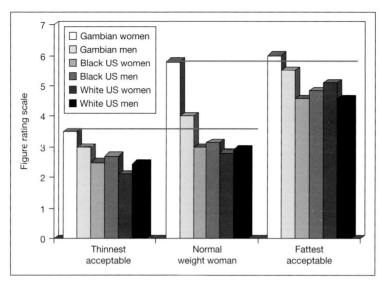

Fig. 4. Acceptability of large body size by urban Gambians in comparison to US white and black men and women. Redrawn from Siervo et al. [14].

Features of the Obesity Epidemic Characteristic of Africa

The fact that Africa has certain characteristics of the obesity epidemic that stand out from other continents may be pertinent both when considering preventative strategies and in predicting the future trends in the epidemic and its likely associated comorbidities. The following are notable differences.

Cultural Acceptability of Obesity in Women
Apart from certain Polynesian islands, Africa is probably the only region in which obesity (especially among women) is viewed culturally as a positive and desirable trait. There is a long and widespread history of fattening ceremonies in Africa, occasionally in men, but much more commonly in marriageable women. Although these are now almost unknown in a ceremonial sense there remain widely discernible echoes that still resonate in modern Africa [7, 13]. These fuel a syndrome of intentional weight gain in young women with fattening and appetite-stimulating drugs widely available in pharmacies, at least in West Africa.

Figure 4 illustrates data gathered from urban Gambians using the Figure Rating Scale (a series of 9 silhouettes of men and women of differing fatness) to examine attitudes towards body size. Men and women were asked to select the 'thinnest acceptable', 'normal' and 'fattest acceptable' images for both their own and the opposite sex [14]. The results are compared to previ-

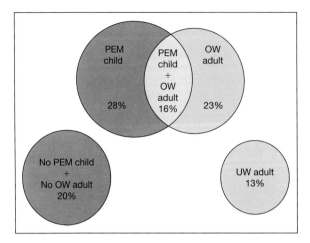

Fig. 5. Coexistence of childhood protein energy malnutrition (PEM) with adult overweight (OW) within families in urban Benin. UW = Underweight. Based on data from Deleuze Ntandou Bouzitou et al. [26].

ously published data from US black and white women. The notable features are that Gambian women are more obesity tolerant than men, but that, on average, Gambians viewed large body size as much more acceptable than Americans. Especially noteworthy is the fact that Gambian women's perception of normal weight is higher than American's views of fattest acceptable weight.

A further factor that has been frequently cited in Africa, though which lacks any formal assessment, is that the high prevalence of AIDS in many sub-Saharan countries also favors fatness because the reverse, i.e. thinness, might be interpreted by peers as a sign of infection.

These cultural drivers have almost certainly lead to major gender differences in obesity rates in many countries described above, and create an uphill slope for health education programs extolling the maintenance of a healthy bodyweight. There are signs, however, that Western ideals associating female slimness with wealth, health, power and influence are starting to penetrate the most educated strata of urban African societies, and gyms and exercise classes for women are starting to proliferate.

Altered Genetic Predisposition to the Major Obesity-Related Chronic Diseases

A general consensus has been that Africans seem genetically prone to higher rates of diabetes and hypertension in association with obesity than Caucasians, but seem to be relatively protected from dyslipidemias [15, 16]. More recent work shows that these interrelationships are more complex and that the role of environmental factors that differ between racial groups has been underestimated [17, 18]. Intriguingly we should reach a much more comprehensive understanding of underlying genetic susceptibilities in the next few years as a result of a vastly increased capacity to analyze large amounts of genetic data. In the past 2 years genome-wide association studies have identified at least 11 new genes linked to type 2 diabetes mellitus [19] and similarly rapid progress is likely to emerge in other complex trait obesity-related diseases such as hypertension. Advances in bioinformatics and the development of new statistical methods using a variety of methods to interrogate haplotype patterns now permit us to test whether individual gene variants have been the subject of recent selective pressure [20, 21], and whether there has been differential selection within each of the major racial groups [22, 23].

High Case-Fatality Rates Associated with Obesity-Related Diseases

The case-specific deaths and disabilities from diabetes and hypertension in Africa are very high due to the paucity of health services and the strain that the 'double burden' of disease places on health systems. For instance, a decade ago McLarty et al. [24] pointed out that death rates from diabetes in Tanzania were higher than in the US and Mauritius where the prevalence of disease was much greater. Similarly rates of detection, treatment and control of hypertension fall far short of those in more advanced countries [25]. There is no reason to conclude that the situation in Tanzania is worse than in most other sub-Saharan countries, indeed it is probably better than many.

The Coexistence of Obesity and Undernutrition within Households

Since the topic of this symposium is 'Emerging Societies – Coexistence of Childhood Malnutrition and Obesity', the literature has been reviewed in a search for data from Africa specifically on this issue. Only a single study was found from urban Benin, the results of which are summarized in figure 5 [26]. The conclusion was that 16% of families had at least one undernourished child coexisting with at least one overweight adult. Note, however, that the definition of overweight was set only at a BMI of 25 rather than the 30 used in some studies from Latin and South America [27], suggesting that, as yet, the problem is not so great in Africa. Nonetheless it is not infrequent to see the mothers of children admitted to therapeutic feeding centers for severely malnourished children looking well-nourished and affluent, emphasizing the dual burden of disease and the fact that malnutrition is frequently precipitated by the high levels of childhood infections (especially diarrhea) in Africa.

39

Conclusions

Like other rapidly emerging areas of the world Africa is feeling the impact of the dual burden of disease often described as 'the unfinished agenda of infectious diseases and the emerging agenda of non-communicable diseases'. There are several features of the developing epidemic of obesity that differ characteristically from other regions. Several of these are detrimental, especially the very high debility and case-fatality rates associated with non-communicable diseases in Africa, but there may be one area in which Africa might hope for a better long-term prognosis than Asia. African women tend to be significantly taller than Asian women and suffer less central obesity. This may be significant in terms of the rate at which Africa can emerge from the nutrition transition. It is arguable that Africa will suffer a lesser burden of chronic disease than Asia in which the 'Developmental Origins of Health and Disease' thesis predicts a major future burden of chronic disease based upon the mismatch between the fetal and adult nutritional environment [28].

References

1 Reddy KS: Regional case study – India; in Kalhan S, Pentice AM, Yajnik C (eds): Emerging Societies – Coexistence of Childhood Malnutrition and Obesity. Nestlé Nutr Workshop Ser Pediatr Program. Vevey, Nestec/Basel, Karger, 2008, vol 63, pp 15–24.
2 Yin S: Regional case study – China; in Kalhan S, Pentice AM, Yajnik C (eds): Emerging Societies – Coexistence of Childhood Malnutrition and Obesity. Nestlé Nutr Workshop Ser Pediatr Program. Vevey, Nestec/Basel, Karger, 2008, vol 63, pp 25–32.
3 Prentice AM, Gershwin ME, Schaible UE, et al: New challenges in studying nutrition-disease interactions in the developing world. J Clin Invest. 2008;118:1322–1329.
4 Mokhtar N, Elati J, Chabir R, et al: Diet culture and obesity in northern Africa. J Nutr 2001;131:887S–892S.
5 March of Dimes Taskforce on Nutrition and Optimal Development: Nutrition Today, Matters Tomorrow. March of Dimes, USA, 2002.
6 Abubakari AR, Lauder W, Agyemang C, et al: Prevalence and time trends in obesity among adult West African populations: a meta-analysis. Obes Rev 2008;9:297–311.
7 Prentice AM: The emerging epidemic of obesity in developing countries. Int J Epidemiol 2006;35:93–99.
8 Sodjinou R, Agueh V, Fayomi B, Delisle H: Obesity and cardio-metabolic risk factors in urban adults of Benin: relationship with socio-economic status, urbanisation, and lifestyle patterns. BMC Public Health 2008;8:84.
9 Popkin BM: Global changes in diet and activity patterns as drivers of the nutrition transition; in Kalhan S, Pentice AM, Yajnik C (eds): Emerging Societies – Coexistence of Childhood Malnutrition and Obesity. Nestlé Nutr Workshop Ser Pediatr Program. Vevey, Nestec/Basel, Karger, 2008, vol 63, pp 1–14.
10 van der Sande MA, Ceesay SM, Milligan PJ, et al: Obesity and undernutrition and cardiovascular risk factors in rural and urban Gambian communities. Am J Public Health 2001;91:1641–1644.
11 van der Sande MA, Milligan PJ, Nyan OA, et al: Blood pressure patterns and cardiovascular risk factors in rural and urban Gambian communities. J Hum Hypertens 2000;14:489–496.
12 Siervo M, Grey P, Nyan OA, Prentice AM: Urbanization and obesity in The Gambia: a country in the early stages of the demographic transition. Eur J Clin Nutr 2006;60:455–463.
13 Webb FM, Prentice AM: Obesity amidst poverty. Int J Epidemiol 2006;35:24–30.

14 Siervo M, Grey P, Nyan OA, Prentice AM: A pilot study on body image, attractiveness and body size in Gambians living in an urban community. Eat Weight Disord 2006;11:100–109.
15 Cappuccio FP: Ethnicity and cardiovascular risk: variations in people of African ancestry and South Asian origin. J Hum Hypertens 1997;11:571–576.
16 Diamond J: The double puzzle of diabetes. Nature 2003;423:599–602.
17 Cappuccio FP, Kerry SM, Adeyemo A, et al: Body size and blood pressure: an analysis of Africans and the African diaspora. Epidemiology 2008;19:38–46.
18 Cooper RS, Wolf-Maier K, Luke A, et al: An international comparative study of blood pressure in populations of European vs. African descent. BMC Med 2005;3:2.
19 Frayling TM: Genome-wide association studies provide new insights into type 2 diabetes aetiology. Nat Rev Genet 2007;8:657–662.
20 Sabeti PC, Schaffner SF, Fry B, et al: Positive natural selection in the human lineage. Science 2006;312:1614–1620.
21 Tang K, Thornton KR, Stoneking M: A new approach for using genome scans to detect recent positive selection in the human genome. PLoS Biol 2007;5:e171.
22 Voight BF, Kudaravalli S, Wen X, Pritchard JK: A map of recent positive selection in the human genome. PLoS Biol 2006;4:e72.
23 Zhang C, Bailey DK, Awad T, et al: A whole genome long-range haplotype (WGLRH) test for detecting imprints of positive selection in human populations. Bioinformatics 2006;22:2122–2128.
24 McLarty DG, Unwin N, Kitange HM, Alberti KG: Diabetes mellitus as a cause of death in sub-Saharan Africa: results of a community-based study in Tanzania. The Adult Morbidity and Mortality Project. Diabet Med 1996;13:990–994.
25 Edwards R, Unwin N, Mugusi F, et al: Hypertension prevalence and care in an urban and rural area of Tanzania. J Hypertens 2000;18:145–152.
26 Deleuze Ntandou Bouzitou G, Fayomi B, Delisle H: Child malnutrition and maternal overweight in same households in poor urban areas of Benin. Sante 2005;15:263–270.
27 Sawaya A-L: Early life malnutrition and later obesity; in Kalhan S, Prentice AM, Yajnik C (eds): Emerging Societies – Coexistence of Childhood Malnutrition and Obesity. Nestlé Nutr Workshop Ser Pediatr Program. Vevey, Nestec/Basel, Karger, 2008, vol 63, pp 95–108.
28 Yajnik CJ: The imperative of preventive measure addressing lifecycle; in Kalhan S, Pentice AM, Yajnik C (eds): Emerging Societies – Coexistence of Childhood Malnutrition and Obesity. Nestlé Nutr Workshop Ser Pediatr Program. Vevey, Nestec/Basel, Karger, 2008, vol 63, pp 177–194.

Discussion of the Forgoing 3 Chapters

Dr. Wickramasinghe: My question is for Dr. Reddy. It is very clear that there is an increased intake of food of animal origin. In your talk you said that there is a decrease in protein consumption. Do you mean that there is a tendency to eat less animal protein?

Dr. Bongga: My question for Dr. Yin is that I didn't see the prevalence of anemia among pregnant and lactating women, and could that perhaps in a way be a risk factor for the high prevalence of anemia in children?

Dr. M.A. Chowdhury: A question for Dr. Prentice: we know that malnutrition is found mainly in lower socioeconomic conditions and overweight in higher socioeconomic conditions, but in your study both undernutrition and obesity are found in the same family. What are the predisposing factors for having both conditions in the same family?

Dr. Balhaj: I have a question for Dr. Prentice. You showed us a striking graph that at the age of 24–32 months there is a big drop in the BMI and the head circumference of these children. Is there any explanation for this? Is it due to the introduction of solid foods after weaning or breastfeeding or are there any other contributing factors?

Dr. Jatana: I have a question for Dr. Yin. The anemia levels improved over the years. Was there a program or was it just dietary intervention which improved anemia in China?

Mrs. Gravereaux: This is a question for Dr. Reddy. I was just wondering whether you know why undernutrition decreases with age in women?

Dr. Mathur: From all the speakers in this session on the epidemiology of the nutrition transition in relation to obesity, it appears that the paramount determinant is economic development. However, when we look at the intervention trials on obesity, behavior modification has been largely attempted [1, 2]. We would have benefited from data and experience being shown for those behavioral risk factors in tackling the obesity epidemic, including the nutritional component of obesity.

Dr. Jaigirdar: This is a question for Dr. Reddy. People from the subcontinent have very low HDL levels. It is one of the great risk factors of ischemic heart disease, especially in the subcontinent. The HDL level can't even be increased with diet, exercise, or drugs. Is there a reason for this?

Dr. Al Waili: To Dr. Yin: you showed us that the subjects have low vitamin A deficiency. Is it because they have a low protein deficiency? Did you look for that, because we know that if they have low protein deficiency they might get vitamin A deficiency, or is it only because of the diet?

Dr. Giovannini: In all the studies did you see any relationship between birthweight and obesity? After the long period of breastfeeding, is the nutritional risk of obesity mostly related to a Western-type diet? These factors may be important. An important point in the Chinese presentation is beef intake, because between the rural and urban areas, beef intake is different. Regarding the Asian study, experience from Cambodia, where children don't receive beef, has shown that beef is the best food for men, secondary for women and least for children. This is also very important, and should be correlated to China where the rate of breastfeeding is traditionally very low.

Dr. Popkin: The critical period is weaning from 6 to 12 months which exists in China. However in India we have both the low birthweight problem and the weaning quality problem. I wonder if we are finding across all 3 countries weaning food changes with economic change and if that is an explanation for some of them? But now I want to turn to the other side of the coin for India. Is there any place in India were healthy normal BMIs can be found for adults? India, for reproductive reasons, has a very long history of women with BMIs of 16–18 producing and feeding babies. Now if suddenly their BMI goes over 18 and 20, are they already at risk of diabetes, and do we have very little room for something that we would call normal weight and normal body composition?

Anonymous: I would like to confirm Dr. Prentice's observation in The Gambia about women and men. The issue of attitude is very important. Do you have any experience with adolescents because Indian girls are now becoming thinner and boys are getting fatter? There seems to be a reversal in adolescents.

Anonymous: This is a question for Dr. Reddy. You said that across India women aged 14–19 are undernourished, and this declines within the age. Why does this happen?*Dr. Bohles:* I have a question for Dr. Prentice. Is there any difference between Eastern and Western Africa? There is a genetic difference in the muscle fiber distribution: in Eastern Africa there is a predominance of type 1 muscle fibers and in Western Africa of type 2 fibers. People with a dominance of type 1 fibers are genetically skinny because type 1 fibers burn up fatty acids as their energetic basis. Is there a difference in the tendency to obesity with respect to East Africa?

Dr. Matthai: Three points. When we define malnutrition we talk in terms of weight for age, and when we talk of obesity we talk in terms of BMI. That seems unscientific. Second, we are bringing down our values for expected BMI, perhaps we should change our standards for defining malnutrition as well. Third, when we say normal requirements for children, for example a 10-year-old child needs 2,000 cal, are we recommending more than what they really need considering genetic background and environmental factors. In other words, when we are preventing or treating malnutrition, are we sowing the seeds for obesity?

Dr. Pandit: It is generally perceived that if there is a shift in the BMI between the age of 6 and 9 years the risk grows considerably, but in the first 2 years of life there is no risk at all as shown by studies from Delhi, Finland, etc. I did not see these patterns in any of the 3 presentations. Could Dr. Reddy elaborate on that? Did you use the Cole standard for BMIs in children, because it is very tricky when the measurements are done.

Dr. Prentice: We have a great number of questions to answer, so I hope you will forgive me if I answer some of these rather rapidly. The first one was the question of what are the predisposing factors within those families who do show the coexistence of malnutrition in a child and obesity in the parents? Hopefully Dr. Sawaya and others will discuss this later, so I will just give a quick answer here. Those that I see, and again this is from the literature, especially a recent paper from Benin [3], is that surprisingly a high socioeconomic status is associated with this coexistence, so there are children in high socioeconomic families who have malnutrition. Generally this is because the mother doesn't know how to look after her child or because the child is HIV-positive and/or because that child has some severe infection that predisposes him to undernutrition. The issue of diet diversity is also being reported as being important. Those families who have this coexistence have a less diverse diet than those who don't.

The next question is related to the rapid decrease in nutritional status in The Gambia. In fact there was a misunderstanding that the x-axis there was weeks, not months, so in fact it is from 3 months to 1 year where there is a precipitant drop, and this is really caused by very poor quality weaning foods. This addresses Dr. Popkin's question also; these foods are very thin nutrient-weak 'monos', as they call them, gruels and porridges. These lead to high rates of infection, as they start to introduce other weaning foods that are highly contaminated.

One questioner stressed that we talked a lot about economy and not a lot about behavior in terms of the risk factors. Those are of course related, the increasing economy allows people the behavior of eating more animal fats, more highly refined oils and carbohydrates, etc. It is enormously complex and it is an agenda that is moving by the month even in Africa. I am going to answer this in relation to the Nigerian question about adolescents as well. One now sees adolescent girls in Africa jogging, going to aerobics and to the gym, something I would have never dreamed of seeing even 5 years ago. They have their TV satellite dishes, they see their models of skinny people from the United States, things are changing. As you said the boys very often want to build muscle and increase body mass. So, yes, things are changing, and in terms of behavior it is difficult to get on top of this because it is such a moving target all the time, but it is clearly something we need to.

There was a question about Eastern vs. Western Africa and the differences in muscle fiber types. An interesting question, and I agree it would be lovely to get some detailed research on this. I am not aware of any, the only thing I can say is that there are lots of very overweight women in East Africa as well.

The final question that was addressed to me was whether in trying to treat the malnutrition issues we are sowing the seeds of obesity. Yes that very often is the case and what we must avoid. There was an interesting case study from Chile where there were very high levels of childhood malnutrition. They had a government-driven institutional supplementation program with high calorie-dense foods, and when after 20 years it was looked at again for the first time, they found that actually they were feeding children who were already overweight and obese so they quickly stopped that.

Dr. Yin: These are very good questions The first was about anemia prevalence. In 2002 we investigated anemia problems for the whole population using sampling, and the highest prevalence is in small children and pregnant women. The averaged national prevalence of anemia was about 28.9 and 30.7% in pregnant and lactating women, respectively [4, 5].

The second question was about the improvement in anemia levels over the years. Iron deficiency and iron deficiency anemia are still serious problems based on the 2002 National Nutrition and Health Survey [5]. This survey showed that the anemia prevalence in children (6–9 years) was 13–14% in cities, indicating that these children are at a high risk of having anemia. For this reason the Chinese government started an iron fortification program. The introduction of fortified soy sauce with EDTA-Fe was carried out 5 years ago, now the fortified soy sauce is sold in markets approved by the Chinese regulation [6].

The third question was about vitamin A deficiency in children. Serious vitamin A deficiency and other forms of malnutrition in children are not very common. However, the incidence of marginal vitamin A deficiency (about 40% in children aged 3–12 years) is relatively high based on the 2002 National Nutrition and Health Survey [5]. The insufficient vitamin A in the diets was the direct cause of the marginal vitamin A deficiency, and most of the retinol equivalents were from plant foods [7].

Another question was about malnutrition and very low breastfeeding in China. But how low; I wonder how to evaluate it. The data show that breastfeeding is about 72% over 4 months, but the problem is the time of weaning. At about 10–11 months of age the children will have stopped breastfeeding; so why do most of the women stop breastfeeding very early. Another problem is the weaning food, the complementary feeding, which needs further work.

Dr. Reddy: Several questions were addressed and I will try to respond as directly and as briefly as possible to each of them. The first question was why protein consumption is decreasing if animal food consumption is increasing? Firstly these are national summary statistics. Animal food consumption is probably increasing in the higher socioeconomic groups, but pulses particularly are becoming overpriced at the moment and pulse consumption is certainly declining all over and mostly affects the lower and middle socioeconomic groups. Therefore one of the major staple sources of protein is actually declining which will result in decreasing protein consumption.

The second question was why women in the younger age group have greater evidence of undernutrition but with increasing age they actually move towards obesity. Again these are the results of cross-sectional studies and do not capture the lifespan experience of a cohort. It will be very difficult to say if this transition is occurring in the life course of a single individual or in the same cohort. However the explanation is likely that in the younger age groups there is a higher level of physical activity, with younger girls particularly taking part in a lot of domestic duties plus of course carrying out other work outside home including schooling and other related activities. By the time the women marry, there is child rearing, which is certainly a physically intense effort, and household chores. By the time they cross the 44-year age barrier, much of these physically arduous duties disappear and then the physical inactivity component rises substantially. This is what I would surmise, but we cannot prove it because there are no cohort studies or multiple behavior type studies.

Coming to behavioral factors, Dr. Mathur raised the question why we talk about economic policy interventions rather than focusing on behavioral indicators, which have been the main focus of attention in various trials. I think the researchers have essentially focused on what they believe they can change, whether they can actually change behaviors or not is a different issue. On the contrary populations are likely to be profoundly impacted by policy interventions even in a short time because they have a population-wide impact. We know this from a variety of interventions, for example how the rationale was changed in Mauritius from palm oil to soya oil and that resulted in a fairly large decline in plasma cholesterol concentrations within a matter of 5 years. Similarly we know what happened in Poland where, for example, the withdrawal of subsidies from animal foods and the import of vegetable oils, and of course of fruits and vegetables, changed the cardiovascular mortality patterns. So we know that through pricing mechanisms, which have a population-wide impact, even if the interventions are non-personal, a considerable impact can be attained in the short-term. But of course we do need to look at the behavioral factors as well and there are multiple studies currently going on which I believe will give a greater indicator. But unless we change the environment to help people make and maintain healthy choices, all the behavioral interventions are unlikely to have a full impact.

In terms of HDL levels, yes Indians seem to be afflicted with a particularly low HDL level. Whether this is a part of the metabolic syndrome complex due to low physical activity, increased insulin resistance, we don't know, but we know that insulin resistance is very high among the people of South Asia. But how much of it is conditioned in utero; how much of it is actually a thrifty gene hypothesis; how much of it is conditioned during the course of adolescence and adult life; it is difficult to tease out. I would speculate that even if we looked at the Barker hypothesis there is a rationale for having a low HDL. If you have intrauterine malnutrition and you want to ensure that your nervous system growth is absolutely ensured for survival then the HDL, which allows more tissue deposition of fat, would have to be lower, and the LDL would have to be higher. I would therefore look at what I call evolutionary survival epidemiology in terms of the Barker or the thrifty gene hypothesis. However I believe that a lack of physical activity is one of the critical events throughout the lifespan and, particularly in adolescence and adulthood, we are increasingly becoming physically inactive, and unless we change that we are not going to be able to change the HDL levels. Whether there are additional factors like low n-3 intake, whether there are additional nutritional factors, I cannot at the moment surmise but these are all areas of research.

In terms of low birthweight and weaning, the pediatricians in the audience keep talking about the very low rates of continued breastfeeding after 6 months and beyond, as well as the low levels of complementary feeding from 6 months onwards and these are two critical factors that need to be corrected if we want to do something about the 0–3 malnutrition. Continued breastfeeding has certainly to be looked at as an important public health intervention.

Dr. Popkin's provocative question, what is normal BMI for adults in India. I suppose in the absence of cohort studies it is going to be a little difficult to say what the adverse outcomes at different BMI levels are. Also in the Indian context it becomes even more challenging when we recognize that at any BMI level the percentage of body fat is quite different from Caucasian populations. Therefore we do need some independent predictors from good cohort studies.

Dr. Pandit asked which criteria were used. In our study we used both the Cole as well as Agarwal criteria, and then we have different levels. As you know in comparison to the Agarwal criteria, the Cole criteria overestimate undernutrition and underestimate overweight, but we used both and we have figures from both. The other question that Dr. Pandit posed: it is generally perceived that cardiovascular disease risk factors considerably increase when the BMI changes between 6 and 9 years but not if it changes between 0 and 2 years, do you agree? From the study that I conducted, the so-called rebound adiposity or catch-up growth, it seems to be coming up much more after 2 years between 2 and 12 or 6 and 9 years, so that could be an important vulnerable age group and we need to consider that. But coming back to the larger question, which is linked to yours, are we setting the stage for obesity and overweight by trying to correct malnutrition? I grapple with this question whenever I have to discuss the Barker hypothesis. I find it very difficult to give a public health recommendation that people who are born small with a nutritional impairment should not have nutritional correction, but adequate nutrition need not be inappropriate nutrition. We need to make sure that fruit and vegetable consumption and fiber components are much more balanced, and not just pump calories into these children. Secondly I believe it is very essential for these children who are at a high risk of insulin resistance to become physically very active. Therefore we need other public health interventions to complement and not just give nutritional corrections to these children. I think we ought to look at the larger picture.

References

1 Plotnikoff RC, Lightfoot P, Spinola C, et al: A framework for addressing the global obesity epidemic locally: the Child Health Ecological Surveillance System (CHESS). Prev Chronic Dis 2008;5:A95.
2 Connelly JB, Duaso MJ, Butler G: A systematic review of controlled trials of interventions to prevent childhood obesity and overweight: a realistic synthesis of the evidence. Public Health 2007;121:510–517.
3 Deleuze Ntandou Bouzitou G, Fayomi B, Delisle H: Child malnutrition and maternal overweight in same households in poor urban areas of Benin (in French). Sante 2005;15:263–270.
4 Yang XG, Zhai FY: The Body Mass and Nutrition Status of Chinese Population – 2002 National Nutrition and Health Survey. Beijing, People's Medical Publishing House, 2006.
5 Yin S, Lai JQ: The Status of Nutrition and Health of Chinese Women – 2002 National Nutrition and Health Survey. Beijing, People's Medical Publishing House, 2008.
6 Chen JS, Zhao XF, Zhang X, et al: The preventing effect of NaFeEDTA on iron deficiency. Population-based intervention trial. J Hyg Res 2003;32:29–38.
7 Zhai FY, Yang XG: The Status of dietary and Nutrient Intakes of Chinese Population – 2002 National Nutrition and Health Survey. Beijing, People's Medical Publishing House, 2006.

Kalhan SC, Prentice AM, Yajnik CS (eds): Emerging Societies – Coexistence of Childhood Malnutrition and Obesity.
Nestlé Nutr Inst Workshop Ser Pediatr Program, vol 63, pp 47–57,
Nestec Ltd., Vevey/S. Karger AG, Basel, © 2009.

Obesity in Emerging Nations: Evolutionary Origins and the Impact of a Rapid Nutrition Transition

Andrew M. Prentice

MRC International Nutrition Group, London School of Hygiene and Tropical Medicine, London, UK, and MRC Keneba, Keneba, The Gambia

Abstract

Here we explore whether there is any evidence that the rapid development of the obesity epidemic in emerging nations, and its unusual coexistence with malnutrition, may have evolutionary origins that make such populations especially vulnerable to the obesogenic conditions accompanying the nutrition transition. It is concluded that any selection of so-called 'thrifty genes' is likely to have affected most races due to the frequency and ubiquity of famines and seasonal food shortages in ancient populations. Although it remains a useful stimulus for research, the thrifty gene hypothesis remains a theoretical construct that so far lacks any concrete examples. There is currently little evidence that the ancestral genomes of native Asian or African populations carry particular risk alleles for obesity. Interestingly, however, there is evidence that a variant allele of the FTO gene that favors leanness may be less active in Asians or Africans. There is also some evidence that Caucasians may be less prone to developing type 2 diabetes mellitus than other races suggesting that there has been recent selection of protective alleles. In the near future, recently developed statistical methods for comparing genome-wide data across populations are likely to reveal or refute the presence of any thrifty genes and might indicate mechanisms of vulnerability.

Introduction

There are many obvious and plausible reasons (and some less obvious ones) that may account for the rapid increase in obesity rates in developing and emerging nations. Changes in diet and activity patterns brought about by the economic transition have been previously discussed in this symposium by Popkin [1]. Later papers will explore the possibility that undernutrition in fetal and early life can reset the metabolic phenotype in ways that make people especially vulnerable to the influences of an obesogenic environment if they escape from the frugality of a subsistence living [2, 3].

Here we seek to answer whether people from developing countries may have a genetic predisposition to obesity and its most common clinical outcome, type 2 diabetes mellitus (T2DM).

Possibility of Evolutionary Selection of Genes Predisposing Populations to Obesity

The concept of 'thrifty genes', first proposed by Neel [4] in the 1960s, has been prominent amongst the various theories proposed to explain the sudden rise in global obesity levels in the late 20th century. The basic premise of the thrifty gene hypothesis is that an ability to rapidly deposit energy as body fat in times of plenty would have assisted individuals to survive periods of starvation, and hence would have been under positive natural selection. Many of the earlier proponents of the theory used it to explain why certain populations had very high levels of obesity and diabetes. For instance, it was suggested that modern Polynesian Islanders are the product of a small founder group that had survived starvation during the long sea journeys across the Pacific as the islands were first colonized. The survivors of these journeys, it was argued, would either have started off as fatter individuals, or would have had mechanisms for conserving their energy when food supplies ran out. Similar arguments have been used as a possible explanation for the high rates of diabetes in the Pima Indians in Arizona, where there is evidence that their forebears may have suffered a famine that greatly depleted a formerly large population [5]. These simplistic interpretations were not those intended by Neel himself whose original theory focused more on the likely mechanism than on the theory's evolutionary origins.

Contemporary interpretations of the evolutionary and ecological implications of the thrifty gene story reappear at frequent intervals. Elsewhere [6–8] I have proposed some modifications to the widely accepted interpretations of Neel's original theory which can be summarized as follows.

First, there is abundant historical evidence to support the view that almost *all* ancient populations have been frequently subjected to selective pressure by famine. Paradoxically such cataclysmic events have been much more common in the past 10,000–12,000 years because the dawn of agriculture permitted the growth of large populations, but also made them vulnerable to climatic and political instability that would have had little significance for hunter-gatherer groups. Agriculture also led to annual hungry seasons in most traditional populations which can also have a selective effect (see below). These arguments suggest that thriftiness, in whatever biological form it might take, is likely to affect all racial groups. Thriftiness is no more likely

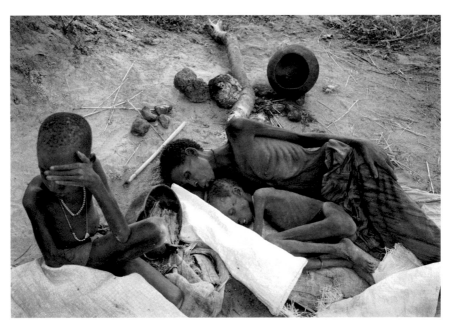

Fig. 1. Famine in contemporary Sudan. Reproduced with permission from Tom Stoddart, Getty Images.

to apply to those populations we associate with having had recent famines (fig. 1), because recent history provides only a snapshot of the longer-term processes of human evolution.

Second, the evidence suggests that transmission of thrifty traits is unlikely to have been strongly selected by mortality within famines (viability selection) and is much more likely to have been due to fertility selection mediated through the powerful effects of regular annual hungry seasons, or episodic starvation, on female fecundity. We have shown in both Bangladesh and The Gambia that birth frequencies show a smooth sinusoidal variation with a two-fold amplitude between peaks and troughs [6]. The data from these and other populations [9] suggest that the variation is driven by a suppression of the hypothalamic-pituitary-ovarian axis when women lose weight in the hungry season. Women who can remain fertile when their peers have stopped ovulating have a greater chance of transmitting their genes and of passing on this trait, which could be considered a form of thriftiness. Modeling such effects easily demonstrates that fertility selection could have had a powerful impact in the 600 or so generations since agriculture started.

Thirdly, we believe that the concept of thriftiness (which is generally interpreted in relation to the saving of energy) should also encompass an element of the 'greedy gene' since disregulated appetite control systems are the most

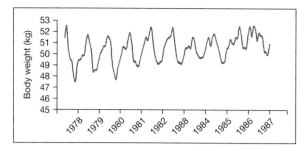

Fig. 2. Seasonal weight loss in rural Gambian women caused by hungry and harvest seasons.

common cause of the genetically based human obesity syndromes so far identified [10]. In primitive conditions, where post-harvest crop losses are high due to inadequate storage systems, it has been calculated that it can be more efficient to store energy in subcutaneous fat rather than to leave crops vulnerable to attack by vermin, insects or moulds. Such a strategy also avoids pressure to share food with others when supplies dwindle in the hungry season. These responses reveal body fat acting as nature intended (fig. 2), namely as a metabolic buffer when external energy supplies are beneath subsistence levels. This adaptation has now become largely redundant in modern societies since the hungry seasons that used to regularly deplete body fat stores seldom, if ever, occur. Hence the famous title of Neel's [4] original paper: Diabetes mellitus: a 'thrifty' genotype rendered detrimental by 'progress'.

Absence of Evidence for Obesity Susceptibility Genes in Different Populations Groups

The fact that certain population groups are highly susceptible to obesity suggests the presence of genetic factors but does not in itself provide any proof of that fact. The most intensively studied group has been the Pima Indians, noted for their very high rates of obesity and T2DM. Extensive genetic analysis of candidate genes known to be involved in susceptibility to obesity at the individual level in various population groups has yielded little evidence in support of a clear genetic susceptibility for Pima Indians as a whole [11–14]. There is similarly a notable absence of publications claiming robust identification of possible 'thrifty' alleles in other obesity-prone populations such as in Nauru.

Recent findings in relation to the FTO gene (the first of the multigenic contributors to human obesity to be identified with certainty [15,16]) reveal some interesting new clues. An FTO variant has been shown, across numerous studies to affect BMI. The effect size is small (at about 0.35 BMI units per copy) but has been confirmed to a very high degree of statistical certainty in several European, Caucasian-American and Hispanic-American populations. The variant allele promotes leanness, not obesity, and hence it is the wild-type that represents the thrifty form. Interestingly our research indicates that the same variant has no effect in native Africans [Fulford, et al., unpublished data] and others have also failed to replicate the findings in non-Caucasians, albeit on small sample sizes. This offers some initial support for the possibility, based on the historical ubiquity of famines and food shortages described above, that most human populations carry genetic mechanisms for thrift.

Although relating to diabetes, rather than obesity per se, there is some evidence that non-Caucasians are more vulnerable to T2DM [17]. It has been controversially suggested by Diamond [17] that susceptible individuals within Caucasian populations must have died out during a previous epidemic of obesity, but no historical evidence supports such a view and it is possible to suggest more cogent mechanisms, based on fertility selection, for their relative protection against T2DM. The likelihood that Caucasians are somewhat protected from T2DM is further suggested by analysis of admixture among the Pima Indians which shows an inverse relationship between the degree of European admixture and susceptibility to T2DM; in other words the greater the proportion of European genes, the lower will be the risk of T2DM [18].

In summary, the concept of the thrifty gene remains nebulous and intangible, and there is very little concrete evidence that even the most obesity-prone populations have any clear-cut genetic susceptibility to obesity, though they may be more prone to diabetes. This has led Joffe and Zimmet [19] to argue that the thrifty phenotype is a more likely explanation. Other possibilities are that susceptibility is driven by cultural 'memes'. Families that have spent generations working extremely hard and consuming a very frugal diet can hardly be blamed for relishing sedentary lifestyles and rich diets when they become available (fig. 3). Such desires are readily apparent among the newly affluent members of developing country societies, and may be propagated further by the notion that a higher BMI is desirable, particularly for women [20, 21].

New Methods in Analysis and Interpretation of Data from Genome-Wide Scans

Exciting times lie ahead with respect to understanding whether or not evolution has endowed any of us with particular susceptibility to obesity and/or diabetes. First the increasing speed and decreasing cost of genome-wide scans have recently opened up the study of multigenic disorders [22]. In 2007, 11 new genes linked to T2DM were added to the 3 that had previously been identified. Second, advances in bioinformatics and the development of new statistical methods using a variety of methods to interrogate haplotype

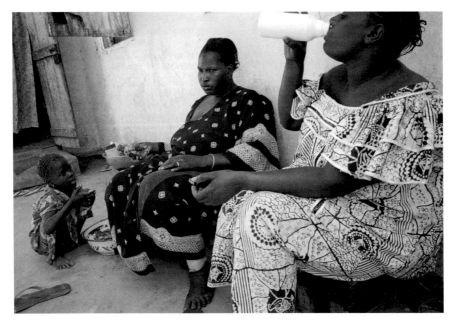

Fig. 3. Obesity in contemporary Gambia. Reproduced with permission from Felicia Webb.

patterns now permit us to test whether individual gene variants have been the subject of recent selective pressure [23, 24]. Similar advances in methods for comparing genome-wide scans between different ethnic/racial groups are starting to pinpoint those genes that show evidence of geographic diversity, and of recent differential selection within each of the major racial groups [25, 26]. Together these new approaches will soon assist in resolving the issues surrounding putative thrifty genes and other evolutionary influences on the obesity epidemic.

Is Understanding the Evolutionary Origins of Obesity Important?

Many readers could be forgiven for asking: So what? Is it really important to understand whether or not different populations have a genetically endowed enhanced risk of becoming fat and contracting the associated chronic diseases? One argument in favor of seeking such knowledge is that it might help to direct interventions. Table 1 lists the primary domains through which thriftiness might operate. Some of them (those listed as metabolic, physiologic and adipogenic) may be non-modifiable except through pharmacologic intervention, but the behavioral domains would be amenable to intervention

Table 1. Examples of the possible manifestations of 'thriftiness'

Metabolic	'Energy-sparing' super-efficient metabolism
Adipogenic	Propensity to rapidly deposit fat
Physiological	Ability to switch off less-essential processes (e.g. adaptive immunity in the short-term)
Gluttony	Tendency to gorge when food is available
Slothfulness	Tendency to conserve energy through inactivity
Behavioral	Hoarding, meanness, theft, etc.

and distinguishing the relative importance of these might therefore be useful. However, the absence of certainty on any of these issues should never inhibit the development and propagation of public health messages and government initiatives to combat obesity. We already have strong evidence that urban populations in developing countries do exhibit high levels of obesity, and this fact alone should drive the public health agenda.

References

1 Popkin BM: Global changes in diet and activity patterns as drivers of the nutrition transition; in Kalhan S, Pentice AM, Yajnik C (eds): Emerging Societies – Coexistence of Childhood Malnutrition and Obesity. Nestlé Nutr Workshop Ser Pediatr Program. Vevey, Nestec/Basel, Karger, 2008, vol 63, pp 1–14.
2 Sawaya A-L: Early life malnutrition and later obesity; in Kalhan S, Pentice AM, Yajnik C (eds): Emerging Societies – Coexistence of Childhood Malnutrition and Obesity. Nestlé Nutr Workshop Ser Pediatr Program. Vevey, Nestec/Basel, Karger, 2008, vol 63, pp 95–108.
3 Whitelaw E: Epigenetic mechanisms linking early exposure to later phenotype; in Kalhan S, Pentice AM, Yajnik C (eds): Emerging Societies – Coexistence of Childhood Malnutrition and Obesity. Nestlé Nutr Workshop Ser Pediatr Program. Vevey, Nestec/Basel, Karger, 2008, vol 63, pp 109–119.
4 Neel JV: Diabetes mellitus: a 'thrifty' genotype rendered detrimental by 'progress'. Am J Hum Genet 1962;14:353–362.
5 Fagan B: Floods, Famines and Emperors. London, Pimlico, 2000.
6 Prentice AM, Rayco-Solon P, Moore SE: Insights from the developing world: thrifty genotypes and thrifty phenotypes. Proc Nutr Soc 2005;64:153–161.
7 Prentice AM: Early influences on human energy regulation: thrifty genotypes and thrifty phenotypes. Physiol Behav 2005;86:640–645.
8 Prentice AM: Starvation in humans: evolutionary background and contemporary implications. Mech Ageing Dev 2005;126:976–981.
9 Ellison PT: On Fertile Ground: A Natural History of Reproduction. Cambridge, Harvard University Press, 2001.
10 Farooqi IS, O'Rahilly S: Monogenic obesity in humans. Annu Rev Med 2005;56:443–458.
11 Ma L, Tataranni PA, Bogardus C, Baier LJ: Melanocortin 4 receptor gene variation is associated with severe obesity in Pima Indians. Diabetes 2004;53:2696–2699.
12 Kovacs P, Ma L, Hanson RL, et al: Genetic variation in UCP2 (uncoupling protein-2) is associated with energy metabolism in Pima Indians. Diabetologia 2005;48:2292–2295.
13 Jenkinson CP, Cray K, Walder K, et al: Novel polymorphisms in the neuropeptide-Y Y5 receptor associated with obesity in Pima Indians. Int J Obes Relat Metab Disord 2000;24:580–584.
14 Norman RA, Permana P, Tanizawa Y, Ravussin E: Absence of genetic variation in some obesity candidate genes (GLP1R, ASIP, MC4R, MC5R) among Pima Indians. Int J Obes Relat Metab Disord 1999;23:163–165.

Prentice

15 Frayling TM, Timpson NJ, Weedon MN, et al: A common variant in the FTO gene is associated with body mass index and predisposes to childhood and adult obesity. Science 2007;316:889–894.
16 Gerken T, Girard CA, Tung YC, et al: The obesity-associated FTO gene encodes a 2-oxoglutarate-dependent nucleic acid demethylase. Science 2007;318:1469–1472.
17 Diamond J: The double puzzle of diabetes. Nature 2003;423:599–602.
18 Williams RC, Long JC, Hanson RL, et al: Individual estimates of European genetic admixture associated with lower body-mass index, plasma glucose, and prevalence of type 2 diabetes in Pima Indians. Am J Hum Genet 2000;66:527–538.
19 Joffe B, Zimmet P: The thrifty genotype in type 2 diabetes: an unfinished symphony moving to its finale? Endocrine 1998;9:139–141.
20 Siervo M, Grey P, Nyan OA, Prentice AM: A pilot study on body image, attractiveness and body size in Gambians living in an urban community. Eat Weight Disord 2006;11:100–109.
21 Siervo M, Grey P, Nyan OA, Prentice AM: Urbanization and obesity in The Gambia: a country in the early stages of the demographic transition. Eur J Clin Nutr 2006;60:455–463.
22 Frayling TM: Genome-wide association studies provide new insights into type 2 diabetes aetiology. Nat Rev Genet 2007;8:657–662.
23 Sabeti PC, Schaffner SF, Fry B, et al: Positive natural selection in the human lineage. Science 2006;312:1614–1620.
24 Tang K, Thornton KR, Stoneking M: A New approach for using genome scans to detect recent positive selection in the human genome. PLoS Biol 2007;5:e171.
25 Voight BF, Kudaravalli S, Wen X, Pritchard JK: A map of recent positive selection in the human genome. PLoS Biol 2006;4:e72.
26 Zhang C, Bailey DK, Awad T, et al: A whole genome long-range haplotype (WGLRH) test for detecting imprints of positive selection in human populations. Bioinformatics 2006;22:2122–2128.

Discussion

Dr. Raju: One thing about the Western population, the Caucasians, is that the incidence of diabetes is very low. Is there a possibility that over a period of several thousands of years they had their share of obesity epidemics and got rid off all those people who have a tendency to become obese and do you think they are more refined and adapted to the modern environment?

Dr. Prentice: That's a very good question. You are, I think, alluding to a paper by Diamond [1] in 2003 in which he described the double puzzle of diabetes. Diamond argues first that diabetes rates for a given level of obesity tend to be lower in Caucasians. His suggestion is that this must have been caused by a previous epidemic of obesity which allowed selection to occur. Now there I disagree profoundly with Diamond. I really cannot see that having been the case. I think there is no historical evidence. The argument that we have made is that actually it is not postnatal viability selection, it is prenatal selection [2]. A colleague, Stephen Corbett from Sydney, has written a paper, which is under review at the moment, suggesting that this may be tied up with fertility selection and polycystic ovary syndrome is part of this story. It may be that insulin sensitivity and resistance were crucial to determining which women would conceive at which BMI and during which periods in the past, and that diabetes may actually be an accidental sequel of a selection that has selected people differently in European and Asian and African populations and which leads to differential susceptibility to diabetes.

Dr. Haschke: Very interesting information on the famine risk in populations living on agricultural products as opposed to the hunting population. What about populations living in coastal areas because this was the first area where people survived.

There should be minimum famine risk. Did you find anything in the literature about the selectivity of change in these populations?

Dr. Prentice: I am not aware of anything.

Dr. Popkin: The lactase gene story is interesting. According to research, 6,000 years ago Northern Europeans adjusted to deal with the lactase enzyme in milk. 3,000 years ago they did that in Southern Africa. We don't really know how long it took in each of these populations to create these genetic adjustments. But does this history give us any hope that perhaps a gene will develop in South Asia so that people will survive with diabetes and be healthy and so forth?

Dr. Prentice: I think there is hope. It is interesting that, as you suggested, there is evidence for independent selection of lactase persistence in both Europe and Africa [3]. Estimates of the time scale for these genetic changes are difficult because they compare the changes within the lactase persistence gene to background variations. First we don't have a good measure of that background; what the natural mutation rate is. Secondly we would have to know how fast populations reproduced, but most importantly the mathematics is profoundly changed by population size and by population growth. So without being able to figure out how populations have changed, it is going to be very difficult to give this an absolute number. So we don't know how fast these things have occurred but I would argue that they probably can occur very fast and I think now we are getting into populations where the obesity rate is so great that it is starting to impact quite significantly on reproductive fitness, and that ultimately may cause a fairly rapid selection of protective genes.

Dr. Whitelaw: I was very interested to see your data about the 9-month lag. As a biologist who often deals with animals and even plants, have you considered the possibility that this is a response to the changes in light/dark cycles and seasonal events that are not necessarily about the availability of food but about other cues that change each year, certainly with mice and certainly with plants, which are known to have long-term effects?

Dr. Prentice: We have. The first thing we can say is that if this was driven by light/dark cycles then we would expect to see this phenomenon in almost all populations – we don't. The phenomenon only occurs in populations where there is seasonal food availability. We tried to look at folate supply and other possibly significant variables such as the frequency and timing of husbands migrating away from the village. It does seem that it is probably very strongly driven by their energy status. We have got data which have also been submitted for publication showing that twinning rates change very radically in these two populations and the increase is in advance of the conception of singletons. This shows us some very clever biology. The woman is able to recognize very quickly when the harvest comes in. Then she is in a good nutritional state and is more likely to conceive twins. This phenomenon may help us to understand why twinning persists in the human genome.

Dr. Ravussin: Speakman [4] has challenged the thrifty genotype and has proposed that a genetic drift over many generations is sufficient to explain the variability in BMI. I'm not siding with Speakman, but on the other hand some geneticists have tried to simulate this, not only with one gene as Speakman did but with many genes, and they also explain this variability as just a random genetic drift over thousands of generations. What is your answer to that?

Dr. Prentice: First of all I would like to say very clearly that I have no definitive answer. As you know I happen to disagree with Speakman and I don't think it is genetic drift. But perhaps he is right; it is intriguing. The answer, I think, will be out within the next 2 years. As you say there are some very clever geneticists doing a lot of modeling at the moment with a lot of data which is going to give us those answers fairly soon.

Dr. Chittal: With the idea that the thrifty gene was indeed determining the survival of the fittest, maybe it should be survival of the fattest. The same gene in times of abundance, could it be a process of natural selection of disasters for the fattest? Is it in any way trying to restrain the human population from overrunning the earth? Is it possible that it is the same gene which is causing destruction now? Do genes work that way? At one time it will be survival, at another time it will be destruction.

Dr. Prentice: I think that would be very difficult to argue. I am going to be very cautious in my response and probably there is someone in the audience who could respond much better. The general thesis I think is that most genetic selection has to occur at the individual level rather than at the population level, and of course there is an interrelationship between those, but I think it would be difficult to model a scenario where what you suggested was true.

Dr. Ray: What is the genetic relation between leptin deficiency and genes?

Dr. Prentice: Leptin deficiency in humans is extraordinarily rare. Dr. Ravussin will probably give me an update on the numbers but I think there are less than 20 individuals in the whole world who are known to have a monogenic leptin deficiency. They are all the offspring of first-cousin marriages, so it is an extraordinarily rare defect which, under most circumstances, is not fatal, but the offspring of those marriages are non-reproductive.

Dr. Ray: Is there any autosomal recessive inheritance?

Dr. Prentice: There is a little bit of evidence I think that it may be beneficial in the heterozygote form.

Dr. Jaigirdar: Bangladesh is a country of disaster, famine, flood, and it is one of the mostly densely populated countries in the world. Don't you think that it satisfies your thrifty gene idea?

Dr. Prentice: I have a lecture I give to the students which is called 'Reproduction against the Odds'. I start off pointing out this paradox that the world's fastest reproductive growth rates are in the most undernourished populations. It is amazing. How do we do it? We are a very efficient species in terms of our ability to reproduce when the chips are down. So yes, I think in a way it is a measure of our thriftiness, but I caution against moving from that general statement, to a specific statement about thrifty genes.

Dr. Popkin: Related to that, I wanted just to follow up with an issue. In India perhaps a third of adult women in rural areas have BMIs of <17–17.5 and very high reproductive efficiency, and high low birthweight rates as well. Does that fit into the talk about the fact that in India and even in South Asia there has been a shift over in the BMI–reproduction ratio for biological adaptation? The BMI is at such a low level that it has to play some role when a BMI of 20 is seen in Ranjan, a body fat level that is equal to a BMI of 35 in the US.

Dr. Prentice: Exactly. This is precisely the thesis that Prof. Stephen Corbett has submitted. Data from the Nurses' Health Study show that there is a U-shaped curve between BMI and fertility in the US, and it's actually a very sharp optimal fertility at a BMI of around 21–22. If a woman is too thin of course we know she will become anovulatory, etc., but also if a woman is too fat, she will also stop reproducing efficiently. Leptin is probably the key driver here; Indians with abdominal obesity even at very low BMI have higher leptin levels, so that story would fit together exactly as you suggested that this is an adaptation to remain fertile under highly energetically deficient conditions.

Dr. Yajnik: This brings us to comparing BMI across populations. We know this is influenced by adiposity. Recently we compared the whole body MRIs of Indian newborns with those of Caucasian newborns. Although lighter by 800 g, the Indian baby has comparable body fat and higher intra-abdominal fat (submitted for publication).

We have also shown that the cord blood leptin concentrations are higher in Indian babies compared with white babies, even after correction for birthweight [5], and adiponectin concentrations are lower. This means the adipocyte function is also different. This might be related to an epigenetic rather than a structural change.

Dr. Prentice: A very important question for which I don't know the answer. We look forward to learning about that in the years to come.

Dr. Raju: You said something tantalizing about whether it is normal to be thrifty or unthrifty. You also said something about being very unthrifty and probably you were referring to oxidative phosphorylase decoupling or whatever, and about human migration up to colder altitudes, thermogenesis. Is that what you are referring to?

Dr. Prentice: Partly those. You have picked up on an important point. There are people who suggest that a high level of mitochondrial fatty acid turnover is important in terms of quenching oxidative damage in the mitochondria; there are people who maintain the other view, and we will be hearing some of that no doubt from Dr. Ravussin in terms of caloric restriction. You have also mentioned the issue of northern latitudes and we can see some evidence of variations in mitochondrial DNA which would support that story. Another important one is the ability to concentrate nutrients, so if you are on a nutrient-poor diet you may need to eat a lot of that food in order to get enough micronutrients, so the trick of being able to burn off calories but hang on to the micronutrients would also be an important adaptation.

References

1   Diamond J: The double puzzle of diabetes. Nature 2003;423:599–602.
2   Prentice AM, Rayco-Solon P, Moore SE: Insights from the developing world: thrifty genotypes and thrifty phenotypes. Proc Nutr Soc 2005;64:153–161.
3   Tishkoff SA, Reed FA, Ranciaro A, et al: Convergent adaptation of human lactase persistence in Africa and Europe. Nat Genet 2007;39:31–40.
4   Speakman JR: A nonadaptive scenario explaining the genetic predisposition to obesity: the 'predation release' hypothesis. Cell Metab 2007;6:5–12.
5   Yajnik CS, Lubree HG, Rege SS, et al: Adiposity and hyperinsulinemia in Indians are present at birth. J Clin Endocrinol Metab 2002;87:5575–5580.

Kalhan SC, Prentice AM, Yajnik CS (eds): Emerging Societies – Coexistence of Childhood Malnutrition and Obesity.
Nestlé Nutr Inst Workshop Ser Pediatr Program, vol 63, pp 59–77,
Nestec Ltd., Vevey/S. Karger AG, Basel, © 2009.

Prenatal Origins of Undernutrition

Parul Christian

Center for Human Nutrition, Department of International Health, Johns Hopkins Bloomberg School of Public Health, Baltimore, MD, USA

Abstract

Undernutrition continues to be high in many regions of the developing world. Birthweight, a common proxy measure of intrauterine growth, is influenced by nutritional, environmental and lifestyle factors during pregnancy and, in turn, affects immediate survival and function, and is a determinant of later life risk of chronic diseases. Maternal pre-pregnancy weight and height are independently associated with birthweight and also modify the effects of pregnancy weight gain and interventions during pregnancy on birthweight and perinatal mortality. Other prenatal factors commonly known to impact birthweight include maternal age, parity, sex, and birth interval, whereas lifestyle factors such as physical activity and maternal stress, as well as environmental toxicants have variable influences. Tobacco and other substance use and infections, specifically ascending reproductive tract infections, malaria, and HIV, can cause intrauterine growth restriction (IUGR). Few studies have examined the contribution of prenatal factors including low birthweight to childhood wasting and stunting. Studies that have examined this, with adequate adjustment for confounders, have generally found odds ratios associated with low birthweight ranging between 2 and 5. Even fewer studies have examined birth length or maternal nutritional status as risk factors. More research is needed to determine the proportion of childhood undernutrition attributable to IUGR so that interventions can be targeted to the appropriate life stages.

Introduction

Childhood undernutrition and its health consequences continue to contribute to the global burden of morbidity and mortality in many regions of the world even as rates of overweight and obesity are on the rise in these same regions. The recent series in the *Lancet* on maternal and child undernutrition estimates that stunting (height for age z score < –2 SD) and severe wasting (weight for age z score < -3 SD) using the World Health Organization (WHO) growth standards and intrauterine growth restriction (IUGR; term low birthweight) are together responsible for 2.2 million deaths and 21% of disability-adjusted life years for children younger than 5 years [1]. More than a decade ago, the synergy between infectious diseases and mild-to-moderate undernutrition in causing childhood deaths was brought to the forefront with an estimate that about half of all deaths in young children (<72 months) could be attributable to undernutrition [2]. The cause-specific population-attributable fractions were 45% for measles, 57% for malaria, 52% for pneumonia, and 61% for diarrhea [3]. Beyond immediate death and disease, childhood undernutrition has also been linked to shorter height and increased blood pressure in adulthood, less schooling, and lower productivity that translates into reduced adult health and human capital in many regions of the world [4]. The link to lower productivity may result from both the effects of undernutrition on physical work capacity and cognitive function. In women, short stature can lead to an increased risk of poor reproductive health, especially increasing the risk of cephalo-pelvic disproportion, and cesarean section [5].

Despite the high levels of undernutrition that continue to exist in the developing world, the burden of chronic diseases is also estimated to be the highest and on the rise in the developing world [6]. The 'developmental origins of health and disease' extends the consequence of fetal growth restriction and suboptimal postnatal growth to well beyond the childhood period to risk of chronic diseases in adulthood and old age. Countries undergoing the nutrition transition with high levels of low birthweight are likely to be faced with the dual burden of under- and overnutrition with each contributing to significant health consequences. This paper reviews the environmental, nutritional, lifestyle and other risk factors of fetal growth restriction and low birthweight. It will also examine the contribution of prenatal nutrition to childhood undernutrition, thereby drawing attention to a perhaps neglected relationship in an attempt to emphasize the need for prevention strategies to begin earlier than in the preschool years of life.

Extent and Magnitude of Child and Maternal Undernutrition and Low Birthweight

Rates of childhood undernutrition continue to be high in many regions of the world, based on analyses recently reported in the *Lancet* nutrition series [1] (fig. 1). Overall, 32% or 178 million children under 5 years of age throughout the developing world are estimated to be stunted and 3.5% or 19 million are severely wasted. Low birthweight (<2.5 kg) is estimated at 16% in developing countries, with rates higher in Asia than in Africa. About 10.8% are estimated to be term low birthweight or IUGR. It is not surprising that maternal undernutrition, which contributes to IUGR in developing

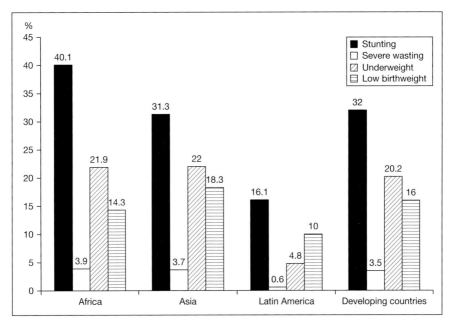

Fig. 1. Childhood (<5 years) stunting, severe wasting, underweight and low birthweight by region [1]. Stunting defined as < –2 height for age z score, severe wasting as <3 weight for height z score, underweight as < –2 weight for age z score. Low birthweight defined as weight <2.5 kg.

countries, is also common and high in both South Asia and sub-Saharan Africa [1] (fig. 2). Unlike in South and parts of Southeast Asia, maternal stunting in Africa ranges between 1 and 2%, except in Madagascar and Mozambique where it is higher at 5%. In Latin America on the other hand, wasting is less common, although stunting continues to affect a higher proportion of women of reproductive age, especially in countries such as Guatemala, Peru, and Bolivia. South Asia harbors the highest rates of maternal wasting and stunting in the world.

Causes and Risk Factors of Fetal Growth Restriction

Birthweight is a common, relatively easy measure of fetal growth taken at the time of birth or soon after. Birthweight is influenced by two biologic processes – growth in utero and the length of gestation. It is common knowledge that low birthweight is predominantly due to fetal growth failure in developing settings whereas preterm (gestational age at birth <37 weeks) contributes to low birthweight in many developed countries [7, 8]. Small for gestational age (SGA), defined as birthweight below the 10th percentile of a reference

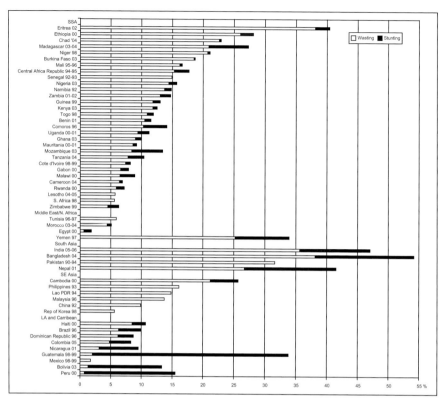

Fig. 2. Prevalence rates of low BMI (<18.5) and low height (<145 cm) among women 15–49 years of age using the most recent national surveys (DHS or WHO) by region [1].

population, is used to classify IUGR, although customized growth curves and birthweight percentiles (www.gestation.net) to define 'customized SGA' have been validated in some settings and are associated with increased risk of morbidity and perinatal and neonatal mortality [9]. This adjustment allows a better estimate of growth restriction vis-à-vis the true growth potential for a fetus taking into consideration factors such as maternal size, ethnicity, parity and fetal sex. The ponderal index (weight/length³), reflecting fetal wasting, is also used to distinguish between symmetric versus asymmetric growth restriction. Causes of fetal growth restriction (or IUGR) are generally nutritional in origin, whereas environmental and lifestyle factors and infections are more likely to result in preterm birth. It is poor fetal growth due to preterm that is more strongly associated with neonatal and infant mortality whereas term low birthweight carries a lower risk [10]. Numerous reviews, summarized below, have examined the determinants of low birthweight.

Biological Factors

Maternal Age and Parity

The optimal age at first birth is a tradeoff between the availability of time for growth during puberty vs. achieving reproductive success as reflected by increased newborn survival. Teen pregnancy is known to increase the risk of low birthweight due to the competing needs for growth of the mother and the fetus, with the youngest adolescent being at the highest risk. Literature to date has not been consistent in describing the risk of adverse birth outcomes related to young age, but this may be due to the diversity of settings and risk factors (behavioral and socioeconomic) under which adolescent pregnancy outcomes have been examined. Confounding due to these factors may attenuate or exaggerate the differences in birth outcomes between adolescent and adult women. In many developing countries, pregnancy in adolescence is a norm resulting from early age at marriage and low contraception prevalence to delay the first pregnancy. Recently it has been demonstrated that adolescents who 'grow' (assessed using knee height changes) and accumulate fat stores during pregnancy are likely to have smaller babies compared to those who cease growth [11], suggesting competition in the partitioning of nutrients between the maternal and fetal compartments. Second, primiparous adolescent girls (<19 years) may have an increased risk of preterm but not SGA compared with primiparous adult women in some settings, a difference that was not apparent between adolescent and adult women for parity 2 or more [12]. Primiparity is a well-known risk factor for low birthweight due to IUGR.

Ethnicity

Ethnicity/race is an interesting risk factor of low birthweight in some settings. In the US, African-American infants are born preterm and weigh on average 200–300 g less at birth than Caucasian babies resulting in an about 2-fold higher rate of low birthweight in this ethnic group. While sociobehavioral factors may underlie this racial/ethnic difference, a genetic component cannot be ruled out. South Asian women living in Europe or the USA are typically known to be at risk of low birthweight, although the low birthweight among them is more likely due to IUGR than preterm birth [13]. Given the intergenerational nature of the consequences of IUGR, only time will tell if low birthweight rates will decline among these ethnic groups over generations.

Other

Sex of the newborn (being female), multiple births, and a short inter-pregnancy interval are other biologic factors known to reduce birthweight, both due to the shorter duration of gestation and IUGR. A meta-analysis revealed that compared with 18–23 months, less than 18 and longer than 59 months are significantly associated with low birthweight, preterm birth and SGA adjusted for maternal age and socioeconomic status [14]. Maternal nutritional depletion due to repeated pregnancies, especially of shorter birth intervals, does not allow catch-up in nutritional status from the high nutrient burden of pregnancy and lactation with the result that women are physiologically and nutritionally ill-prepared for the next pregnancy. It has been shown that women who are severely malnourished tend to gain more weight during a reproductive cycle at the same time as showing lower birthweight for the second compared to the first birth relative to marginally malnourished or well-nourished women who have lower weight gain but higher birthweight for the second offspring [15]. Few intervention strategies exist, especially in developing countries, to target women between pregnancies, especially those that are closely spaced. The increased risk of a long birth interval (>59 months) is hypothesized to be related to a gradual decline in reproductive capacity, resulting in the women becoming similar to primigravidae or perhaps due to confounding by factors related to low fertility such as reproductive tract infections which can also result in adverse birth outcomes [15].

Lifestyle Factors

Smoking is a well-known risk factor sharing a dose-response relationship with both the risk of low birthweight and preterm delivery [16]. Adjusted for confounders, even passive smoking is known to elevate the risk of IUGR [17]. The risk of fetal alcohol syndrome including IUGR are well known, whereas drug consumption including cocaine results in an increased risk of both preterm and IUGR, as well as other complications such as congenital malformations. Smoking, caffeine, alcohol and drug consumption behaviors tend to cluster and may have additive if not synergistic effects on adverse pregnancy outcomes.

Various elements of physical activity during pregnancy have been examined for their association with low birthweight and preterm delivery, although confounding is commonly not well considered. In a systematic review of studies from developed countries no more than a moderate effect size (relative risk ≤1.4) was found for the risk of low birthweight and preterm related to prolonged work hours, shift work, lifting, standing, and heavy physical workload [18]. Generally, moderate levels of work/exercise may be beneficial during pregnancy, but higher intensity of work may be harmful [17]. In settings where malnutrition, poverty, and morbidity are high, the relationship between physical work and birth outcomes tend to suffer from reverse causation; healthier women with better pregnancy outcomes may in fact report performing higher levels of physical activity compared to those who were ill and experienced adverse outcomes [19] resulting in what has been termed as the 'healthy pregnancy/worker' phenomenon.

Maternal psychosocial stress during pregnancy caused by a myriad of factors may result in poor birth outcomes and obstetric complications. Elevated levels of anxiety and depression may be associated with increased odds of low birthweight, preterm and SGA, although inadequate control for confounders, and low precision and inaccuracy in assessments of anxiety and depressive moods, including assessment of their levels rather than a diagnosis of disorders of mood/anxiety are of concern [20]. The most likely biologic pathway underpinning this relationship is an altered hypothalamic-pituitary axis in pregnancy. Research is needed to elucidate the exact mechanism by which maternal stress (psychosocial or other) leads to poor pregnancy outcome. Indeed, nutritional deprivation, hunger, micronutrient deficiencies as well as inflammatory conditions can be viewed as 'stressors' and can lead to altered maternal-placental-fetal pathways that cause adverse outcomes. However, psychosocial support interventions in the past have failed to show significant reductions in birthweight, perhaps because many of the trials reviewed had methodology issues [21]. There is weak evidence for prenatal care and its various current components, even in the context of developed countries, to either adequately identify pregnancies at risk of preterm delivery or IUGR or to prevent these birth outcomes [22]. Few developing countries have adequate antenatal care delivery in place as reflected by low coverage for antenatal iron-folate supplementation and screening for malaria during pregnancy.

Infection

Globally sexually transmitted infections, HIV-1, and malaria may be the largest infectious causes of low birthweight and preterm [17, 23]. These infections also tend to coexist exacerbating pregnancy-related outcomes. Reproductive tract infections, especially ascending infections leading to endometritis can result in preterm and low birthweight. Untreated sexually transmitted infections such as gonorrhea, chlamydia and syphilis as well as bacterial vaginosis are well linked to an increased incidence of preterm and low birthweight. Malaria in pregnancy due to altered immunity to the infection results in severe anemia, placental parasitemia, and low birthweight, especially in primigravidae [1]. The risk of IUGR is higher if infection occurs towards the end of pregnancy [1].

Subclinical infection may also be associated with preterm birth [24]. Labor initiation normally involves inflammatory cascades, thus, determining if labor is induced by intrauterine infection would be difficult. Furthermore, pregnancy itself is considered an inflammatory state, and it is known that C-reactive protein normally increases throughout normal pregnancy. Yet, a recent study in Nepalese women reported finding that higher α_1-acid glycoprotein in the third trimester was associated with lower birthweight [25].

Maternal HIV-1 infection needs special mention in the context of sub-Saharan Africa and increasingly in some parts of Asia. Infants of infected mothers have an increased risk of low birthweight, prematurity, and perinatal and neonatal mortality [26] but treatment with zidovudine is efficacious in reducing the risk of low birthweight as indicated by results from five placebo-controlled trials (pooled RR 0.75, 95% CI 0.57–0.99) [27].

Finally, in settings where geohelminths, especially hookworm, and low birthweight are common, deworming is associated with reductions in the incidence of low birthweight [28].

Environment

Epidemiologic evidence is convincing that maternal exposure to airborne particulate matter is associated with adverse outcomes including preterm and IUGR. Although the risk may be small and varies widely [29], some of the suggested biologic pathways include oxidative stress, inflammation, endothelial function and hemodynamic mechanisms that could potentially be modified by nutrition including intakes of vitamin- and mineral-rich foods [30]. Few studies have examined the risk in the context of the developing world, especially measuring different types of pollutants (CO, NO_2, SO_2, particulate matter, O_3, etc.) and their levels in the ambient air. Among other environmental pollutants, arsenic in drinking water needs further investigation in countries such as Bangladesh, whereas lead exposure either directly or through mobilization of that accumulated in the bones during pregnancy can cross over to the placenta leading to IUGR and preterm.

Maternal Nutrition and Diet

Kramer [7] showed more than two decades ago that maternal nutritional factors may account for more than 50% of the etiology of low birthweight in developing countries. These factors included low pre-pregnancy weight, short stature, and low caloric intake during pregnancy (or weight gain) as well as maternal low birthweight. It is not a coincidence that rates of low birthweight are high in settings where maternal malnutrition is common. The intergenerational cycle of growth failure has long been used as a framework for considering the appropriate life stages for intervening. The following concepts and knowledge have emerged from years of research in this area: (a) food supplementation trials during pregnancy, targeting a narrow window in life, have shown limited efficacy and modest increments in birth weight; (b) nutrition interventions that begin earlier in pregnancy are likely to have stronger effects; (c) maternal short stature, which is strongly correlated with uterine volume, is independently associated with IUGR; (d) maternal stunting is also a risk factor for cesarean section deliveries and cephalo-pelvic disproportion; a meta-analysis found a 60% (95% CI 50–70%) increase in delivery assistance in the lowest quantile of maternal height compared with the highest quantile [5], an association that is likely to be modified by newborn size, and (e) finally, pre-periconceptional nutrition may be a strong determinant of the fetal growth trajectory, the cues for which may be derived early on through processes involving placentation, placental vascularization and genetic imprinting. And yet, few studies examine interventions targeted during this period of the life.

Adequate caloric intake and weight gain are critical during pregnancy. Balanced energy protein supplementation in pregnancy based on randomized controlled trials has been shown to reduce IUGR by 32% (26–44%) [31]. Chronic micronutrient deficiencies, specifically those of iron, calcium, magnesium and other micronutrients, may contribute to IUGR [32]. The efficacy of multiple micronutrient interventions for a range of outcomes is reviewed elsewhere in this book.

Fruit and vegetable intake during pregnancy has been associated with improved birthweight in both developed [33] and developing countries [34] as has consumption of dairy (Chile, Denmark), perhaps due to increased micronutrient intake, although in the case of milk, IGF-1 concentrations in the blood of children were found to be higher [35]. Findings from these observational studies do not prove causality despite adjustment for confounders. Food-based micronutrient intervention trials during pregnancy are currently ongoing in India and are likely to shed light on their benefits for developing dietary guidelines, policy and programs for interventions beyond calories and proteins during pregnancy.

Maternal nutritional status, both pre-pregnancy and during pregnancy may also modify the effect of other risk factors and stressors associated with preterm and low birthweight. For example, there is evidence that high maternal BMI or vitamin and mineral intakes may ameliorate the risk of adverse outcomes due to psychosocial stress, smoking, and environmental pollutants, underscoring the importance of maternal nutrition in reproductive function.

Childhood Undernutrition: Contribution of IUGR

Factors contributing to growth faltering and undernutrition are diverse and complex and include factors such as inadequate exclusive breastfeeding, frequency, energy density and micronutrient levels of complementary foods, diarrheal and acute lower respiratory infections, malaria, and increasingly, HIV in the context of Africa [1] where rates of stunting for the first time have superseded those in South Asia. Other factors that may contribute to undernutrition include parity, birth interval, maternal work and maternal education. The latter may take away from child care or bring in earned income that is spent on child nutrition and health. Improving linear growth in infancy and childhood is possible but food/nutritional interventions seem to be efficacious only before 2 or perhaps 3 years of age but not beyond. Growth during

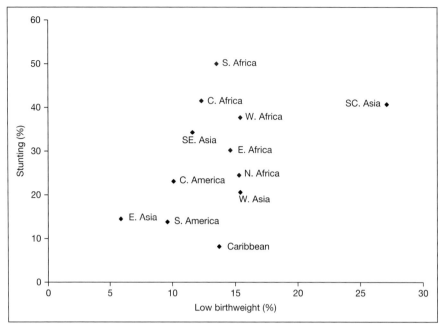

Fig. 3. Rates of stunting among under 5-year-old children and low birthweight by region [1]. Stunting defined as < –2 height for age z score. Low birthweight defined as weight <2.5 kg.

adolescence in developing countries may be prolonged by up to 3 years with the onset of puberty often delayed. This results in some (but not all) catch-up for the early growth deficit in height [36].

Although it is well known that high rates of low birthweight and childhood stunting tend to coexist (fig. 3), few analyses have carefully examined the role of prenatal factors in influencing later life nutritional status. The contribution of fetal growth restriction among various other factors influencing childhood undernutrition is not well defined. While growth generally tends to track, 'decanalization' or 'centile crossing' or 'catch-up' will commonly occur among almost half of infants during infancy and early childhood which is considered a normal pattern of growth to meet one's genetic potential following gestation [37] when fetal growth is more constrained. Mechanisms signaling catch-up or catch-down growth are not well understood but may involve programming of appetite [38]. The period of catch-up growth is also the time when growth is most responsive to food interventions [36].

Observational studies that examine birthweight as a risk factor for childhood nutritional status require a longitudinal design. Adjustment for confounding is critical as there are many factors that can predict low birthweight and are also associated with childhood undernutrition including maternal age, parity, birth interval, socioeconomic status, and literacy among others. Table 1 describes such studies presenting adjusted odds ratios linking low birthweight to stunting, and in some cases, wasting and underweight among under 5-year-olds. Adjustment was done for anywhere up to 22 variables or in some studies for statistically significant confounders. Adjusted odds ratios ranged from 2 to 5 for stunting. The positive correlation between the rates of low birthweight and stunting observed in some settings such as Asia and Africa was not observed in Brazil where catch-up growth appeared to be higher. Studies also found this association to exist beyond preschool age. One study (not shown) showed a significant positive association between weight taken at birth and height and weight for age z scores at a later age of 5–12 years [47]. In the Philippines low birthweight was associated with more severe stunting in the first 2 years of life, and it also significantly reduced the likelihood of 'recovery' from stunting up to 12 years of age [48]. Among a cohort of children born very preterm (<32 weeks gestation) and very low birthweight (<1,500 g) followed at 10 years, SGA children (especially those very preterm) continued to experience stunting compared to adequate for gestational age children who experienced catch-up growth [49]. The cause and type of fetal growth restriction will determine catch-up in childhood as demonstrated in a study where symmetrically smaller infants at birth among smoking mothers showed complete catch-up growth in infancy as did infants of primiparous pregnancies who were thin at birth but became heavier and taller than infants of multiparous women [38].

Few studies have examined the prevalence of stunting at birth and whether it predicts stunting in childhood or later, although shortness at birth may be a strong predictor and even better than low birthweight or IUGR [36]. In a study among West Javanese infants, neonatal weight and length in multivariable analyses were the strongest positive predictors of nutritional status of infants and the strongest negative predictors of increases in weight and length during infancy [50].

In a follow-up study of rural Nepali children (n ~1,000) whose anthropometry was assessed at a mean age of 12 days (SD 8.6), stunting, wasting, and underweight were prevalent at 63, 53, and 13%, respectively, at 30–59 months of age. Both neonatal and maternal factors in this study were associated with the risk of undernutrition (table 2). The adjusted odds ratios ranged from 2 to 3 for low neonatal weight and height, both of which were independently associated with the risk of stunting and wasting. Neonatal weight was a stronger predictor of wasting relative to neonatal length which was more strongly associated with childhood stunting. Maternal nutritional status variables were tested in a separate model. While maternal BMI was associated with stunting and wasting in children, maternal height was only predictive for stunting. These data are unique in that they simultaneously examined neonatal and maternal factors both of which are reflective of the prenatal environment.

Christian

Table 1. Adjusted odds ratios for childhood stunting, wasting and underweight related to low birthweight

Study	Population n	LBW %	Age	Stunting %	Stunting AOR (95% CI)	Wasting %	Wasting AOR (95% CI)	Underweight %	Underweight AOR (95% CI)
Ricci and Becker [39]	Philippines, 2,885	15.0	12–29 months	34.1 (U) 39.8 (R)	1.7 (U) 1.9 (R)	11.8 (U) 8.6 (R)	1.5 (U) 2.0 (R)		
Marins and Almeida [40]	Brazil, 2,194	9.0	14–59 months	5.1–8.1	2.9 (1.9–4.3)			3.5–7.0	2.6 (1.6–4.1)
Aerts et al. [41]	Brazil, 3,389	18.8	<5 years	6.8	3.8 (2.4–6.0)				
Chopra [42]	South Africa, 868	16.3	3–59 months	26.3	5.2 (3.1–8.9)			12.0	8.3 (4.4–15.8)
Ukwuani and Suchindran [43]	Nigeria, 5,331	15.4 (small)[1]	<5 years	42.6	1.3*	8.9	1.6*		
Mamiro et al. [44]	Tanzania, 378	11.0	2–23 months	35.0	5.1 (2.3–11.2)				
Hong [45]	Ghana, 3,077	15.8	<5 years	29.6	1.7 (1.4–2.5)				
Ergin et al: [46]	Turkey, 1,400	4.4	<5 years	10.9	2.5 (1.2–5.3)				

U = Urban; R = rural; AOR = adjusted odds ratio; CI = confidence interval.
* p < 0.05.
[1] Collected during the Demographic Health Surveys by asking mothers whether their baby was small, large or very large.

Table 2. Adjusted odds ratios and 95% confidence intervals for stunting, wasting, and underweight by neonatal and maternal nutritional status among 30- to 59-month-old children in rural Nepal

Neonatal status	Stunting	Wasting	Underweight
Weight <2.5 kg	1.7 (1.2, 2.5)	2.4 (1.5, 3.7)	2.9 (2.0, 4.1)
Length <50 cm	2.4 (1.7, 3.3)	1.8 (1.0, 3.1)	2.0 (1.4, 2.8)
Maternal status	Stunting	Wasting	Underweight
BMI	0.89 (0.82, 0.97)	0.77 (0.68, 0.87)	0.77 (0.71, 0.84)
Height, cm	0.90 (0.87, 0.93)	NS	0.92 (0.89, 0.94)

Adjusted for significant (p < 0.05) covariates in each logistic regression model. Models for the neonatal measurements included both weight and length in the same model. Models for the maternal measurements included both BMI and height in the same model.
NS = Not significant.

Maternal weight and to some extent height were also related with undernutrition in Indonesia [50] and the Philippines [51]. These prenatal predictors of childhood undernutrition are considered 'constitutional' to separate them from time-dependent and more proximate factors such as infection and feeding practices among others [51]. In Nepal we adjusted for socioeconomic variables in the model, some of which remained significant such as maternal literacy, housing material, and asset ownership. Previous work has suggested that socioeconomic determinants of undernutrition in children may operate in two ways: economic status or maternal schooling may work through prenatal factors whereas dwelling factors are likely to influence children's nutritional status more directly [52]. More work is needed to better understand the contribution of prenatal factors to childhood undernutrition in different environments.

References

1 Black RE, Allen LH, Bhutta ZA, et al: Maternal and child undernutrition: global and regional exposures and health consequences. Lancet 2008;371:243–260.
2 Pelletier DL, Frongillo EA Jr, Schroeder DG, Habicht JP: The effects of malnutrition on child mortality in developing countries. Bull World Health Organ 1995;73:443–448.
3 Caulfield LE, de Onis M, Blossner M, Black RE: Undernutrition as an underlying cause of child deaths associated with diarrhea, pneumonia, malaria, and measles. Am J Clin Nutr 2004;80:193–198.
4 Victora CG, Adair L, Fall C, et al: Maternal and child undernutrition: consequences for adult health and human capital. Lancet 2008;371:340–357.

5 WHO: Maternal anthropometry and pregnancy outcomes. A WHO Collaborative Study. Bull World Health Organ 1995;73(suppl):1–98.
6 WHO: Preventing Chronic Disease: A Vital Investment: A WHO Global Report. Geneva, World Health Organization, 2005.
7 Kramer MS: Intrauterine growth and gestational duration determinants. Pediatrics 1987;80:502–511.
8 Ramakrishnan U: Nutrition and low birth weight: from research to practice. Am J Clin Nutr 2004;79:17–21.
9 Gardosi J: Fetal growth: towards an international standard. Ultrasound Obstet Gynecol 2005;26:112–114.
10 Christian P: Infant mortality; in Semba RD, Bloem MW (eds): Nutrition and Health in Developing Countries. Totowa, Humana Press, 2008, in press.
11 Scholl TO, Hediger ML, Schall JI, et al: Maternal growth during pregnancy and the competition for nutrients. Am J Clin Nutr 1994;60:183–188.
12 Stewart CP, Katz J, Khatry SK, et al: Preterm delivery but not intrauterine growth retardation is associated with young maternal age among primiparae in rural Nepal. Matern Child Nutr 2007;3:174–185.
13 Goldenberg RL, Culhane JF: Low birth weight in the United States. Am J Clin Nutr 2007;85:584S–90S.
14 Conde-Agudelo A, Rosas-Bermudez A, Kafury-Goeta AC: Birth spacing and risk of adverse perinatal outcomes: a meta-analysis. JAMA 2006;295:1809–1823.
15 King JC: The risk of maternal nutritional depletion and poor outcomes increases in early or closely spaced pregnancies. J Nutr 2003;133:1732S–1736S.
16 Kramer MS: The epidemiology of adverse pregnancy outcomes: an overview. J Nutr 2003;133:1592S–1596S.
17 de Bernabe JV, Soriano T, Albaladejo R, et al: Risk factors for low birth weight: a review. Eur J Obstet Gynecol Reprod Biol 2004;116:3–15.
18 Bonzini M, Coggon D, Palmer KT: Risk of prematurity, low birthweight and pre-eclampsia in relation to working hours and physical activities: a systematic review. Occup Environ Med 2007;64:228–243.
19 Christian P, Katz J, Wu L, et al: Risk factors for pregnancy-related mortality: a prospective study in rural Nepal. Public Health 2008;122:161–172.
20 Alder J, Fink N, Bitzer J, et al: Depression and anxiety during pregnancy: a risk factor for obstetric, fetal and neonatal outcome? A critical review of the literature. J Matern Fetal Neonatal Med 2007;20:189–209.
21 Lu Q, Lu MC, Schetter CD: Learning from success and failure in psychosocial intervention: an evaluation of low birth weight prevention trials. J Health Psychol 2005;10:185–195.
22 Lu MC, Tache V, Alexander GR, et al: Preventing low birth weight: is prenatal care the answer? J Matern Fetal Neonatal Med 2003;13:362–380.
23 Bergstrom S: Infection-related morbidities in the mother, fetus and neonate. J Nutr 2003;133:1656S–16560S.
24 Lockwood CJ, Kuczynski E: Markers of risk for preterm delivery. J Perinat Med 1999;27:5–20.
25 Hindle LJ, Gitau R, Filteau SM, et al: Effect of multiple micronutrient supplementation during pregnancy on inflammatory markers in Nepalese women. Am J Clin Nutr 2006;84:1086–1092.
26 Brocklehurst P, French R: The association between maternal HIV infection and perinatal outcome: a systematic review of the literature and meta-analysis. Br J Obstet Gynaecol 1998;105:836–848.
27 Suksomboon N, Poolsup N, Ket-Aim S: Systematic review of the efficacy of antiretroviral therapies for reducing the risk of mother-to-child transmission of HIV infection. J Clin Pharm Ther 2007;32:293–311.
28 Christian P, Khatry SK, West KP Jr: Antenatal anthelmintic treatment, birthweight, and infant survival in rural Nepal. Lancet 2004;364:981–983.
29 Sram RJ, Binkova B, Dejmek J, Bobak M: Ambient air pollution and pregnancy outcomes: a review of the literature. Environ Health Perspect 2005;113:375–382.
30 Kannan S, Misra DP, Dvonch JT, Krishnakumar A: Exposures to airborne particulate matter and adverse perinatal outcomes: a biologically plausible mechanistic frame-

work for exploring potential effect modification by nutrition. Environ Health Perspect 2006;114:1636–1642.

31 Bhutta ZA, Ahmed T, Black RD, et al: What works? Interventions for maternal and child undernutrition and survival. Lancet 2008;371:417–440.

32 Keen CL, Clegg MS, Hanna LA, et al: The plausibility of micronutrient deficiencies being a significant contributing factor to the occurrence of pregnancy complications. J Nutr 2003;133:1597S–1605S.

33 Mikkelsen TB, Osler M, Orozova-Bekkevold I, et al: Association between fruit and vegetable consumption and birth weight: a prospective study among 43,585 Danish women. Scand J Public Health 2006;34:616–622.

34 Rao S, Yajnik CS, Kanade A, et al: Intake of micronutrient-rich foods in rural Indian mothers is associated with the size of their babies at birth. Pune Maternal Nutrition Study. J Nutr 2001;131:1217–1224.

35 Olsen SF, Halldorsson TI, Willett WC, et al: Milk consumption during pregnancy is associated with increased infant size at birth: prospective cohort study. Am J Clin Nutr 2007;86:1104–1110.

36 Schroeder DG: Malnutrition; in Semba RD, Bloem MW (eds): Nutrition and Health in Developing Countries. Totowa, Humana Press, 2008, in press.

37 Demerath EW, Choh AC, Czerwinski SA, et al: Genetic and environmental influences on infant weight and weight change: the Fels Longitudinal Study. Am J Hum Biol 2007;19:692–702.

38 Ong KK, Preece MA, Emmett PM, et al, ALSPAC Study Team: Size at birth and early childhood growth in relation to maternal smoking, parity and infant breast-feeding: longitudinal birth cohort study and analysis. Pediatr Res 2002;52:863–867.

39 Ricci JA, Becker S: Risk factors for wasting and stunting among children in Metro Cebu, Philippines. Am J Clin Nutr 1996;63:966–975.

40 Marins VM, Almeida RM: Undernutrition prevalence and social determinants in children aged 0–59 months, Niteroi, Brazil. Ann Hum Biol 2002;29:609–618.

41 Aerts D, Drachler Mde L, Giugliani ER: Determinants of growth retardation in Southern Brazil. Cad Saude Publica 2004;20:1182–1190.

42 Chopra M: Risk factors for undernutrition of young children in a rural area of South Africa. Public Health Nutr 2003;6:645–652.

43 Ukwuani FA, Suchindran CM: Implications of women's work for child nutritional status in sub-Saharan Africa: a case study of Nigeria. Soc Sci Med 2003;56:2109–2121.

44 Mamiro PS, Kolsteren P, Roberfroid D, et al: Feeding practices and factors contributing to wasting, stunting, and iron-deficiency anaemia among 3–23-month old children in Kilosa district, rural Tanzania. J Health Popul Nutr 2005;23:222–230.

45 Hong R: Effect of economic inequality on chronic childhood undernutrition in Ghana. Public Health Nutr 2007;10:371–378.

46 Ergin F, Okyay P, Atasoylu G, Beser E: Nutritional status and risk factors of chronic malnutrition in children under five years of age in Aydin, a western city of Turkey. Turk J Pediatr 2007;49:283–289.

47 Sekiyama M, Ohtsuka R: Significant effects of birth-related biological factors on pre-adolescent nutritional status among rural Sundanese in West Java, Indonesia. J Biosoc Sci 2005; 37:413–426.

48 Adair LS: Filipino children exhibit catch-up growth from age 2 to 12 years. J Nutr 1999;129:1140–1148.

49 Knops NB, Sneeuw KC, Brand R, et al: Catch-up growth up to ten years of age in children born very preterm or with very low birth weight. BMC Pediatr 2005;5:26.

50 Schmidt MK, Muslimatun S, West CE, et al: Nutritional status and linear growth of Indonesian infants in west java are determined more by prenatal environment than by postnatal factors. J Nutr 2002;132:2202–2207.

51 Adair LS, Guilkey DK: Age-specific determinants of stunting in Filipino children. J Nutr 1997;127:314–320.

52 Delpeuch F, Traissac P, Martin-Prevel Y, et al: Economic crisis and malnutrition: socioeconomic determinants of anthropometric status of preschool children and their mothers in an African urban area. Public Health Nutr 2000;3:39–47.

Discussion

Dr. Agarwal: I am now talking about an Indian Council of Medical Research study which I conducted for over 7 years. This was for the Integrated Child Development Services (ICDS) and we observed data on over 6,000 deliveries in rural areas. One thing was very interesting and is associated with your Nepal study on preterm births: those undernourished anemic rural women had more preterm births than those who were undernourished but had less or no anemia. The brain development and growth of these babies was followed up to 18 years of age. So the stunting you have shown is continuous up to pre-adolescence, but when adolescence starts the undernourished as well as the well-nourished control children gain the same height during the adolescent period that normally one should gain. Although the nutrition supplementation by the ICDS was poor, it was still effective, effective in the length gained as well as the weight gained. The iron and folate distributed by the Ministry of Health were good enough to gain the weight reduced by low birthweight. Your studies support that anemia is more related to preterm and undernutrition, and more related to low birthweight babies.

Dr. Genuino: In your talk you mentioned that a child who is born small will stay small and I am particularly interested in whether you have come across any data showing an association between the final adult height of these children who are born small and adult chronic diseases?

Dr. Christian: Because I was focusing on childhood undernutrition I did not actually show the data that link birth size with adulthood height and stunting. In fact the data are there, and there is a linkage across life in terms of tracking. Regarding your second question on adult disease, somebody else will be talking about this and I specifically limited my discussion to undernutrition. Other speakers are going to talk about low birthweight and chronic diseases.

Dr. Chittal: The female fetus will have IUGR. Is IUGR intrauterine growth retardation or low birthweight?

Dr. Christian: Females are born with low birthweight but they also have IUGR more often.

Dr. Chittal: Would interventions help a female fetus?

Dr. Christian: From what I have seen interventions tend to help female fetuses more, but the effects are variable. So not all interventions have a better impact on females.

Dr. Chittal: Why were cheese and ice cream excluded from dietary supplementation as milk products?

Dr. Christian: I don't know. Perhaps they are just considered not good sources.

Dr. Chittal: What dairy products were utilized? Milk alone or milk and yoghurt?

Dr. Christian: Milk and perhaps yoghurt.

Dr. Prentice: I would like to carry on from that previous question. This issue of whether we have more IUGR babies that are girls, is rather a matter of semantics. Girls are smaller, so if we present the data according to a growth chart for girl babies then we would not expect to see more IUGR. We do see more girl babies below 2.5 kg because that is a single cutoff that is used for both sexes. One of the important things we need to understand is the concept of an 'appropriateness', a 'harmony' of growth between the mother and the baby. When we say that shorter, smaller mothers have more IUGR, thank goodness they do, because, as you demonstrated, the difficulties in terms of obstetric outcome occur when you get a mismatch between a small mother and a big baby. This is one of the issues that in particular Dr. Yajnik is trying to get around. How do we break this cycle, how do we move to a bigger baby without breaking that inherent biological harmony between the size of the baby and the size of the mother.

Dr. Christian: With the customized percentile [1], the adjusted references, I think that is part of trying to characterize fetal growth a little better and perhaps we should do that more. Of course the factors that they take into account are maternal size as well as BMI and the sex of the fetus. Perhaps I am not a hundred percent sure but, apart from female babies being low birthweight, they are also more likely to be IUGR, but you can challenge me on that.

Dr. Yajnik: Can I make a comment? I was approached by someone in Fiji because they got very excited that all the IUGR babies in Fiji were Indian and all the LGA babies were Pacific Islander babies. They thought it was an ethnic difference. I suggested correction for maternal size and this explained a large part of the difference. So I think maternal size is not being considered in the definition of appropriateness of birthweight, which is a major problem. The second issue is that we are concentrating only on birthweight and sometimes on length. But we are not talking about body composition. For example a female child is more adipose than a male child, and has a different cord blood hormonal profile [2]. Hattersley and Tooke [3] recently published on this, and there is a gender insulin hypothesis. The complexities increase as we go from weight to BMI to body composition and physiology.

Dr. Christian: I wish we had better ways to assess fetal development because MRIs are very hard to do in communities, so how do we measure body composition? Measuring length is one step ahead and we have a long way to go.

Dr. Yajnik: Recently we showed in the Pune Maternal Nutrition Study that smaller leg length seems to predict a metabolic problem [4]. This was demonstrated by Leitch [5] about 5 years ago when she related short legs to cardiovascular risk. Thus there is complexity within length also and implications for the windows of opportunity.

Dr. Shahkhalili: I would like to make a comment. Fetal undernutrition is a consequence of placental insufficiency and not maternal nutritional status. A condition that is common in developed countries and also needs to be addressed.

Dr. Whitelaw: As a geneticist I am just interested that you don't raise the issue of genetics as being involved in any of these studies. For example, when you correlate maternal BMI or size with fetal or newborn size, surely genetics is likely to play a contributing role. I realize it must be quite complicated to put that into the equation, but it seems likely.

Dr. Christian: In the nutritional community, at least in the context of developing countries, our understanding is that most of the stunting in adults has nutritional origins. If you take the example of a malnourished child being adopted into a well-nourished setting, then he/she experiences some catch-up growth, and when you talk about migrations of people from a developing country to a better setting, over generations an increase in height is actually seen. I think that the genetic component to explain stunting in a developing country is very low because when certain ethnic groups have lived for a substantially long period of time in a well-nourished setting, they tend to gain height.

Dr. Pandit: Nature always tries to correct itself in adverse situations by creating something favorable. For example the studies by Dr. Yajnik in Pune have demonstrated that gestational diabetes has now become a necessary evil for increasing birthweight. In your study did you see this effort of nature to have more gestational diabetes in all these IUGR?

Dr. Christian: In the two places in which I have worked, Nepal and Bangladesh, we find very little evidence of gestational diabetes. We did some standard measures of proteinuria and hypertension and did not find any evidence.

Dr. Kayal: Is there a laboratory model of specific micronutrient deficiency with low birthweight in animals?

Christian

Dr. Christian: Folate and B_{12} deficiency has been looked at in sheep. I am not quite sure if I understand your question, but there are lots of studies in humans which have looked at specific micronutrient deficiencies.

Dr. Kayal: The results of human studies have been inconclusive. Are there any animal studies linking specific micronutrient deficiencies to low birthweight in the offspring, because we will be able to control those things?

Dr. Christian: The studies that I am aware of are human studies.

Dr. Yajnik: Over the last 5 years there have been a number of models. There are models for magnesium and calcium deficiency and also for protein deficiency. Recently a B_{12} and folate model has been developed. Dr. Christian referred to the recently published sheep model for periconceptional B_{12} and folate deficiency which actually replicated what we have shown in humans, that there is a growth restriction followed by higher adiposity and insulin resistance in the offspring. There are a number of models.

Dr. Matthai: You said that there is an association between low birthweight and subsequent smallness in adulthood. How much of this is environmental and how much of it is because the person started with a low birthweight?

Dr. Christian: To the extent that the environment influences low birthweight; I think it is environmental. What I was trying to show is that there is a certain fraction of variation in stunting or wasting in children that is explained by being born with a low birthweight which we cannot do anything about once the child is 2–5 years of age. That was the purpose of examining that association. I showed all the environmental factors that actually contribute to low birthweight and those would still be there as risk factors.

Dr. Matthai: Do you think that this person's growth potential would be similar to someone with normal birthweight?

Dr. Christian: Yes, but they have to be corrected before childhood; prenatally or even when the mother is growing as a child or in adolescence. So you are talking about a reproductive life stage approach for interventions but the data that I presented do not tell you the attributable fraction, which is what I said at the end; we should try to figure out what the fraction of risk is that is attributable to the prenatal factors.

Dr. Bhattacharya: Have you come across any syndromes, such as Down's syndrome or others, that can be linked to nutrition?

Dr. Christian: In our studies we have mostly assessed gross congenital malformations and defects. We have only been able to pick these up because these are community-base studies. Births are happening in the women's homes and getting to them on time is always a challenge. In a lot of instances when a congenital malformation is severe the baby dies. So if we reach and find them on time, they have to be surviving babies. This is of concern because we are only capturing survivors. But the congenitally malformed babies tend also to have lower birthweight.

Dr. De Curtis: In the last few years the rate of prematurity has increased in many developed countries. In the USA it has reached about 12–13% and in Italy it is about 7–8%. Is there a similar increase in developing countries? Have developing countries adopted local neonatal reference growth charts or are they using charts from developed countries? It is important to use local neonatal charts to rule out the possibility that many infants are considered SGA when they are actually normal for that region.

Dr. Christian: From what I understand the increasing trend in the US with regard to preterms is mostly associated with the indicated cesarean section preterm rate. It is not the spontaneous preterm rates that have gone up. There is a recent paper by Goldenberg and Culhane [6] showing the different kinds of preterms, and the increase is mostly indicated preterm cesarean sections which are considered for adverse pregnancies. Your second question regarding growth charts is actually a very controversial topic. If you take fetal growth references or standards and if you use Caucasian or European standards for fetuses in developing countries, then you are comparing apples and oranges. No, I don't think that we have adequate references and that is why adjustment for various factors is something that is recommended.

References

1   Gardosi J: Fetal growth: towards an international standard. Ultrasound Obstet Gynecol 2005; 26:112–114.
2   Yajnik CS, Godbole K, Otiv SR, Lubree HG: Fetal programming of type 2 diabetes: is sex important? Diabetes Care 2007;30:2754–2755.
3   Hattersley AT, Tooke JE: The fetal insulin hypothesis: an alternative explanation of the association of low birthweight with diabetes and vascular disease. Lancet 1999;353:1789–1792.
4   Kulkarni SR, Fall CH, Joshi NV, et al: Determinants of incident hyperglycemia 6 years after delivery in young rural Indian mothers: the Pune Maternal Nutrition Study (PMNS). Diabetes Care 2007;30:2542–2547.
5   Leitch I: Growth and health. 1951. Int J Epidemiol 2001;30:212–216.
6   Goldenberg RL, Culhane JF: Low birth weight in the United States. Am J Clin Nutr 2007;85: 584S–590S.

Kalhan SC, Prentice AM, Yajnik CS (eds): Emerging Societies – Coexistence of Childhood Malnutrition and Obesity.
Nestlé Nutr Inst Workshop Ser Pediatr Program, vol 63, pp 79–94,
Nestec Ltd., Vevey/S. Karger AG, Basel, © 2009.

Postnatal Origins of Undernutrition

Marc-André Prost

MRC International Nutrition Group, London School of Hygiene and Tropical Medicine, London, UK

Abstract

Obesity and nutrition-related chronic disorders are fast rising in developing countries. But undernutrition – stunting, underweight, wasting and micronutrient deficiencies – still affect millions of preschool children in both rural and urban settings increasing the risks of morbidity and mortality, impairing cognitive development, reducing productivity and increasing the risk of chronic diseases in later life. In addition undernutrition has a transgenerational effect. Here I review the evidence for a synergistic effect of inadequate nutrition (breastfeeding, complementary feeding), infection, and inappropriate mother–child interactions on growth and nutritional deficiencies. Underlying socioeconomic, environmental and genetic factors are also explored. Finally some perspectives on how urbanization and globalization may affect the prevalence and distribution of undernutrition are discussed. Fighting child undernutrition is still an urgent necessity and a moral imperative.

Introduction

Developing countries are undergoing a rapid nutrition transition characterized by changes in diet and physical activity patterns. These changes are occurring at such a fast rate that the rising burden of obesity and nutrition-related chronic diseases is compounding the secular problems of undernutrition rather than displacing them [1], creating the so-called 'double burden of malnutrition'. Stunting and overweight have been found to coexist not only at the community level [2] but also within individual households [3] and even within individuals [4]. Moreover, early childhood stunting is now recognized as a risk factor for obesity in later life [4]. Although non-communicable diseases are now the leading cause of death and disability in most developing countries, underweight together with iron, zinc and vitamin A deficiencies are still among the leading 15 causes of death worldwide [5].

The determinants and consequences of childhood undernutrition have been studied for several decades. There is considerable evidence that early nutritional insults are strongly associated with impaired physical growth, increased morbidity and mortality, impaired cognitive development, reduced economic productivity through diminished physical work capacity, increased risk of chronic disease in adulthood and, for women, lower offspring birthweight [6]. Questions remain, however, regarding the precise mechanisms governing malnutrition, such as linear growth faltering [7]. The relationships between proximal and distal factors leading to childhood malnutrition were sketched out nearly 20 years ago in the UNICEF's classical framework for malnutrition, which is still the reference today [8].

Here I examine how proximal etiological factors for undernutrition, namely inadequate nutrition, infection and maternal–child interactions, can work synergistically to impair child growth. The relative contribution of socioeconomic and demographic factors as well as other environmental factors is also explored. Finally, I discuss how urbanization and globalization may modify the pattern of risk factors.

Effects of Nutrition and Feeding Practices on Infant and Young Child Nutritional Status

Breastfeeding

The WHO recommends breastfeeding exclusively for 6 months and throughout the second year [9]. In Asia and Africa, 75–80% of infants are exclusively or predominantly breastfed for the first 2 months of life [10]. In most women, breast milk provides enough energy and protein to cover the needs of their offspring for normal growth during the first 6 months of life [11]. Wasting or kwashiorkor seldom occur in early infancy and when they do are usually associated with maternal or child inability to breastfeed (famine, maternal physical or mental illness, child cleft lip or cleft palate) in very poor communities.

The worldwide timing of growth faltering (fig. 1) suggests that linear growth retardation starts before 3 months of age and possibly inside the womb [12]. In normal birthweight babies however, weight faltering does not seem to occur until 3–6 months of age [12], suggesting that prenatal influences are more strongly exerted on length than weight accretion. However, caution is in order since antenatal multiple micronutrient supplementation trials have shown a greater effect on birthweight than length [13]. The mechanisms of linear growth retardation are not fully understood, but the timing of initiation of length and weight faltering suggest very different etiologies.

There is empirical evidence for a compounding effect of inadequate breast milk quality coupled with suboptimal infant stores at birth in the etiology of early linear growth faltering. Low birthweight is frequently reported as the

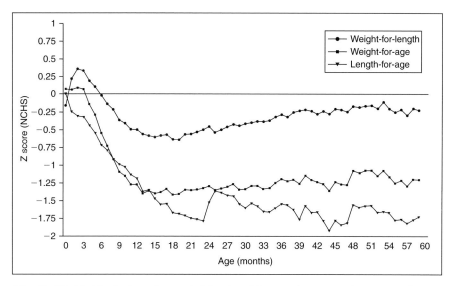

Fig. 1. Worldwide timing of growth faltering. Mean anthropometric z scores by age relative to the NCHS reference (0–59 months) in 39 nationally representative surveys conducted in Latin America, Asia, and Africa from 1987 to 1997. Reproduced with permission from Shrimpton et al. [12].

strongest determinant of stunting in the first year of life [14]. In addition, breast milk concentrations of vitamin A, B_6, and B_{12} are strongly influenced by maternal status and diet [11]. Iron, zinc and vitamin D are provided in inappropriate amounts in breast milk regardless of maternal status or intake, and the infant's needs are met by endowment at birth (or sunlight exposure for vitamin D) until an exogenous source is supplied [11]. It is therefore likely that in deficient populations, infants' stores at birth together with intake (through breast milk) of several micronutrients fail to meet the requirements for growth and development, contributing to linear growth retardation and micronutrient deficiencies.

Complementary Feeding: Timing of Initiation

The attrition rate beyond 2 months for exclusive breastfeeding in Africa and Asia is very important. The proportion of infants exclusively or predominantly breastfed falls to ~50% in the 2–5 months age group indicating that untimely exposure to potentially contaminated or qualitatively inadequate foods is widespread [10]. Introduction of complementary foods increases the risk of diarrhea. Brown et al. [15] in Peru observed a doubling of the prevalence of diarrhea in infants receiving liquids in addition to breast milk compared to those exclusively breastfed. The risk of dehydration from diarrhea was 7 times greater when food was introduced between 3 and 5 months among Brazilian infants [16]. Early introduction of complementary foods has also been consistently associated with an increased incidence of respiratory illnesses [16].

The introduction of complementary foods displaces breast milk intakes [17]. Although infants are able to self-regulate their energy intake, they are constrained by a small gastric capacity. In addition, the low energy density of mostly plant-based infant porridges in developing countries contributes to a reduction in energy and other nutrient intakes due to their poor availability and bioavailability compared to that in breast milk [17]. Although the availability of micronutrients in human milk can be low, they are generally well absorbed.

Early introduction of complementary foods affects growth directly by reducing the quality and quantity of the diet, and indirectly through increased incidence of diarrheal and other diseases.

Dietary Quality versus Quantity of Complementary Foods

From 6 months, breast milk alone is no longer sufficient to meet the requirements for normal biological functions and growth in increasingly active and mobile infants [9]. Most cultures introduce complementary foods in the second half of infancy (e.g., solid family food) and in environments with poor water quality and traditionally low nutrient density diets, infants are at increased risk of nutritional deficiencies [18], in particular moderate and severe acute malnutrition (severe wasting, kwashiorkor) and stunting. It is during this period that growth trajectories deviate markedly from the reference in developing countries. On a global scale, weight-for-age and weight-for-length falter sharply between 3 and 12 months with a some catch-up thereafter, particularly in terms of weight-for-length, more pronounced in Africa. Length-for-age continues to falter throughout infancy and childhood until about 3 years [12].

The initial attention of the research community focused primarily on the influence of weaning on severe acute malnutrition, since the short-term prognosis is highly unfavorable if left untreated. The debate has shifted from protein deficiency, initially hypothesized by Williams [19] in the etiology of kwashiorkor, to energy deficiency. More recently the focus has shifted to multiple deficiencies due to the reduced availability and bioavailability of nutrients in complementary foods [18].

In most developing countries infant porridges are plant-based with a low proportion of energy provided from animal sources [20]. Consequently the bioavailability of nutrients and energy density are reduced and these foods often fail to meet the increasing needs for growth, physical activity, and health. There is strong evidence that wasting, but not stunting, is associated with an energy-deficient diet or one with a low protein to energy ratio [21]. This can be observed at its extreme in anorexic children suffering severe infections, or in times of famine. There is, however, evidence of stunting in children from deprived communities with appropriate energy intakes [22]; Mexican children with energy and protein intakes comparable to those of North American infants displayed a marked prevalence of stunting, suggesting that other nutrients may be limiting [23]. In the Huascar longitudinal study in Peru, the diet of infants in the second semester averaged 70–75% of energy requirements [18]. Brown [18] calculated that even if these infants would eat larger quantities to satisfy their energy requirements, their diet would remain below the recommendations for protein, vitamin A, calcium, iron, and zinc intakes most of the time. Recently, a review of growth-limiting nutrient intakes from complementary feeding in Bangladesh, Ghana, Guatemala, Mexico, Peru, and the USA revealed that although protein density is adequate, iron, zinc and calcium fail to meet desired intakes across all countries and age groups from 6 to 11 months, and in all countries but the USA between 12 and 23 months [17]. In the 1998 WHO report on complementary feeding, iron and zinc were identified as 'problem nutrients' [20]. The bioavailability of zinc and iron is further affected by high concentrations of anti-nutrients (phytates, dietary fibers) in cereal-based preparations as observed in Malawi with maize-based porridges [24].

Poor nutrient quality and quantity in complementary food has an indirect effect on appetite. Growth-retarded Mexican children left over 25% of the food offered suggesting a qualitative rather than a quantitative problem [25]. Several nutritional factors drive appetite in children including the organoleptic properties and viscosity of the food offered [18], but also micronutrient composition. This has been suggested by Golden and Golden [26] who refer to the fact that anorexia is a key feature of zinc deficiency in experimental human and animal studies.

Infections and Growth

Effect of Common Childhood Illnesses on Growth
There is a clear association between infection and growth faltering. Diarrhea is the most strongly related illness but other acute infections such as pneumonia, malaria, acute febrile illnesses and measles, as well as chronic infections, can impact on growth even at a subclinical stage.

Diarrheal diseases are the most prevalent illnesses in infancy and childhood. Peak incidence occurs in the second half of infancy, coinciding with the introduction of complementary foods and the period when weight faltering is most acute [27]. Diarrheal episodes seem to have a transient effect on weight gain. In studies compiled by Bhan et al. [28], reporting a significant growth impairment due to diarrheal diseases, 8–80% of the short-term weight deficit was explained by diarrhea. The proportion explained was greater in African studies as well as in the context of higher diarrhea prevalence. Long-term effects (beyond 6 months intervals) were somewhat smaller ranging from 6 to 24% of the weight deficit associated with diarrhea, suggesting some catch-up growth. The impact of diarrhea on length velocity was smaller: only 8–15% of the length deficit across nine studies was explained by this type of infection [28].

Lower respiratory tract infections have been associated with a 6–35% deficit in short-term weight gain but no long-term effects beyond 6 months apart from a small effect of severe pneumonia in Brazilian infants [29]. No effect has been reported on length. Malaria and measles have also been reported to have a significant effect on weight [28]. Measles epidemics in very low income countries are frequently associated with subsequent peak admissions of severely malnourished children in rehabilitation centers.

Chronic infections have also been investigated in relation to growth and show different patterns of interaction. Guinean infants infected by *Cryptosporidium parvum*, a protozoan that causes severe and persistent diarrhea, suffered permanent retardation in both weight and length growth [30]. In The Gambia, colonization of the gastrointestinal tract by *Helicobacter pylori* in the first half of infancy was significantly associated with shorter, thinner and lighter infants in later infancy [31]. HIV, even subclinical, has been shown to impair linear growth from the first trimester of life and throughout infancy and childhood [32]. It has also been associated with wasting in developing countries but not developed countries, highlighting the importance of appropriate nutritional support [28].

Albendazole trials conducted to investigate the impact of helminthiasis on growth reported inconsistent effects on weight gain, with greater effects in areas of high prevalence. No significant impact on length gain was observed; however, all but one trial was conducted in school-age children where changes in length are unlikely [28].

The variability in the measured effect of various infections as well as the mechanisms by which infections act on weight and length accretion are not fully understood. Effects are greater in high prevalence settings as well as in nutritionally compromised children. Clearly the severity, duration, frequency, and type of infection are key factors mediating the effect on growth by increasing nutrient requirements, losses, and provoking anorexia. Enteropathies affect gut mucosal integrity hence reducing nutrient absorption. In The Gambia, long-term intestinal lesions explain 43% of growth faltering among 2- to 15-month-old children [33].

Synergism of Malnutrition and Infections

The potentiating effect of malnutrition on infection has been recognized for years. Inappropriate dietary energy and micronutrient intake increases susceptibility to and delays recovery from infection. Infection in turn increases the nutrient requirements necessary to contain and combat pathological assaults. Furthermore, infection increases losses (diarrhea) and reduces intakes by affecting appetite, therefore further compromising nutritional status, delaying recovery, and impairing growth [34].

New estimates on the role of undernutrition as an underlying cause of child deaths from infectious diseases were given in the *Lancet* series on Maternal and Child Undernutrition [10]. Underweight was implicated in 19% of all deaths, stunting and wasting in approximately 15%, and vitamin A deficiency in 6.5%. Caution is in order when interpreting these figures since the combined effect of multiple deficiencies is less than the crude sum of individual deficiencies as some deaths may be attributable to multiple deficiencies.

Mother–Child Interactions

UNICEF first promoted the importance of maternal care in its 1990 conceptual framework for malnutrition to explain differences in nutritional outcomes between communities and households with comparable resources [8].

The level of care provided to infants and children is the result of maternal endogenous factors and societal values, constraints, and policies interacting with each other. Maternal factors determining the quality of the mother–child relationship comprise education and beliefs, physical and mental health, nutritional status and self-confidence. At the interface between maternal and societal determinants are workload and time available for care, and time spent on care, and maternal autonomy and control of resources, highlighting the pivotal influence of the father on the mother–child relationship. Finally the provision of care to children is influenced by the level of social support received by mothers. It is not possible here to review the evidence available for the effect of each of these determinants on the care and feeding practices and ultimately on the child's nutritional status. Instead, I will highlight key findings related to two aspects: maternal education and maternal mental health. For a complete review one can refer to the excellent report by Engle et al. [35].

Maternal Education

Children born of women with higher schooling status are less likely to be malnourished. The results of a very large cross-sectional study in Indonesia and Bangladesh recently published in the *Lancet* estimated that each additional year of maternal education decreases the odds of stunting by 4–5% in their offspring [36]. Parental education impacts on child health and nutritional status through three behavioral mechanisms, namely feeding practices, home health practices, and child–caregiver interaction [35].

Maternal education has been associated with a greater commitment to care. In Mexico, mothers from higher education levels were more vocal, had a more stimulating style of interaction with their infant, and were more likely to adapt responsive practices to the age of their infant [37].

Educated mothers adopt better home healthcare provision behaviors in the form of preventative healthcare (immunization, use of antenatal care) and health-seeking behavior for curative medicine. In Metro Cebu, the Philippines, the odds of full immunization of infants rose by 10–15% for each additional year of maternal education [38].

The interaction between feeding practices and maternal education is complex. In Pakistan, the timing of introduction of complementary foods was associated with maternal education [39]. In a study in Bangladesh, maternal education correlated positively not only with feeding frequency and duration, but also with the quality of feeding (less distraction while feeding, cleaner environment, fresher foods, etc.) [40]. In contrast, higher maternal education is consistently associated with earlier termination of breastfeeding in developing countries [35], possibly because better educated mothers engage more in income-generating activities, have less time to dedicate to caring and have wider access to breast milk substitutes due to higher incomes.

Maternal Mental Health

A recent *Lancet* series on mental health highlighted the burden of postnatal depression in developing countries [41]. Postnatal depression affects 10–15% of mothers in developed countries and the proportion is probably higher in low and middle income countries. Prevalences of 23 and 20% have been reported in India, and 28% in Pakistan [42]. Consistent associations between postnatal mental disorders, child undernutrition and diarrheal episodes have been reported. Infants of antenatally depressed mothers were around 4 times more likely to be underweight and stunted at 6 months and around 2.5 times at 12 months [43]. The risk of having 5 or more diarrheal episodes per year was 2.4.

There is compelling evidence from both developed and developing countries that postnatal depression correlates with long-term cognitive and behavioral problems in children, and failure to thrive [42]. Three mechanisms have been proposed. First, maternal depression is associated with inappropriate healthcare seeking behaviors (full immunization, antenatal care attendance) [43], suboptimal breastfeeding practices and risk-taking behaviors (smoking, drinking alcohol, unhealthy eating) [41, 42]. Second, depressive symptoms impact negatively on the emotional quality of parenting. Depressed mothers provide less quantity and poorer quality of stimulations and are less responsive to their child. Third, maternal depression could increase psychosocial adversity in infancy, which has been linked with stunting [42].

Socioeconomic and Demographic Factors

Socioeconomic

Malnutrition is a disease of poverty. Socioeconomic status expressed at the household level (income, expenditure, asset ownership, etc.) has been consistently associated with indices of malnutrition in a variety of studies, but the pathways and mechanisms by which it impacts on child nutritional status are complex, numerous, and highly variable between household, communities and countries. Analysis of the global determinants of stunting and wasting

86

by Frongillo et al. [44] have highlighted the fact that child undernutrition is as much a consequence of factors at national and provincial levels as at the individual household level. In their model, three quarters of the variability of stunting between countries and two thirds of that of wasting were explained by factors at national and provincial levels. Stunting was more strongly associated with lower energy availability, lower female literacy rates and lower gross domestic product. Wasting was negatively correlated with vaccination coverage and, in Asia, energy availability.

The relationship between poverty and undernutrition at the country level is not linear. For instance Zimbabwe and Kenya have achieved lower rates of underweight and stunting than India, although their gross national income per head is much lower. Mexico has a higher prevalence of stunting than China despite being nearly 4 times more wealthy [45]. The Green Revolution and sustained economic growth in Asia over the past decades contributed to the eradication of famines and brought self-sufficiency in many countries. But in countries like India, mild to moderate undernutrition remain staggeringly high probably due to large inequities in income distribution. Conversely, countries like Panama and Costa Rica have seen a steady decrease in child undernutrition from 1970 to 2000 despite economic stagnation [46].

Other socioeconomic factors associated with child undernutrition in various contexts include: access to safe water (through the incidence and duration of diarrheal diseases); access to healthcare (incidence and duration of infections); dwelling characteristics (wealth, indoor air pollution, etc.); access to latrines (incidence of diarrheal and other diseases due to fecal contamination), and many more.

Demographic Factors
The word 'kwashiorkor' used by Cecily Williams in her seminal 1933 article was borrowed from the Ga language to designate the disease of 'the displaced child' [21] since kwashiorkor was more frequently observed in weanlings experiencing a sudden decline in maternal care and attention due to the arrival of a new sibling. Parity, birth spacing and birth order are among factors frequently associated with child undernutrition. In Thailand, Indonesia and the Philippines, these as well as mortality of the previous child were risk factors for child mortality [47]. Parental marital status and maternal age also seem to exert an influence on child nutritional status. Demographic factors may be partly mediated through socioeconomic status and education.

Environmental, Genetic and Other Factors

Sex
A higher prevalence of stunting has been reported in boys in several African studies showing a ~15% difference in the prevalence between boys

and girls and a 1.5- to 2-fold increase in the risk of stunting for boys [14, 48]. In a meta-analysis of 16 demographic and health surveys conducted in sub-Saharan African countries, Wamani et al. [49] concluded that the odds of stunting were 18% higher in boys than girls, suggesting that males are more vulnerable to health inequities.

No data were compiled for Asia or Latin America but studies in Bangladesh consistently report higher rates of stunting in girls than boys [50].

Intergenerational Effect on Undernutrition

The typical intergenerational cycle of growth failure was described in UNICEF's State of the World Children 1998: 'young girls who grow poorly become stunted women and are more likely to give birth to low-birth-weight babies. If those are girls, they are likely to continue the cycle by being stunted in adulthood and so on ...' [8]. Ramakrishnan et al. [51] reviewed the evidence from developed countries and reported on new data from Guatemala. Correlation coefficients of 0.42–0.5 between adult height of parents and their offspring were reported in developed countries. For each 100-gram increase in maternal birthweight, a 10- to 20-gram increase was reported in their offspring. In Guatemala, the increase in child's birthweight was nearly twice as much (29 g/100 g maternal birthweight) and birth length was increased by 0.2 cm/1 cm increase in maternal birth length. These findings highlight the importance of addressing undernutrition now for future generations but also that it may take several generations to completely eradicate stunting.

Seasonality, Food Availability and Infections

Seasonal variations in growth patterns among agro-pastoral communities have been described in many countries, with weight showing greater seasonal variability than height. The nadir of weight faltering has been correlated with the timing of lowest food availability (pre-harvest period) in Bangladesh and Kenya [50, 52] or the period of highest diarrhea incidence in Uganda and Bangladesh [50, 53]. Resumption of height growth seems to lag 3–4 months behind that of weight accretion in line with Golden's [54] observation that during catch-up growth (recovery from severe acute malnutrition) weight takes precedence over length.

Perspective on Urbanization, Globalization and Undernutrition

The United Nations' Population Division estimates that in 2008 the proportion of the urban population will equal the rural population and be urbanized in its majority thereafter [55]. These changes have taken place increasingly rapidly in the last two decades in the context of the globalization of trade, technology, information, and labor resources.

Over a third of the urban population in the developing world live in shanty towns and are exposed to a lack of access to safe water, poor housing conditions, overcrowding, poor hygiene conditions due to lack of drainage, and environmental pollution. Consequently children are exposed to higher transmission rates of respiratory and diarrheal diseases than in rural areas [56]. Urbanization affects not only the environment but behaviors. Rates and duration of breastfeeding are lower in urban than rural areas in Africa and Latin America [57], and the ability and, often, the necessity of mothers to work impacts on the time and quality of health and nutrition care. It is not surprising that children from urban slums in India have a higher prevalence of underweight, stunting and wasting than those living in rural areas [58].

A feature of trade globalization has been a sustained integration of national markets to the global economy. For poor, often urban populations in developing countries, this has meant greater stability in food availability thus a better resilience against adverse local climatic and man-made disasters, but also a greater vulnerability to global price fluctuations. The price of oil and basic food commodities is rising rapidly nowadays, pulled by a booming demand from China and diversion of agricultural productions into biofuel generation reducing global food availability and accessibility. Riots erupted recently in Cameroon (February 2008), Burma (July 2007), and Iran (June 2007) over the price of oil. In China, a harsh winter characterized by gigantic floods has meant a sharp increase in basic food products and a steep decline in rice exports, affecting global prices. Whether or not this may signal the return of famines in Asia and elsewhere is unknown, but low income countries already suffering a disproportionate share of the burden are ill equipped to face a global competition for dwindling resources.

Conclusion

The increasing prevalence of obesity and nutrition-related chronic disease compounds rather than displaces traditional health problems due to undernutrition in developing countries. Trends indicate that, if left unchecked, stunting will remain the most prevalent nutritional disorder in childhood, and underweight, wasting and micronutrient deficiencies will continue to affect children throughout their lives and across generations. The burden of child undernutrition remains so great that there is a renewed moral urgency to find integrated solutions to tackle the problem. Over- and undernutrition are now seen as different manifestations of a global phenomenon rather than extremes of the malnutrition spectrum. Since they are linked, fighting undernutrition should impact positively on both outcomes.

Prost

References

1 Uauy R, Kain J, Mericq V, et al: Nutrition, child growth, and chronic disease prevention. Ann Med 2008;40:11–20.
2 Duran P, Caballero B, de Onis M: The association between stunting and overweight in Latin American and Caribbean preschool children. Food Nutr Bull 2006;27:300–305.
3 Doak CM, Adair LS, Bentley M, et al: The underweight/overweight household: an exploration of sociodemographic and dietary factors in China. Public Health Nutr 2002;5:215–221.
4 Sawaya AL, Roberts S: Stunting and future risk of obesity: principal physiological mechanisms. Cad Saude Publica 2003;19(suppl):S21–S28.
5 World Health Organization: The World Health Report 2002: Reducing Risks, Promoting Healthy Life. Geneva, WHO, 2002.
6 Martorell R, Haschke F (eds): Nutrition and Growth. Nestlé Nutr Workshop Ser Pediatr Program. Philadelphia, Lippincott William & Wilkins, 2001, vol 47.
7 Frongillo EA: Symposium: Causes and etiology of stunting. Introduction. J Nutr 1999;129(suppl):529S–530S.
8 UNICEF: The State of the World's Children 1998: Focus on Nutrition. New York, UNICEF, 1998.
9 World Health Organization: The Optimal Duration of Exclusive Breastfeeding. Report of an Expert Consultation. Geneva, WHO, 2001.
10 Black RE, Allen LH, Bhutta ZA, et al: Maternal and child undernutrition 1: global and regional exposures and health consequences. Lancet 2008;371:243–260.
11 Butte NF, Lopez-Alarcon MG, Garza C: Nutrient Adequacy of Exclusive Breastfeeding for Term Infants during the First Six Months of Life. Geneva, WHO, 2002.
12 Shrimpton R, Victora CG, de Onis M, et al: Worldwide timing of growth faltering: implications for nutritional interventions. Pediatrics 2001;107:e75.
13 Vaidya A, Saville N, Shrestha BP, et al: Effects of antenatal multiple micronutrient supplementation on children's weight and size at 2 years of age in Nepal: follow-up of a double-blind randomised controlled trial. Lancet 2008;371:492–499.
14 Espo M, Kulmala T, Maleta K, et al: Determinants of linear growth and predictors of severe stunting during infancy in rural Malawi. Acta Paediatr 2002;91:1364–1370.
15 Brown KH, Black RE, Lopez de Romana G, et al: Infant-feeding practices and their relationship with diarrheal and other diseases in Huascar (Lima), Peru. Pediatrics 1989;83:31–40.
16 Victora CG: Infection an disease: the impact of early weaning. Food Nutr Bull 1996;17. Accessed online March 9, 2008: http://www.unu.edu/unupress/food/8F174e/8F174E0i.htm#Infection%20and%20disease:%20The%20impact%20of%20early%20weaning.
17 Dewey KG, Brown KH: Update on technical issues concerning complementary feeding of young children in developing countries and implications for intervention programs. Food Nutr Bull 2003;24:5–28.
18 Brown KH: The importance of dietary quality versus quantity for weanlings in less developed countries: a framework for discussion. Food Nutr Bull 1991;13. Accessed online March 9, 2008: http://www.unu.edu/unupress/food/8F132e/8F132E02.htm#The%20importance%20of%20dietary%20quality%20versus%20quantity%20for%20weanlings%20in
19 Williams CD: A nutritional disease of children associated with maize diet. Arch Dis Child 1933;8:423–433.
20 World Health Organization: Complementary Feeding of Young Children in Developing Countries: A Review of Scientific Knowledge. Geneva, WHO, 1998.
21 Waterlow JC: Protein-Energy Malnutrition. London, Edward Arnold, 1992.
22 Waterlow JC (ed): Linear Growth Retardation in Less Developed Countries. Nestlé Nutr Workshop Ser Pediatr Program. Vevey, Nestec, 1988, vol 14.
23 Butte NF, Villapando S, Wong WW, et al: Human milk intake and growth faltering of rural Mesoamerindian infants. Am J Clin Nutr 1992;55:1109–1116.
24 Hotz C, Gibson RS: Complementary feeding practices and dietary intakes from complementary foods amongst weanlings in rural Malawi. Eur J Clin Nutr 2001;55:841–849.
25 Lutter CK, Rivera JA: Nutritional status of infants and young children and characteristics of their diets. J Nutr 2003;133(suppl):2941S–2949S.
26 Golden BE, Golden MHN: Relationship among dietary quality, children's appetite, growth stunting, and efficiency of growth in poor populations. Food Nutr Bull 1991;13:105–109.

27 Allen LH: Nutritional influences on linear growth: a general review. Eur J Clin Nutr 1994;48(suppl):S75–S89.
28 Bhan MK, Bahl R, Bhandari N: Infection: how important are its effects on child nutrition and growth?; in Martorell R, Haschke F (eds): Nutrition and Growth. Vevey, Nestec/Philadelphia, Lippincott Williams & Wilkins, 2001, vol 47, pp 197–221.
29 Victora CG, Barros FC, Kirkwood BR, et al: Pneumonia, diarrhea, and growth in the first 4 y of life: a longitudinal study of 5914 urban Brazilian children. Am J Clin Nutr 1990;52:391–396.
30 Molbak K, Andersen M, Aaby P, et al: Cryptosporidium infection in infancy as a cause of malnutrition: a community study from Guinea-Bissau, West Africa. Am J Clin Nutr 1997;65:149–152.
31 Thomas JE, Dale A, Bunn JEG, et al: Early *Helicobacter pylori* colonisation: the association with growth faltering in the Gambia. Arch Dis Child 2004;89:1149–1154.
32 Arpadi SM: Growth failure in children with HIV infection. J Acquir Immune Defic Syndr 2000;25(suppl):S37–S42.
33 Lunn PG, Northrop-Clewes CA, Downes RM: Intestinal permeability, mucosal injury, and growth faltering in Gambian infants. Lancet 1991;338:801–810.
34 Schrimshaw NS, Taylor CE, Gordon JE: Interaction of Nutrition and Infection. Geneva, WHO, 1968.
35 Engle PL, Menon P, Haddad LJ: Care and Nutrition: Concepts and Measurements. Washington, IFPRI, 1997.
36 Semba RD, de Pee S, Sun K, et al: Effect of parental formal education on risk of child stunting in Indonesia and Bangladesh: a cross-sectional study. Lancet 2008;371:322–328.
37 LeVine RA, LeVine SE, Richman A, et al: Women's schooling and child care in the demographic transition: a Mexican case-study. Popul Dev Rev 1991;17:459–496.
38 Becker S, Peters DH, Gray RH, et al: The determinants of use of maternal and child health services in Metro Cebu, the Philippines. Health Transit Rev 1993;3:77–89.
39 Liaqat P, Rizvi MA, Qayyum A, et al: Association between complementary feeding practice and mothers education status in Islamabad. J Hum Nutr Diet 2007;20:340–344.
40 Guldan GS, Zeitlin MF, Beiser AS, et al: Maternal education and feeding practices in rural Bangladesh. Soc Sci Med 1993;36:925–935.
41 Prince M, Patel V, Saxena S, et al: No health without mental health. Lancet 2007;370:859–877.
42 Patel V, Rahman A, Jacob KS, et al: Effect of maternal mental health on infant growth in low income countries: new evidence from South Asia. BMJ 2004;2004:820–823.
43 Rahman A, Iqbal Z, Bunn J, et al: Impact of maternal depression on infant nutritional status and illness. Arch Gen Psychiatry 2004;61:946–952.
44 Frongillo EA, de Onis M, Hanson KMP: Socioeconomic and demographic factors are associated with worldwide patterns of stunting and wasting of children. J Nutr 1997;127:2302–2309.
45 UNICEF: The State of the World's Children 2008: Child Survival. New York, UNICEF, 2007.
46 Commission on the Nutritional Challenges of the 21st Century: Ending malnutrition by 2020: an agenda for change in the millennium. Final report to the ACC/SCN. Food Nutr Bull 2000;21(suppl):1–87.
47 Greenspan A: Changes in fertility patterns can improve child survival in Southeast Asia. Asia Pac Pop Policy 1993;27:1–4.
48 Zere E, McIntyre D: Inequities in under-five child malnutrition. Int J Equity Health 2003;2:7–17.
49 Wamani H, Astrøm NA, Peterson S, et al: Boys are more stunted than girls in sub-Saharan Africa: a meta-analysis of 16 demographic and health surveys. BMC Pediatr 2007;7:17.
50 Brown KH, Black RE, Becker S: Seasonal changes in nutritional status and the prevalence of malnutrition in a longitudinal study of young children in rural Bangladesh. Am J Clin Nutr 1982;36:303–313.
51 Ramakrishnan U, Martorell R, Shroeder DG, et al: Role of intergenerational effects on linear growth. J Nutr 1999;129(suppl):544S–549S.
52 Kigutha HN, van Staveren WA, Veerman W, et al: Child malnutrition in poor smallholder households in rural Kenya: an in-depth situation analysis. Eur J Clin Nutr 1995;49:691–702.
53 Vella V, Tomkins A, Borghesi A, et al: Determinants of child nutrition and mortality in north-west Uganda. Bull World Health Organ 1992;70:637–643.
54 Golden MHN: The role of individual nutrient deficiencies in growth retardation of children as exemplified by zinc and protein; in Waterlow JC (ed): Linear Growth Retardation in Less

Prost

Developed Countries. Nestlé Nutr Workshop Ser Pediatr Program. New York, Raven Press, 1988, vol 14, pp 143–163.
55 United Nations: World Urbanization Prospects. The 2007 Revision. New York, UN/DESA, 2007. Accessed online March 9, 2008: http://www.un.org/esa/population/unpop.htm.
56 Gracey M: Child health implications of worldwide urbanization. Rev Environ Health 2003;18:51–63.
57 Perez Escamilla R: Breastfeeding and the nutritional transition in the Latin American and Caribbean region: a success story? Cad Saude Publica 2003;19(suppl):S119–S127.
58 Ghosh S, Shah D: Nutritional problems in urban slum children. Indian Pediatr 2004;41:682–696.

Discussion

Dr. Haschke: My comment is related to the growth curves which you showed. You are still using the NCHS growth curves as the reference. Since the arrival of the WHO growth curves, we know that the NCHS references are completely outdated because they overestimate weight and length during the second 6 months of life. Therefore if the NCHS curves indicate that disabled populations have a z score of –1.25 for weight for age, the new WHO curves would indicate a z score of between –0.6 or 0.7. This would be less dramatic. The new WHO growth curves provide a much better estimate of the growth of infants who are breastfed according to the present recommendations. A second short comment: you showed the growth of infants with HIV until 22 years; I assume it is 22 months.

Dr. Prost: The graph showing the growth of children according to their HIV status is over the 2 first years of life, so it is 22 months. Coming back to your comment about the WHO growth standards, I completely agree with you but with caution because the implications of the new WHO standards are not fully understood with regard to how they compare with the NCHS references that were widely used until then. In very early infancy using the WHO growth standards will increase the prevalence of stunting, wasting and underweight, and in later infancy, in childhood, it is likely to be fairly similar to the NCHS references. In my opinion the issue of using the new WHO standards and how they will impact on our estimation of undernutrition has not yet been sorted out.

Dr. Haschke: The differences between the 2 growth curves are substantial. During the first 3 months the new WHO growth curves show exactly the same pattern you showed in breastfed infants, weight and length are above the NCHS. However, from 4 to 12 months the new WHO standards for weight and length are 0.6 z scores lower than indicated by the NCHS references.

Dr. Pandit: You mentioned iron, zinc and vitamin A deficiencies among the leading causes of death. How is the cause-and-effect relationship established between the iron, zinc and vitamin A deficiencies? What indicators have been used?

Dr. Prost: The data I have presented were from the World Health Report 2002, so these are WHO estimates and I am not aware of how they calculated these.

Dr. Christian: I think the vitamin A estimates are based on randomized placebo-controlled trials of vitamin A supplementation in young children and their impact on child mortality. With zinc what they have done for the recent estimate in the *Lancet* series [1] is to use the two trials of zinc supplementation also using a placebo-controlled randomized study design to estimate the relative contribution of zinc deficiency to childhood mortality. With regard to iron, I think those estimates are based on two randomized control trials of iron supplementation but actually in the malarious setting they have shown a negative impact of iron on morbidity and mortality.

92

Dr. Ganapathy: The Nepal study [2] which involved about 65,000 children has given zinc a questionable role. Are we dealing more with food faddism which is contributing to zinc and iron deficiencies or are we overestimating the problem? Is there a role for zinc?

Dr. Christian: The question about whether zinc plays a role is related to using or promoting zinc supplementation to prevent childhood mortality. A program would actually have to be developed that targets all children of that age group for daily zinc supplementation, and it is questionable whether that is really possible given the modest effects on mortality that were observed in that study.

Dr. Shetty: I completely agree with Dr. Haschke that the numbers of undernourished, all categories, are going to change, particularly stunting and underweight, because the new WHO standards have produced growth references for children which are based on data from exclusively breastfed children from developing countries and India is part of this database. With the changes in both bodyweight and length, the numbers and prevalence of stunting and underweight will change [3]. The second point I want to make is with regard to your comments on the rise in food prices. There is no doubt that there has been an increase in food prices over the last 12 months or so, largely because of the increased food being diverted to feed animals (a lot of soya production in Brazil goes straight to China to feed animals), and also maize for instance going to biofuel production in the USA. But if you look at the changes in food prices over the last 20 years there has been a remarkable drop in food prices that what we are paying now for food does not even cover the production costs of that food. So this increase since 1980 is a very small increase in food price. I know it will affect a lot of low income people but the same low income people have benefited from extremely low food prices over the last 20 years. We may hence be misleading when we state that the cause of undernutrition in children is because of the increase in food prices over the last 12 months.

Dr. Prost: I completely agree with you, this is a very short period of time to look at an increase in food prices, but if we look at the larger picture, the conclusion might be a little bit different. However, I think that over a very short period of time there has been a substantial increase, but nobody here can say whether it really has increased child undernutrition or not because we don't have the data. Obviously when there is a 50% increase in food prices, it will very strongly affect the poor. We might not be affected as much by that, but the poor will certainly feel it, and I think it is linked to the price of oil as well. As you said, we have a short view here on food prices, and all the prices are increasing and nobody would actually dare to say that they are going to decrease. In the long-term food prices will continue to increase, and if they continue to increase at the present rate there will be a problem, there is no doubt about it.

Dr. Shetty: If you look at undernutrition in Indonesia, for instance, you can see how the economic crisis in East Asia has had an impact on undernutrition. So when you talk about global factors, food is just one component. If there is an economic recession, even if food prices do not change because they are subsidized, there will still be an impact on child undernutrition, and therefore to highlight just the rise in food prices as being the main causative driver of undernutrition is something that I do not agree with.

Dr. Sirajul Islam: As far as the food price is concerned, I think the food prices have risen very alarmingly. Two years back the price of rice was 21 taka/kg and it is now more than 50 taka/kg, pulses were 30 taka/kg, now they are 140 taka/kg, and this has happened in the last couple of months. For a man who earns 150 taka/day, has a family of 5 children and isn't working regularly, it is a devastating situation. We must not underestimate the food price at the present time.

Dr. Wharton: Can I ask you to enlarge a bit on your views on the effects of urbanization? The current ideas are that urbanization in developing countries generally isn't good, and yet historically in other communities urbanization is being associated with a reduction in mortality rates, with employment, and easier access to sources of education, and so on. Could you just say a bit more about what you think about urbanization?

Dr. Prost: The first thing I should highlight is that my field is epidemiology, so I am not very knowledgeable about the effect of urbanization on child undernutrition. Dr. Popkin could answer that question better than me. Urbanization as such is not a problem, it is uncontrolled urbanization. Urbanization is associated generally with an increase in income and that has a positive effect on child undernutrition. But uncontrolled urbanization leads to an increased exposure to risk, particularly for children, and this is what I wanted to highlight in my talk, the extent to which it has a negative impact on the health of children.

Dr. Agarwal: I have only two comments to make. One is in the case of India. Undernutrition has remained the same, wasting as well as stunting, for the last 7 years, and therefore this marginal rise in prices has not had an affect. The second thing I have seen in rural areas where I have done some interventions is that the weaning food is contaminated, the bottles, the utensils and the water are all contaminated. We have to solve two problems: one is water control and the other is bringing down the bacterial content of the water, and the cleaning of things. In dealing with infections, such as diarrhea and respiratory infections, it should be taken into account that the weaning foods are contaminated. I think the Gambian experience also shows the same.

Dr. Matthai: You made the point that there is still a very high burden of malnutrition in India. I think it is important to remember that what we now see in most parts of India is not the severe malnutrition that we used to see about 20 years ago. Most of what we see is the milder grades – grades 1 or 2. I suspect if we apply the new WHO standards and growth curves many of those who we have been classified as having malnutrition by our earlier standards would now be classified as normal. So, yes, there still is malnutrition in India, but I think the prevalence and severity are probably much less than what is commonly thought.

Dr. Christian: I just wanted to point out that both the NFHS-3 and the *Lancet* series' estimates of the global burden of undernutrition have used the new standards and rates that we were discussing earlier on, the 51% of stunting is based on using the new standards, so I don't think that we are misclassifying malnutrition, that is not really happening.

References

1   Black RE, Allen LH, Bhutta ZA, et al: Maternal and child undernutrition: global and regional exposures and health consequences. Lancet 2008;371:243–260.
2   Tielsch JM, Khatry SK, Stoltzfus RJ, et al: Effect of daily zinc supplementation on child mortality in southern Nepal: a community-based, cluster randomised, placebo-controlled trial. Lancet 2007;370:1230–1239.
3   de Onis M, Onyango AW, Borghi E, et al: Comparison of the World Health Organization (WHO) Child Growth Standards and the National Center for Health Statistics/WHO international growth reference: implications for child health programmes. Public Health Nutr 2006;9:942–947.

Kalhan SC, Prentice AM, Yajnik CS (eds): Emerging Societies – Coexistence of Childhood Malnutrition and Obesity.
Nestlé Nutr Inst Workshop Ser Pediatr Program, vol 63, pp 95–108,
Nestec Ltd., Vevey/S. Karger AG, Basel, © 2009.

Malnutrition, Long-Term Health and the Effect of Nutritional Recovery

Ana Lydia Sawaya, Paula Andrea Martins,
Vinicius José Baccin Martins, Telma Toledo Florêncio,
Daniel Hoffman, Maria do Carmo P. Franco, Janaína das Neves

Department of Physiology, Section Physiology of Nutrition, Federal University of São Paulo, São Paulo, Brazil

Abstract

It is estimated that over 51 million people in Brazil live in slums, areas where a high prevalence of malnutrition is also found. In general, the population of 'slum dwellers' is growing at a faster rate than urban populations. This condition is associated with poor sanitation, unhealthy food habits, low birthweight, and stunting. Stunting is of particular concern as longitudinal and cross-sectional studies of stunted adolescents have shown a high susceptibility to gain central fat, lower fat oxidation, and lower resting and postprandial energy expenditure. In addition, higher blood pressure, higher plasma uric acid and impaired flow-mediated vascular dilation were all associated with a higher level of hypertension in low birthweight and stunted children. In particular, stunted boys and girls also showed lower insulin production by pancreatic β cells. All these factors are linked with a higher risk of chronic diseases later in life. Among stunted adults, alterations in plasma lipids, glucose and insulin have also been reported. However, adequate nutritional recovery with linear catch-up growth, after treatment in nutritional rehabilitation centers, can moderate the alterations in body composition, bone density and insulin production.

Health, Nutrition and Life Conditions

It has become clear that, for a real understanding of diseases and their etiology, the influence of the anthropological aspects, the psychological dynamism and the social context on the regulation of body metabolism must be considered. A reasonable amount of scientific findings offer ever more examples of an integrated approach to studying medical problems, such as studies on the effects of happiness on the overall health of elderly people. For example, a study of catholic nuns in the United States concluded that writings with a positive emotional content at 22 years of age were associated with health and longevity at 60 years of age [1]. Thus, one may ask, as far as physiology is concerned, what goes on in a person who considers him or herself happy? There are strong relationships between that kind of statement, life expectancy and the frequency and intensity of chronic diseases, such as cardiovascular, inflammatory and self-immune ones [2]. Such studies identified an inversely correlate biological marker of that happiness declaration: cortisol, the stress hormone. The higher its levels in the saliva when the person wakes up, the greater the stress level and the worse the life quality in the long-term. The quality of a human life depends on what he feels and on the meaning he gives to things, both of which are associated with physiological status.

These same mechanisms are activated when a person receives insufficient nutrition in quantitative terms or inadequate nutrition in qualitative terms (when there is a lack of necessary nutrients, such as good quality of protein, vitamins and minerals), mainly early in life. In this case, the nervous system seems to permanently program itself to conserve energy as fat and to reduce growth to guarantee survival in adverse conditions. One of the essential hormones for fat conservation that is released during stress, such as periods of undernutrition, is cortisol, aptly named a stress hormone. The vicious cycle of inadequate food intake and infectious diseases stimulate the release of cortisol, a factor that plays a very important role in the association of malnutrition with chronic diseases in the adult phase [3, 4].

Malnutrition is responsible for over 50% of childhood mortality worldwide and is associated with many other diseases of children under 5 years of age [5]. Worldwide, as well as in Brazil, the prevailing type of malnutrition is stunting, an indicator not only of poor nutrition but also of poverty, as environmental factors are more significant than genetics in determining a person's adult height [6]. The causes for stunting range from poor maternal diet, intrauterine growth restriction secondary to placental insufficiency, not breastfeeding until the child is 6 months old, late introduction of complementary foods, inadequate quantity and quality of complementary foods, nutrient absorption impaired by infections and intestinal parasitic diseases [7].

In Brazil, approximately 52 million people live in slums [8], areas with an annual growth rate greater than urban areas. For example, in São Paulo, the growth rate of slums was estimated at 2.97% in 2000, while that of the city was 0.78% [9]. According to data from the municipality of São Paulo, there are over 2,000 slums with the greatest concentration in the southern zone of the city (1,107) [9]. Data on malnourished children under treatment at a center for recovery from malnutrition in São Paulo (CREN) located in that zone [10] found that over 70% of the children were born with low or insufficient weight. CREN is a center that offers treatment to children from the slums who are reported to have mild to severe malnutrition. Pediatricians, nutritionists, social workers and psychologists participate in the treatment. The pediatrician monitors the clinical status, laboratory findings and anthropometric progress of each child. The nutritionist follows the child's diet and corrects the problems identified during treatment. Laboratory tests (blood and stools) are done each semester and the children also receive Fe and vitamin (A, B, C and D) supplements in prophylactic doses. The children are either treated in an outpatient clinic or in a day-hospital. The children treated in the day-hospital are more severely malnourished. Data from CREN show that, among the moderately malnourished children under treatment, about 80% had at least one infectious episode in the previous month, and among the severely malnourished ones, that prevalence rose to about 90%. The difference in the severity of malnutrition referred mainly to the rate of infections. Besides, 60% of them had parasites. Another very common occurrence was anemia, verified in 62% of the children [11].

With regard to infections, it is important to note that most acute infections are often not life-threatening for a healthy child, but can jeopardize not only weight gain but also linear growth in a malnourished child. This observation is confirmed by the work at CREN where the recovering children stay all day (from 7.30 a.m. to 17.30 p.m.), eat 5 balanced meals/day, receive adequate treatment for the infections, and where both they and their families have the necessary medical and psychological care. Yet despite these interventions, normal childhood infections, such as otitis media, pharyngitis or the flu, have been found to retard normal growth. One can only speculate that if they were at home with no access to these interventions they would most certainly suffer more serious growth retardation and slip down the growth charts toward being severely stunted (fig. 1).

What Are the Long-Term Consequences of Malnutrition?

One important consequence of chronic malnutrition is that the body programs itself to store energy. We have previously shown that children who have been malnourished and who have not recovered in terms of height present a greater fasting respiratory quotient than those who have never been malnourished [12]. This means that the organism is physiologically prone to accumulate body fat, especially truncal fat [13]. Therefore, the child will grow less, have a lower fat-free mass, impaired bone growth, and will tend to use more excess energy ingested for fat accumulation [14]. Such findings are also associated with a greater susceptibility to accumulate body fat when the malnourished children consume a diet richer in fats [15].

By comparing the rate of weight gain of stunted adolescent girls to a control group, a longitudinal study showed that the malnourished girls presented faster weight gain, at the expense of a reduction in resting energy expenditure. That reduction in energy expenditure to gain weight was associated with an increase in body fat, mainly in the waist region where fat accumula-

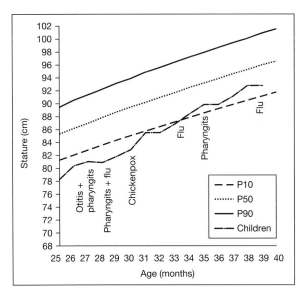

Fig. 1. Height gain of a child under treatment at CREN. Reprinted with permission from Revista de Estudos Avançados [11].

tion is most dangerous since it is closely related to chronic diseases such as diabetes and cardiovascular diseases in the adult life [16].

In a recent study comparing stunted adolescents to controls with normal height, we observed a reduction in insulin production by the β-pancreas cells (HOMA-β) and, as a response to this deficiency, a greater insulin sensitivity (HOMA-S). These alterations may lead to pancreatic failure and to a greater risk of diabetes in adult life (fig. 2) [17].

Our studies also showed higher diastolic blood pressure levels in boys and girls living in slums, which indicated greater risk of hypertension and cardiovascular diseases in adult life [18]. Further studies have shown that malnourished children with low birthweight have vascular alterations (a reduction of the vessel elasticity) and higher plasma uric acid, which might be the cause of the alterations observed in blood pressure and the pancreas (fig. 3) [19].

Combining all that information (fig. 4), we can then say that insufficient consumption during growth causes a stress in the organism, leading to an increase in the cortisol-to-insulin ratio. As is well known, malnutrition and/or hunger are powerful stimulators of stress and can prompt an increased secretion of cortisol and its catabolic action to direct energy as glucose to brain. In addition, energy restriction reduces the anabolic action of insulin-dependent tissue synthesis, resulting in wasting. This hormonal balance leads to a reduction in key hormones responsible for growth, such as insulin-like growth factor-1 (IGF-1) [20]. The high cortisol-to-insulin ratio and low IGF-1 also reduce the gain of muscle mass and linear growth, as well as increasing the waist-to-

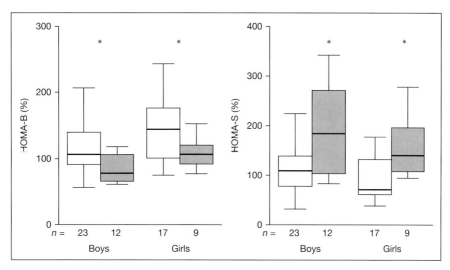

Fig. 2. Homeostasis model assessment for pancreatic β-cell function (HOMA-B) and for insulin sensitivity (HOMA-S) values of stunted (shaded boxes) and non-stunted (white boxes) boys and girls. Significant difference between groups: * $p < 0.05$. Reprinted with permission from the British Journal of Nutrition [17].

hip ratio and reducing body fat oxidation. If a child in that condition starts to ingest a 'modern' diet and presents physical inactivity due to urban living conditions, an excessive fat gain will take place, which can result in an association between stunting, obesity, hypertension and diabetes.

In fact, a study of individuals living in slums of Maceió, Brazil, showed an association between stunting and diabetes in the adult population [21]. Table 1 shows the biochemical profiles of overweight/obese women and men of short and average stature. In comparison to women of average stature, short women presented statistically higher levels of glycosylated hemoglobin, total and LDL cholesterol, insulin, HOMA-IR (an indication of insulin resistance) and HOMA-%β (β-cell function), whereas their HDL cholesterol levels were significant lower, as well as the T_3 levels. Among men higher levels of glycosylated hemoglobin, insulin, HOMA-IR and HOMA-%β, were found, indicating a risk of diabetes.

What Happens after Nutritional Recovery?

When a child has received appropriate treatment for malnutrition at a day-hospital, their chances of full recovery of weight and maintenance of normal growth rate are high [11]. In fact, at CREN, children recover height faster than weight [11] and we have observed a recovery of height-for-age of about 1

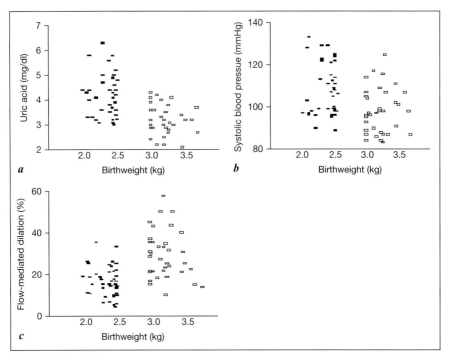

Fig. 3. Children with normal (opens symbols) and low (solid symbols) birthweight. Correlations between birthweight and uric acid (**a**; r = –0.498, p > 0.001), systolic blood pressure (**b**; r = –0.320, p = 0.004), and flow-mediated dilation (**c**; r = 0.427, p < 0.001). Reprinted with permission from Hypertension [19].

standard deviations among the most severely malnourished per year. Another important finding is that children with low weight at birth often recover better than those with normal weight at birth. Thus, it appears as though the human organism is potentially prepared to recover what was lost in the beginning of life, especially among intrauterine growth-restricted children who receive adequate treatment during the first years of life [11].

Recently, when studying children who recovered from malnutrition and were discharged from CREN, we observed normal body composition unlike what is found in malnourished children who were never treated and who remained stunted throughout their childhood and until their adolescence, as described previously. Among the recovered girls, the lean mass and body fat mass were similar to that observed in the control group (children with no history of weight or height deficits; table 2). Among the boys, body composition was normal, even though their values were lower in comparison to those of the control group. Similar findings have also been reported with respect to bone mineral density as outlined in figure 5 [10].

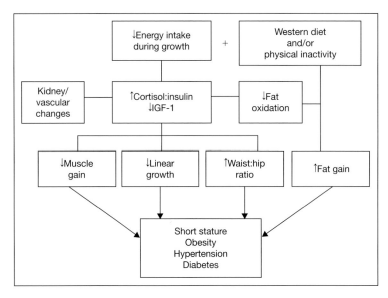

Fig. 4. Association between short stature, obesity, hypertension and diabetes.

Table 1. Biochemical profile of overweight/obese women and men of short and average stature

Stature	Women			Men		
	short	normal	p	short	normal	p
Glucose, mmol/l	04.76	04.68	0.16	05.04	05.00	0.72
Glucosylated hemoglobin, %	07.70	07.34	0.02*	07.96	07.72	0.03*
Cholesterol, mg/dl	186.0	166.2	0.03*	187.8	191.2	0.22
LDL, mg/dl	116.0	103.2	0.02*	114.6	112.8	0.12
HDL, mg/dl	044.0	048.3	0.05*	044.1	043.6	0.61
Total cholesterol/HDL, mg/dl	04.23	03.44	0.02*	04.25	04.38	0.25
T_3, ng/ml	01.22	01.48	0.04*	01.49	01.41	0.57
Insulin, µg/ml	11.34	09.26	0.02*	09.72	08.58	0.05*
HOMA-IR	02.39	01.93	0.01*	02.17	01.91	0.04*
HOMA-β%	180.0	156.9	0.002*	126.2	114.4	0.03*

Data obtained from a very low income population in Maceió, Alagoas, northeastern Brazil.

Recently, we studied how glucose metabolism and insulin levels changed in children who received adequate treatment at nutritional rehabilitation centers and showed linear catch-up growth. The results of the recovered group, consisting of children who were treated in their early years of life (0–6 years),

Table 2. Body composition of control, outpatient, and day-hospital groups of girls and boys at follow-up, including only prepubertal children

	Girls				Boys			
	control (n = 15)	outpatient (n = 12)	day-hospital (n = 18)	p value	control (n = 15)	outpatient (n = 12)	day-hospital (n = 18)	p value
Body fat, kg	6.9±2.6	3.8±0.9[a]	4.0±1.0[a]	0.006	6.2±2.2[b]	3.9±1.4[a]	3.6±0.7[a]	0.001
Body fat, %	26.4±4.5[b]	19.9±3.4[a]	19.8±2.8[a]	0.016	20.5±5.0[a]	17.7±3.4[a]	15.4±2.4[b]	0.007
Lean mass/ height, g/cm	145±13	130±10	131±14	0.112	173±18[b]	146±26[a]	151±17[a]	0.003
Fat-free mass, kg	18.7±3.2	15.3±1.8	16.1±2.5	0.104	23.8±4.4[b]	18.4±5.3[a]	19.9±3.2[a]	0.012
Fat-free mass index, kg/m²	12.5±0.3	11.9±0.7	11.8±1.1	0.259	13.9±0.7[b]	12.7±1.3[a]	12.8±0.9[a]	0.002

Values are means ± SD. Means in a row without a common superscript differ: $p < 0.05$. Reprinted with permission from the Journal of Nutrition [10].

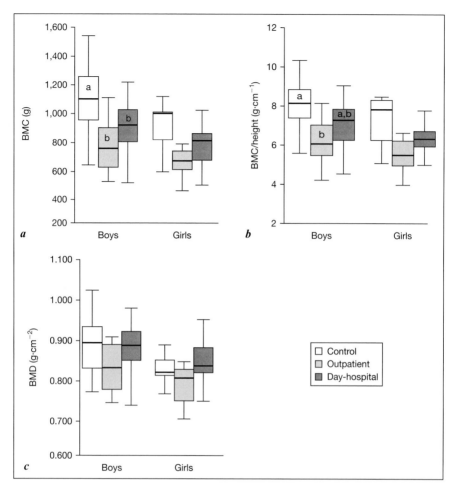

Fig. 5. Whole body bone mineral content (BMC; **a**), BMC/height (**b**) and bone mineral density (BMD; **c**) of the control, outpatient, and day-hospital groups, including only prepubertal children. The boxes represent the interquartile ranges (50% of the values), the whiskers are the highest and lowest values (excluding outliers), and the lines are the medians (n = 5–18). Medians without a common letter differ: p < 0.05. Reprinted with permission from the Journal of Nutrition [10].

showed insulin and insulin-sensitivity values similar to the control group (well-fed) [22]. Thus, what was once considered to be a metabolic alteration now appears to be reversible under favorable dietary and medical conditions.

These findings can be explained by the treatment offered at CREN, which consists of a balanced diet with protein of high biological value, nutrition education, and medication for parasites, infections and anemia. Parents and children receive nutrition education, which is an important source of information on what should be consumed in terms of food in order to recover nutritionally and develop healthier life habits. This education is very important for the slum population who live in poor urban areas, tend to consume cheap industrialized or out-of-home prepared food, and face a high level of unemployment or irregular jobs leading to lower physical activity.

Conclusion

We have presented data suggesting that children who experience energy restriction early in life may be metabolically programmed to deposit more fat, under specific conditions, and suffer from a number of metabolic pathologies. However, we also presented data suggesting that undernourished children exposed to proper dietary and medical environments can reverse these pathologies and return to normal growth trajectories. These findings, taken together, show that nutritionally recovered children foster a normalization of body composition, bone density and insulin metabolism and, therefore, reduce the risk of chronic diseases in adulthood.

References

1 Danner D, Snowdon D, Friesen W: Positive emotions in early life and longevity: findings from the nun study. J Pers Soc Psychol 2001;80:804–813.
2 Steptoe A, Wardle J, Marmot M: Positive affect and health-related neuroendocrine, cardiovascular, and inflammatory processes. Proc Natl Acad Sci USA 2005;102:6508–6512.
3 Rosmond R: The glucocorticoid receptor gene and its association to metabolic syndrome. Obes Res 2002;10:1078–1086.
4 Fernald LC, Grantham-McGregor SM: Stress response in school-age children who have been growth retarded since early childhood. Am J Clin Nutr 1998;68:691–698.
5 Repositioning Nutrition as Central to Development – A Strategy for Large-Scale Action. Washington, International Bank for Reconstruction and Development/ World Bank, 2006, p 9.
6 Florencio TT, Ferreira AS, França APT, et al: Obesity and undernutrition in a very-low-income population in the city of Maceió, northeastern Brazil. Br J Nutr 2001;86:277–283.
7 Allen LH, Gillespie SR: What Works? A Review of the Efficacy and Effectiveness of Nutrition Interventions. Geneva, ACC/SCN/Manila, Asian Development Bank, 2001.
8 Davis M: Planeta Favela. São Paulo, Boitempo, 2006, p 34.
9 Marques E, Torres H: Segregação, pobreza e desigualdades sociais. São Paulo, Senac, 2005.
10 Neves J, Martins PA, Sesso R, Sawaya AL: Malnourished children treated in day-hospital or outpatient clinics exhibit linear catch-up and normal body composition. J Nutr 2006;136:648–655.
11 Sawaya AL: Desnutrição: conseqüências em longo prazo e efeitos da recuperação nutricional. Revta Estud Avanç 2006;20:147–158.
12 Hoffman DJ, Sawaya AL, Verreschi I, et al: Why are nutritionally stunted children at increased risk of obesity? Studies of metabolic rate and fat oxidation in shantytowns children from São Paulo, Brazil. Am J Clin Nutr 2000;72:702–707.
13 Hoffman DJ, Martins PA, Roberts SB, Sawaya AL: Body fat distribution in stunted compared with normal-height children from the shantytowns of São Paulo, Brazil. Nutrition 2007;23:640–646.

14 Martins PA, Hoffman DJ, Fernandes MTB, et al: Stunted children gain less lean body mass and more fat mass than their non-stunted counterparts: a prospective study. Br J Nutr 2004;92:819–825.
15 Sawaya AL, Grillo LP, Verreschi I, et al: Mild stunting is associated with higher susceptibility to the effects of high fat diets: studies in a shantytown population in São Paulo, Brazil. Am Soc Nutr Sci 1998;128:415S–420S.
16 Grillo LP, Siqueira AFA, Silva AC, et al: Lower resting metabolic rate and higher velocity of weight gain in a prospective study of stunted vs nonstunted girls living in the shantytowns of São Paulo, Brazil. Eur J Clin Nutr 2005;59:835–842.
17 Martins PA, Sawaya AL: Evidence for impaired insulin production and higher sensitivity in stunted children living in slums. Br J Nutr 2006;95;996–1001.
18 Sawaya AL, Sesso R, Florencio TT, et al: Association between chronic undernutrition and hypertension. Matern Child Nutr 2005;1:155–163.
19 Franco MCP, Chrisitofalo DMJ, Sawaya AL, et al: Effects of low birth weight in 8-to-13-year-old children. Implications in endothelial function and uric acid levels. Hypertension 2006;48:45–50.
20 Thissen JP, Underwood LE, Ketelslegers JM: Regulation of insulin-like growth factor-1 in starvation and injury. Nutr Rev 1999;67:167–176.
21 Florêncio TT, Ferreira HS, Cavalcante JC, et al: Short height, obesity and arterial hypertension in a very low income population in North-eastern Brazil. Nutr Metab Cardiovasc Dis 2004;14:26–33.
22 Martins VJB, Martins PA, Das Neves J, Sawaya AL: Children recovered from malnutrition exhibit normal insulin production and sensitivity. Br J Nutr 2008;99:297–302.

Discussion

Dr. Yajnik: Your studies have shown that stunting is associated with bad metabolic outcomes. It is impressive that they did quite well after treatment. It seems you improved other things, but not blood pressure. At what age did you supplement them? When did you study them again? Was there any relationship to their early life experiences?

Dr. Sawaya: We treat these children, not only with supplementation, until they recover their stature. The most severe ones are treated in hospital and the less severe ones are treated as outpatients. They receive education, medication, but not food, and they receive treatment between 0 and 6 years. I did not show the data, but the only difference between the children less than 2 and more than 2 years of age is the speed with which they recover. Children recover from malnutrition also during puberty. Obviously it depends on the mother, the parents, and the life situation of the children. Treatment should not only include the child, but the whole family. Not only should food be given but also nutritional education. In our experience nutritional education works so well that the children take the good habits home to their families and they start teaching their parents that they want to sit at the table, they want to have vegetables, they want to eat fruits, and they want to eat at a certain time of the day.

Dr. Yajnik: Is there a window of opportunity? What do you think is the ideal time to intervene?

Dr. Sawaya: If they are treated before 2 years of age, they recover much faster in the features I showed. I am not sure about hypertension.

Dr. Yajnik: What was the age during the repeat study?

Dr. Sawaya: It depends on the age of the child because in general they stay in this treatment for 2 years until they recover. When they have caught up and their stature has normalized, they are discharged. We studied the children 3–6 years after they left the center. So the age at the repeat study was 8, 9, 10 years and even up to puberty.

Dr. Shetty: I just want to confirm that the classical thinking is that stunting is not reversed beyond 2 years of age. It is very interesting that you show that in fact stunting can be reversed even after 2 years of age. To my knowledge there are studies with micronutrient supplements showing that stunting can be reversed to some extent. Have you measured cortisol, insulin and IGF in the children who recovered? Are you changing the environment such that the endocrine response at that time has changed?

Dr. Sawaya: I personally believe that cortisol is a key issue. When I think about cortisol, I am not thinking about hunger, famine or whatever, I am thinking about stress, all kinds of stress. It is false to separate the stress of these children because living in a slum with a high score of depression is by itself a stressful condition, and we definitely measured higher cortisol levels. The cortisol levels decreased but I did not measure it in these children. Especially abdominal fat has normalized; they didn't have the accumulation of abdominal fat that is so typical with high cortisol.

Dr. Popkin: First I want to disagree. We have had a lot of population studies in the last 4–5 years showing catch-up growth in South Africa, the Philippines and elsewhere. Rolland-Cachera et al. [1] did a number of studies in France on children and hypothesized that increased protein intake would be associated with reduced adiposity. Now your research is leading to the protein side, because you seem to show that the stunted children who got the higher protein diet were the ones who reduced their risk of obesity. Or am I reading your results wrong?

Dr. Sawaya: No, not exactly. We give them good nutritional education, and during treatment they receive supplementation of vitamins, especially iron. We also treat the diseases related to malnutrition, all infections, parasites, etc., the whole treatment. I think the most important finding is that the good food education we give them is retained. We also found that protein intake was significantly higher compared to control slum dwellers, and the protein intake was of good quality because they are taught to avoid processed food and to eat natural foods, and therefore decrease the cost of the feeding.

Dr. Ravussin: What is the likelihood of misclassification because height is one of the most heritable traits? Do you adjust the height or the percentile height of the child for the parents, or at least the mothers when the fathers are missing?

Dr. Sawaya: About genetic background, yes we do measure the height of the mothers and they are low. But in a population with this standard of living I don't believe at all that stunting is not due to nutritional deficits over generations. I do know that if the bodies of these children are given the opportunity to catch up in height, then they do reach the normal range. So the body or the brain sees that the genetic potential is not there, and if the opportunity is there they catch up, for example the results with the supplements. If food is given they eat more, they don't control the daily food intake as the non-stunted control children do. If we measure IGF1, for me this is the most important thing, it is below the normal range. So these children are stunted because they have lower IGF1 levels, below the normal range.

Dr. Ravussin: My second question is more about energy metabolism in these children. You showed, at least in adult women, that there was a very low T3, and a low metabolic rate. There was also no difference in food or energy intake. First of all, do you trust the food intake measurements? In small numbers I would not trust them myself. Can you account for the low metabolic rate; does it account for the weight gain that is seen during this catch-up period?

Dr. Sawaya: Yes, I believe that a lower energy expenditure is causing the actual data in adolescents; we don't have data in adults. What we saw in these stunted adolescents, mainly girls, over the 36-month follow-up period was a lower energy expenditure associated with higher weight gain over time. So in the adult population I am implying that these lower T3 levels are also related to lower energy expenditure.

Dr. Ajayi: I just want to link up the earlier lecture to this one with regard to income and malnutrition. I believe that it is purely coincidental that income does not lead to malnutrition, because if a person has the ability to buy food and eat it, it does not mean they have the knowledge of what to buy and what to eat. I think this is reflected in this particular presentation as well, because it is only when a person has the knowledge, the understanding of what to use, even when it is not expensive, that they actually come out of the cycle of malnutrition. This is also true for people with high incomes because having a high income does not necessarily mean that they do not have malnutrition or are not malnourished. It is just coincidental, a person buys something, it happens to be good food and it is eaten, not because they have the knowledge of what to buy, what to eat, and how to prepare and how to consume it. We must not forget to look at education; educating those who have the resources as well as educating those who do not have the resources. When people have a sound understanding and know what to apply, then the right results will be obtained.

Dr. Ganapathy: There are a lot of articles on changing urban lifestyle and the metabolic syndrome [2–4]. You showed us your work on the metabolic syndrome: low growth hormone, lean body mass, low muscle mass, adiposity, insulin resistance, along with a rather low T3 for that age. Do you feel that you should have evaluated the TSH status? During rehabilitation was there a change in the environment of the slum child? Was is it only rehabilitation that brought the child back to normal? Did you ever think of endocrine disruptors in that slum area?

Dr. Sawaya: Yes, the condition of the family in general changes. What does not change, because it requires a big change, is the place where they live. To be able to move from a slum to a house, to be able to pay a rent is a big step upwards in terms of income, and that is difficult, at least in our environment. But if you think about the life within the family, yes, it has improved. We have data about the stability of jobs, the ability to shop and to choose the proper food. The comparison between the nutritional education given to these families and the drop in the obesity rate among very rich Brazilian women is due to the return to the natural staple Brazilian diet. So if cheaper food is supplied, at least in Brazil, by avoiding processed foods that are more expensive, good nutritional education and good nutritional outcome can be achieved, even if the person lives in a slum.

Dr. Ganapathy: Was there a change in the environment? I just want to know whether they were institutionalized, hospitalized, or something of that sort.

Dr. Sawaya: It is a daycare center. We don't take the children out of their families. If they need hospitalization we send them to the hospital, but this is for a few days or a few weeks, due to other infections like pneumonia.

Dr. Ganapathy: So they were not hospitalized, only receiving nutritional rehabilitation. What about TSH?

Dr. Sawaya: We have not measured TSH here.

Dr. Ganapathy: When there is stunting and obesity, it is prudent to think of an endocrine cause such as hypothyroidism.

Dr. Sawaya: You are a pediatrician, so I understand your concern. In our situation it is so obvious that these people don't have enough money to buy food, and it is so obvious that the whole family is short due to nutritional problems. When there is a high prevalence of stunting as in this situation, we are talking about 20% of the slum population, hormonal problems are something that we don't think of as the first cause of stunting, so we have not measured TSH.

Dr. Shetty: I just want to follow-up on the role of cortisol. In the West Indies they conducted studies during stress in children and showed that the cortisol responses were much higher in stunted as compared to non-stunted children [5]. I believe this is a very simple noninvasive method, looking at stress and its relationship to salivary cortisol and may be worth looking at in your subjects.

Dr. Wharton: The other thing that they did in Jamaica was to get the children to play much more. You mentioned psychological input to the mother but you did not mention anything about psychological input into the children or play. Did you do that as well in the daycare?

Dr. Sawaya: It is very important for the children to be in a positive environment. Very often they are not in a positive environment at home, and so the day hospital treatment for the most severely affected children with the most severe problems in their family is very important. In our center the social workers say that when they see that the mother is well-dressed and happy, the growth curve of the child is better. So a very positive environment for these children is definitely very important.

Dr. Shahkhalili: In your control group the energy intake is still not adequate. Thus you are comparing stunted children with undernourished but non-stunting children, is that true?

Dr. Sawaya: You are correct; I am comparing slum-dwelling children. The controls had lower IGF1, higher blood pressure; so they are not healthy either, they are slum children. So I am comparing control non-stunted slum children with stunted slum children.

Dr. Shahkhalili: You demonstrated the health and growth improvements in your treated group, except for the kidney problem. Do you know if your study group suffered from IUGR which has an irreversible impact on kidney development?

Dr. Sawaya: This is a good question; I don't know and would like to study this more. As far as I know, the number of nephrons in the kidney is mainly set up prenatally. 73% of our children have low or insufficient birthweight, and that is why I think it starts before birth and continues after birth, it is a continuing problem. I would like to see what happens after puberty for example.

References

1 Rolland-Cachera MF, Deheeger M, Akrout M, Bellisle F: Influence of macronutrients on adiposity development: a follow up study of nutrition and growth from 10 months to 8 years of age. Int J Obes Relat Metab Disord 1995;19:573–578.
2 Caballero B: The global epidemic of obesity: an overview. Epidemiol Rev 2007;29:1–5.
3 McLaren L: Socioeconomic status and obesity. Epidemiol Rev 2007;29:29–48.
4 Kelishadi R: Childhood overweight, obesity, and the metabolic syndrome in developing countries. Epidemiol Rev 2007;29:62–76.
5 Fernald LC, Grantham-McGregor SM: Growth retardation is associated with changes in the stress response system and behavior in school-aged Jamaican children. J Nutr 2002;132:3674–3679.

Mechanisms of Metabolic Damage

Kalhan SC, Prentice AM, Yajnik CS (eds): Emerging Societies – Coexistence of Childhood Malnutrition and Obesity.
Nestlé Nutr Inst Workshop Ser Pediatr Program, vol 63, pp 109–119,
Nestec Ltd., Vevey/S. Karger AG, Basel, © 2009.

The Role of Epigenetics in Mediating Environmental Effects on Phenotype

Daniel K. Morgan[a,b], Emma Whitelaw[a]

[a]Division of Population Studies and Human Genetics, Queensland Institute of Medical Research, Brisbane, and [b]School of Medicine, University of Queensland, Brisbane, Australia

Abstract

Epigenetics is being suggested as a possible interface between the genetic and environmental factors that together give rise to phenotype. In mice there exists a group of genes, known as metastable epialleles, which are sensitive to environmental influences, such as diet, and undergo molecular changes that, once established, remain for the life of the individual. These modifications are epigenetic and in some cases they survive across generations, that is, through meiosis. This is termed transgenerational epigenetic inheritance. These findings have led to the idea that similar processes might occur in humans. Although it is clear that the lifestyle of one generation can significantly influence the health of the next generation in humans, in the absence of supporting molecular data it is hard to justify the notion that this is the result of transgenerational epigenetic inheritance. What is required first is to ascertain whether genes of this type, that is genes that are sensitive to the epigenetic state, even exist in humans.

Copyright © 2009 Nestec Ltd., Vevey/S. Karger AG, Basel

Introduction

The term 'epigenetics' was coined by Waddington in the 1950s to describe the mechanism by which multicellular organisms develop different tissue types from one genotype. Today, we recognize that this process is associated with detectable molecular marks on genes, known as epigenetic marks. These epigenetic marks take various forms, such as DNA methylation and modifications to the chromatin proteins that package the DNA, but they do not alter the primary sequence of the DNA. They do, however, affect the transcriptional activity of the underlying genes; for example, cytosine methylation of DNA correlates with transcriptional silencing, whereas methylation and/

109

or acetylation of some histones is associated with transcriptional activity. Epigenetics is the study of changes in gene expression that are not due to DNA sequence changes and that are relatively stable through cell division.

In mice, genes have been identified that display variable expressivity among genetically identical littermates and these variations in gene expression have been shown to correlate with differences in the epigenetic state of the locus. Once established, these differential expression states last for the life of the individual. One example of this in mice is the *agouti viable yellow* (A^{vy}) locus. Of particular interest is that this locus is sensitive to environmental factors.

Metastable Epialleles in the Mouse

Some genes in the mouse are particularly sensitive to epigenetic state and exhibit variegation (that is, different expression patterns among cells of the same type), variable expressivity in an isogenic context and transgenerational epigenetic inheritance. These are known as metastable epialleles. The A^{vy} allele and the *axin-fused* $(Axin^{Fu})$ allele are two examples. The A^{vy} allele is a dominant mutation of the murine *agouti (A)* locus, caused by the insertion of an intracisternal A-particle (IAP) retrotransposon approximately 100 kb upstream of the agouti coding exons [1]. Contained within this IAP is a cryptic promoter which, when active, can drive constitutive expression of the *agouti* gene, resulting in a yellow coat color. When the cryptic promoter is silenced, a pseudoagouti coat color is produced (fig. 1). Many mice have both yellow and agouti patches, called mottled, indicating a clonal pattern of silencing, that is, variegation, in these mice. It has been shown that methylation at this promoter correlates with silencing of *agouti* gene expression [2]. An interesting phenotype of A^{vy} mice is that yellow mice become obese and are more likely to become insulin-resistant [3], whereas pseudoagouti mice remain lean throughout their lifetime. This implies that, for mice carrying the A^{vy} allele, an individual's propensity to become obese is influenced by epigenetic gene-silencing processes.

Metastable epialleles, such as A^{vy}, have been shown to be sensitive to environment. As discussed above, inbred mice carrying the A^{vy} allele show a range of coat colors and the proportions of yellow, mottled and pseudoagouti mice depends on their genetic background. Experiments have shown that changing the dam's diet before and during pregnancy can significantly alter these proportions. For example, when pregnant mothers' diets were supplemented with methyl donors, there was a shift in the colors of their offspring away from yellow and towards pseudoagouti [4]. This shift was correlated with a shift towards a more highly methylated state (that is, silencing) of the A^{vy} locus [5]. Similar experiments found that feeding genistein, found in soy milk, to heterozygous A^{vy} mothers shifted coat color towards pseudoagouti [6]. In

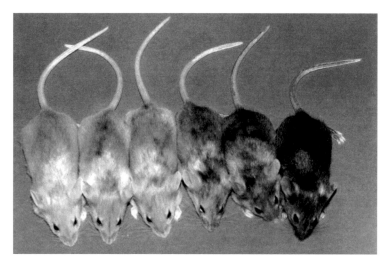

Fig. 1. Isogenic mice carrying the A^{vy} allele display a range of phenotypes, from completely yellow (pale in figure), through degrees of yellow/agouti mottling, to completely agouti (darker in figure; termed pseudoagouti). Yellow coat color correlates closely with adult body weight.

other words, in both cases the dietary change led to decreased disease (that is, obesity and insulin resistance) susceptibility by permanently altering the epigenome.

It has also been reported that the epigenetic state of a locus can be modified by behavioral programming. Postnatal maternal behavior in rats has been shown to alter the offspring's response to stress and this correlates with a change in the epigenetic state of the glucocorticoid receptor gene promoter in the hippocampus [7]. This is a second instance in which it appears that the epigenetic state of a gene can be influenced by environment, and that once established this state is mitotically heritable throughout the lifetime of the organism. In such a case, the epigenetic state is a record of environmental history, providing an opportunity to estimate disease risk and improve preclinical diagnosis.

Transgenerational Epigenetic Inheritance in Mice

Although epigenetic states, once established, are maintained for the life of the organism, it is rare for these states to be passed to the next generation. Between generations, the epigenetic state of the genome undergoes two dynamic reprogramming events: once in the gametes of the parent and again in the zygote. In spite of this, however, there is clear evidence in mice for transmission of an epigenetic state at a small number of loci through the gametes to the next generation. This is known as transgenerational epigenetic inheritance and was initially demonstrated at the A^{vy} locus [2] following strong evidence for such a phenomenon obtained from a number of independent studies at other loci [8–10]. Morgan et al. [2] showed that the distribution of phenotypes among offspring was related to the phenotype of the dam. A^{vy} dams that displayed the agouti phenotype were more likely to produce agouti mice; the converse was also true for A^{vy} dams displaying the yellow phenotype. This effect was interpreted as the result of incomplete erasure of the epigenetic mark as it passed through the female germline. Similar transgenerational epigenetic inheritance has now been reported at two other loci [11, 12].

Sensitivity to environment, combined with transgenerational epigenetic inheritance at the A^{vy} locus [2, 4], imply that the diet of a pregnant mother could not only affect her offspring's coat color and propensity for obesity, but that of their offspring as well, via transgenerational epigenetic inheritance. This was, in fact, recently demonstrated by Cropley et al. [13]. They showed that methyl donor diet supplementation can change the epigenetic state of the A^{vy} allele in the germline and that these modifications can be retained through the epigenetic reprogramming that occurs during early embryogenesis. However, these results have been somewhat tempered by the failure of another study to detect this transgenerational effect [14]. Although information in addition to DNA sequence can be inherited from parent to offspring in mice, what is the evidence that this occurs in humans?

Evidence for Transgenerational Epigenetic Inheritance in Humans

There is little direct evidence for transgenerational epigenetic inheritance in humans, despite a number of reports describing effects that superficially appear similar. The evidence is predominantly indirect and based on epidemiological studies. One frequently cited example, the Dutch Famine Birth Cohort Study [15], reported that offspring born during times of famine in World War II were smaller than average if maternal undernutrition occurred in the third trimester. Furthermore, the offspring of the second generation of individuals also weighed less than expected when the initial undernutrition occurred during the first trimester. Hence, the effects of the maternal undernutrition were observed in both the first *and* second generations.

More recently, Pembrey et al. [16] reported transgenerational responses in humans, using the Avon Longitudinal Study of Parents and Children and Överkalix cohorts. They found that paternal smoking prior to 11 years of age was associated with greater BMI at 9 years of age in their sons, but not daughters. It was also found that the paternal grandfather's food supply in the slow growth period was linked to the mortality risk ratio of grandsons only, while the paternal grandmother's food supply was associated with the mortality risk ratio of only the granddaughters. Hence, while transgenerational effects of maternal nutrition and environment are well recognized, this report described sex-specific, *paternal* transgenerational effects.

It is pertinent to note that, although the above epidemiological studies appear to demonstrate transgenerational effects induced by environmental and dietary factors, these data have not been supported by any molecular evidence. This is despite the hypothesis put forward by Pembrey et al. [16] that the reported transmissions are mediated by the X and Y sex chromosomes. Although the epidemiological evidence is tantalizing, we should resist the temptation to extrapolate from mice to humans without more convincing evidence. If, however, even a small number of human genes are found to be subject to transgenerational epigenetic inheritance, it would signal a paradigm shift in the way we think about the inheritance of phenotype. So how might we set about identifying transgenerational epigenetic inheritance in humans at the molecular level?

Identifying Metastable Epialleles in Humans

In the mouse, both of the alleles that display transgenerational epigenetic inheritance at a molecular level, A^{vy} and $Axin^{Fu}$ [2, 17], are metastable epialleles. Correlations between expression and epigenetic state have been observed at these alleles. It follows, then, that loci that demonstrate these characteristics of metastable epialleles in humans would be good candidates for transgenerational epigenetic inheritance. But how do we find metastable epialleles in humans?

Unlike laboratory mice, human populations are generally outbred, with the inherent genetic differences making it difficult to definitively determine phenotypic variation due to epigenetic causes. One way to circumvent this 'genetic noise' is to study monozygotic (MZ) twin pairs, which are considered to be genetically identical, and look for epigenetic variation between individuals in a twin pair. One could then study these loci in the general population, in particular, looking for inheritance of phenotype associated with epigenetic state. Many complex diseases, including cancer, diabetes mellitus, tuberculosis and schizophrenia display high levels of discordance among MZ twins [18, 19] and, as such, provide a convenient place to start in the search for metastable epialleles in humans. Once a cohort of twins discordant for particular phenotypes is available, what technology is available to observe epigenetic variation via a candidate gene approach?

DNA methylation, which occurs on cytosine residues in CpG dinucleotides, is the most extensively studied epigenetic modification to date, in part because of the excellent methods that have been developed to detect this change, such as bisulfite sequencing [20]. This technique enables determination of the methylation state of a DNA sequence and involves treating the

DNA of interest with sodium bisulfite, which converts unmethylated cytosine residues to thymine, while methylated cytosine residues remain unchanged. Sequencing of the products allows the methylation state of the original DNA to be determined. Bisulfite sequencing has been the driving force behind recent advances in epigenetics.

Following are examples in which disruption of the normal epigenetic state of the locus of interest has been implicated in the associated disease state.

Human Disease Resulting from Aberrant Epigenetic State

A pair of Dutch MZ twin girls discordant for caudal duplication anomaly has been described in which one twin was normal, except for clinodactyly of her fifth fingers and a preauricular pit, while the other twin had complete spinal duplication from the L4 vertebrate down, as well as many other associated birth defects [21]. *AXIN1* was suspected as being involved because reduced levels of Axin1 in the mouse results in a similar phenotype [22]. However, sequencing of the coding exons showed no difference between the twins. When the methylation state of the *AXIN1* promoter was analyzed it was found that both twins had significantly higher methylation levels than normal controls. In addition, the affected twin had significantly higher methylation levels than her unaffected co-twin [23], implying that methylation at the *AXIN1* gene may play an important role in this disease, in the absence of genetic mutation. It is important to note that correlation does not imply causation, but nevertheless, such findings will have value in preclinical diagnosis as indicators of disease risk.

Independent of MZ twin studies, there have been reports that also indicate that disruptions in epigenetic state can result in disease, for example, obesity. Prader-Willi syndrome is a rare genetic disease that is characterized by, among other symptoms, decreased mental capacity, obesity, insatiable appetite and an increased risk of diabetes. This syndrome is generally associated with genetic mutation in a set of genes on chromosome 15, but there have been some cases reported where there is no mutation, but instead, aberrant methylation, that is, an epimutation [24]. This epimutation appears to be the result of an allele that has passed through the male germline without clearing of the silent epigenetic state previously established in the grandmother, indicative of transgenerational epigenetic inheritance. Other cases of diseases resulting from disruptions in epigenetic state have been described, such as hereditary non-polyposis colorectal cancer [25] and α-thalassemia [26], however, these are not known to be associated with transgenerational epigenetic inheritance.

It has also been reported that assisted reproductive technologies, such as in vitro fertilization, are associated with an increased risk of the rare congenital imprinting disorders Beckwith-Wiedemann syndrome and Angelman syndrome in the offspring [27]. These diseases are normally associated with disruption to epigenetic gene silencing on either the paternal or maternal allele. It has been suggested that the increased risk may be due to disruption of epigenetic processes in the zygote, leading to disease. However, it remains possible that it is the result of genetic differences in the parents associated with the infertility, causing the parents to employ assisted reproductive technologies. Evidence that disruption to the epigenetic reprogramming associated with in vitro embryo manipulation can alter phenotype has come from nuclear cloning experiments carried out in mice, sheep and cattle. In many cases, the cloned offspring display large offspring syndrome [28–30]. An interesting report has shown that although mice cloned by in vitro embryo manipulation have an obese phenotype, they did not have an increased appetite, nor did they pass this obesity on to their offspring [31], suggesting that, at least with respect to this phenotype, transgenerational epigenetic inheritance is not occurring.

Conclusion

Our understanding of epigenetics is rapidly expanding and through mouse models and new technologies, we are learning that the inheritance of phenotype is more than simply the transmission of DNA sequence from one generation to the next. It is now clear that environmental factors play a bigger role in phenotypic inheritance than was once thought. However, the evidence for transgenerational epigenetic inheritance in humans is scant. While it remains possible that sporadic or complex diseases, for example, schizophrenia and obesity, could be caused by epimutations, the notion that these epimutations are passed down from one generation to the next remains unsubstantiated.

Acknowledgements

E.W. is supported by the National Health and Medical Research Council (NHMRC), the Queensland Institute of Medical Research (QIMR) and the Australian Research Council (ARC). D.K.M. is supported by an Australian Postgraduate Award from the University of Queensland.

References

1 Duhl DMJ, Vrieling H, Miller KA, et al: Neomorphic agouti mutations in obese yellow mice. Nat Genet 1994;8:59–65.
2 Morgan HD, Sutherland HE, Martin DIK, Whitelaw E: Epigenetic inheritance at the agouti locus in the mouse. Nat Genet 1999;23:314–318.
3 Miltenberger RJ, Mynatt RL, Wilkinson JE, Woychik RP: The role of the agouti gene in the yellow obese syndrome. J Nutr 1997;127:1902S–1907S.

4   Wolff GL, Kodell RL, Moore SR, Cooney CA: Maternal epigenetics and methyl supplements affect agouti gene expression in A^{vy}/a mice. FASEB J 1998;12:949–957.
5   Waterland RA, Jirtle RL: Transposable elements: targets for early nutritional effects on epigenetic gene regulation. Mol Cell Biol 2003;23:5293–5300.
6   Dolinoy DC, Weidman JR, Waterland RA, Jirtle RL: Maternal genistein alters coat colour and protects Avy mouse offspring from obesity by modifying the fetal epigenome. Environ Health Perspect 2006;114:567–572.
7   Weaver ICG, Cervoni N, Champagne FA, et al: Epigenetic programming by maternal behaviour. Nat Neurosci 2004;7:847–854.
8   Allen ND, Norris ML, Surani MA: Epigenetic control of transgene expression and imprinting by genotype-specific modifiers. Cell 1990;61:853–861.
9   Hadchouel M, Farza H, Simon D, et al: Maternal inhibition of hepatitis B surface antigen gene expression in transgenic mice correlates with de novo methylation. Nature 1987;329:454–456.
10 Roemer I, Reik W, Dean W, Klose J: Epigenetic inheritance in the mouse. Curr Biol 1997;7:277–280.
11 Herman H, Lu M, Anggraini M, et al: Trans allele methylation and paramutation-like effects in mice. Nat Genet 2003;34:199–202.
12 Rassoulzadegan M, Grandjean V, Gounon P, et al: RNA-mediated non-Mendelian inheritance of an epigenetic change in the mouse. Nature 2006;441:469–474.
13 Cropley JE, Suter CM, Beckman KB, Martin DIK: Germ-line epigenetic modification of the murine A^{vy} allele by nutritional supplementation. Proc Natl Acad Sci USA 2006;103:17308–17312.
14 Waterland RA, Travisano M, Tahiliani KG: Diet-induced hypermethylation at agouti viable yellow is not inherited transgenerationally through the female. FASEB J 2007;21:3380–3385.
15 Lumey LH, Stein AD: In utero exposure to famine and subsequent fertility: the Dutch Famine Birth Cohort Study. Am J Public Health 1997;87:1962–1966.
16 Pembrey ME, Bygren LO, Kaati G, et al: Sex-specific, male-line transgenerational responses in humans. Eur J Hum Genet 2006;14:159–166.
17 Rakyan VK, Chong S, Champ ME, et al: Transgenerational inheritance of epigenetic states at the murine Axin(Fu) allele occurs after maternal and paternal transmission. Proc Natl Acad Sci USA 2003;100:2538–2543.
18 Vogel F, Motulsky A: Human Genetics: Problems and Approaches, ed 3. Berlin, Springer, 1997.
19 Gottesman II: Schizophrenia Genesis – The Origins of Madness. New York, Freeman, 1991.
20 Clark SJ, Harrison J, Paul CL, Frommer M: High sensitivity mapping of methylated cytosines. Nucleic Acids Res 1994;22:2990–2997.
21 Kroes HY, Takahashi M, Zijlstra RJ, et al: Two cases of the caudal duplication anomaly including a discordant monozygotic twin. Am J Med Genet 2002;112:390–393.
22 Zeng L, Fagotto F, Zhang T, et al: The mouse Fused locus encodes Axin, an inhibitor of the Wnt signaling pathway that regulates embryonic axis formation. Cell 1997;90:181–192.
23 Oates NA, van Vliet J, Duffy DL, et al: Increased DNA methylation at the AXIN1 gene in a monozygotic twin from a pair discordant for a caudal duplication anomaly. Am J Hum Genet 2006;79:155–162.
24 Buiting K, Gross S, Lich C, et al: Epimutations in Prader-Willi and Angelman syndromes: a molecular study of 136 patients with an imprinting defect. Am J Hum Genet 2003;72:571–577.
25 Suter CM, Martin DIK, Ward RL: Germline epimutation of MLH1 in individuals with multiple cancers. Nat Genet 2004;36:497–501.
26 Tufarelli C, Stanley JA, Garrick D, et al: Transcription of antisense RNA leading to gene silencing and methylation as a novel cause of human genetic disease. Nat Genet 2003;34:157–165.
27 Gosden R, Trasler J, Lucifero D, Faddy M: Rare congenital disorders, imprinted genes, and assisted reproductive technology. Lancet 2003;361:1975–1977.
28 Eggan K, Akutsu H, Loring J, et al: Hybrid vigor, fetal overgrowth, and viability of mice derived by nuclear cloning and tetraploid embryo complementation. Proc Natl Acad Sci USA 2001;98:6209–6214.
29 Farin PW, Farin CE: Transfer of bovine embryos produced in vivo or in vitro: survival and fetal development. Biol Reprod 1995;52:676–682.
30 Sinclair KD, McEvoy TG, Maxfield EK, et al: Aberrant fetal growth and development after in vitro culture of sheep zygotes. J Reprod Fertil 1999;116:177–186.

31 Tamashiro KL, Wakayama T, Akutsu H, et al: Cloned mice have an obese phenotype not transmitted to their offspring. Nat Med 2002;8:262–267.

Discussion

Dr. Kalhan: When do we say that methylation has become permanent? Why doesn't it disappear? When demethylation occurs in the blastocyste stage, how does this affect heritable markers? Does the transcriptional regulation also involve some methylation?

Dr. Whitelaw: So the first question and the last question can perhaps be combined. How do we know which methylation marks will last and which ones won't, and we don't know. We were under the assumption that all methylation of C residues lasted for the lifetime of an organism. But environmental studies have shown that development can be modified later with respect to these things. A recent paper has come out looking at methylation occurring during transcriptional pulses down a gene [1]. In this amazing paper they show that transient methylation is seen for a matter of minutes at a promoter when the RNA polymerase comes and runs down the gene, and then that methylation pattern changes, and then when the next polymerase comes and produces a transcript, there is another change. I don't know how we are going to decipher the difference between those two types of methylation but I have no doubt that we will. As I said I think the underlying critical events are the changes to the histone molecules on the chromatin proteins and the methylation of DNA is tightly linked to those events. But those events are very heterogeneous and they have been harder for us to study. Because of the development of antibodies to say methylated histone, H3 or antibodies to methylated something else, we are starting to have the ability to better understand the relationship. So I think both are true and we will have to work hard to understand that. Now why doesn't everything get demethylated? I think the reason is twofold, and we are not really sure about this, but at the moment we think that the telomeres and the centromere of a chromosome are heavily methylated and they are silenced transcriptionally, and this is part of the structure overall of epigenetic molecules. So chromatin is not just involved in transcription, it is also involved in packaging a chromosome, and that chromosome has to have its ends, it has to line up at cell division and so on. I think there are some parts of the genome, and I would say centromeres and telomeres, where the epigenetic state must not change, you cannot release that tight chromatin state. Now genes that lie in what we call pericentromeric, peritelomeric regions adjacent to these heterochromatic ends on the center of chromosomes, I think might be the kinds of positions where you might get a metastable epiallele, you are getting kind of double signaling. There is a desire to keep you methylated and heterochromatinized, but nevertheless you are a gene and maybe you want to come on and maybe they have to clear you. So these are the kinds of regions where I think we will see metastable epialleles. The other parts of the chromosome that I think we do not want to have in an active form are retrotransposons. I don't know if you are aware that about 40% of your genome is the result of ancient retrotransposition. These are parasitic DNA elements that integrate into your genome and then get silenced epigenetically followed by mutation. Once a mutational event has happened at the retrotransposon it is permanently silent. But in the interim, before it undergoes a mutational event that inactivates it, it is good to have evolved a system which will silence that retrostransposon even in the gametes, even during this period where you want to reprogram the majority of your genome. It is very dangerous to have retrotransposons that are active because they then insert themselves throughout the genome and break up critical genes.

Dr. Ravussin: You gave us two examples of genes which are clearly methylated, basically the agouti viable yellow as well as the glucocorticoid receptor. In the twin studies you referred to, I remember reading a study in which it was shown that twins discordant for obesity had basically larger differences in total methylation. We have so few candidate genes when it comes to epigenetics, what does total methylation tell you about this? How far are we from having an epigenetic map?

Dr. Whitelaw: We are a long way from having an epigenetic map and there are a number of reasons for that. One is that there has to be a map for every different tissue type because the maps will be different. The epigenome project is orders of magnitude larger than the genome project. But the epigenome project is being undertaken now in the NIH and there is an international consortium of countries that is doing this. Regarding the twin studies, I think doing a twin study and finding that the global methylation level between the two twins is different, is not helpful. I would find it very hard to know how to interpret that.

Dr. Ravussin: It was in published in *PNAS*, and one of the things that they showed was that the older the pairs, the more the differences. Does this mean that things can happen later on?

Dr. Whitelaw: If you look very carefully at that paper, they had one older pair of twins. In fact it is now being studied at a different level by a group in Cambridge who are looking at the epigenome. They have some data in twins, and they see no increase in the level of difference within twin pairs with aging. So the biggest problem with that paper was that they didn't look at the same individuals that had the same underlying genotype as they aged. That is the right experiment, you can do it in a mouse; perhaps it is hard in a human. You have got to be quite careful about interpreting experiments like that.

Dr. Raju: Are we going back to the theory of Lamarck that acquired features can be inherited? Is there enough proof that epigenetics can result in certain features being acquired during one generation and passed on later? Are we validating that?

Dr. Whitelaw: I think there is very little evidence for that, and I tried to make that clear. So this is the debate really and it is very important. People get carried away with the idea that the marks that are laid down can last, in a Lamarckian sense, and be inherited through the gametes to the next generation. There are metastable epialleles where that hasn't been induced as a result of an environment. Independently, other people have shown that you can change the probability by environment. There are two papers in which they tried to combine those two studies to see whether Lamarck was right at that locus, and they both conclude differently. So one of the studies, which is in *PNAS*, says that there is inheritance to the next generation, but they acknowledge that that could have been because when the environmental event occurred the generation two's gametes were developing at that stage in the early fetus. So that is not really Lamarckian; it depends how you interpret Lamarck. So I think there is very poor evidence. Another paper did not even find the effect.

Dr. Yajnik: David Barker postulated that DOHaD has an epigenetic basis, thus nutritional programming is epigenetic. In the Pune Maternal Nutrition Study for the first time we have evidence of a maternal nutrient status predicting adiposity and insulin resistance in the child [1]. The two nutrients are vitamin B_{12} and folate, the two methyl donors. Could you advise us how we could investigate whether this association has an epigenetic basis? We have DNA samples and have the opportunity to collect them every 6 years. We have also collected DNA sample before and after a vitamin B_{12}-folic acid intervention.

Dr. Whitelaw: My advice to people in this position is to wait, because I think very soon we will have better technologies for interrogating candidate genes. Yes, in theory we can do genome-wide analysis but I think it is too early. I would hold on to that precious DNA and wait 3 or 4 years and then I think there will be better candidates, in part based on mass models in which there has been a change in folate. For example the *agouti viable yellow* is one reported gene, but those individual genes that have been made in various laboratories can then be interrogated genome-wide, and then you know the kind of genes that you might look at and that are involved in the phenotypes you are interested in. I think that is the safest thing.

Dr. Yajnik: There is a recent paper in on the sheep models [2]. They produced methionine deficiency in sheep by dietary manipulation of vitamin B_{12}, folate, etc., and demonstrated high homocysteine levels in blood and granulose cells and follicular fluid. The eggs were fertilized in vitro, and blastocysts were transferred to a normally nourished mother. The offspring had normal birthweights, but the male sheep grew rapidly, became adipose and insulin-resistant. Molecular investigations showed altered methylation at over 50 sites, half of which were male-specific. The phenotype of male offspring is very similar to our human findings. This is a very clear demonstration that periconceptional nutrition influences epigenetic changes.

References

1   Yajnik CS, Deshpande SS, Jackson AA, et al: Vitamin B_{12} and folate concentrations during pregnancy and insulin resistance in the offspring: the Pune Maternal Nutrition Study. Diabetologia 2008;51:29–38.
2   Sinclair KD, Allegrucci C, Singh R, et al: DNA methylation, insulin resistance, and blood pressure in offspring determined by maternal periconceptional B vitamin and methionine status. Proc Natl Acad Sci USA 2007;104:19351–19356.

Kalhan SC, Prentice AM, Yajnik CS (eds): Emerging Societies – Coexistence of Childhood Malnutrition and Obesity.
Nestlé Nutr Inst Workshop Ser Pediatr Program, vol 63, pp 121–133,
Nestec Ltd., Vevey/S. Karger AG, Basel, © 2009.

Metabolism of Methionine in Vivo: Impact of Pregnancy, Protein Restriction, and Fatty Liver Disease

Satish C. Kalhan

Departments of Gastroenterology and Pathobiology, Cleveland Clinic, Cleveland Clinic Lerner College of Medicine, Case Western Reserve University, Cleveland, OH, USA

Abstract

The coexistence of intrauterine and neonatal malnutrition and the development of obesity, type 2 diabetes and related comorbidities have been confirmed in a number of studies in humans and animal models. Data from studies in animals suggest that epigenetic changes as a result of altered methylation of the genomic DNA may be responsible for such metabolic patterning. Methionine, an essential amino acid, plays a critical role in the methyltranferases involved in the methylation by providing the one-carbon units via the methionine transmethylation cycle. Because of its interaction with a number of vitamins (B_{12}, folate, pyridoxine), its regulation by hormones, i.e. insulin and glucagon, and by the changes in redox state, methionine metabolism is effected by nutrient and environmental influences and by altered physiological states. In the present review the impact of human pregnancy, dietary protein restriction and fatty liver disease on methionine metabolism is discussed. The role of methionine in metabolic programming in a commonly used model of intrauterine growth retardation and in propagation of fatty liver disease is briefly described.

Introduction

The rapid urbanization and improving economic wellbeing in emerging societies has been associated with high rates of obesity, insulin resistance, type 2 diabetes and coronary heart disease. At the same time, low birthweight or intrauterine growth retardation (malnutrition) remains a persistent problem, accounting for as many as 30% of the births in several countries, including India [1]. Almost 75% of low birthweight infants are born at full term. A number of epidemiological studies in humans from different parts of the world have shown a correlation between intrauterine growth restriction (IUGR), resulting in thinness or small size at birth (low birthweight) and chronic disease in adults. Data from animal studies, particularly in the rodent, show that alterations in the intrauterine environment caused by nutrient interventions in the mother, e.g. protein or calorie restriction, iron deficiency or by hypoxemia, result in restricted growth of the fetus and long-term consequences. The latter include, amongst others, changes in hypothalamic pituitary axis, altered expression of glucose transporters and changes in glucose uptake by the fetus and neonate, chronic hypertension, changes in vascular reactivity, obesity and type 2 diabetes [2–5]. The mechanism of the 'permanent' effect, also termed imprinting or programming, remains a subject of investigation.

In the commonly used model of IUGR, i.e. dietary protein restriction of the mother, Rees et al. [6] have shown hypermethylation of the genomic DNA in the fetal liver. Methylation of cytosine in the DNA has been related to the activities of a number of mammalian genes, somatic inheritance and cellular differentiation [7]. The activation of some genes has been attributed to the demethylation of critical CpG loci. However, as reviewed by Jones and Takai [8], this is an oversimplification. Methylation changes the interactions between protein and DNA, leading to alterations in chromatin structure and in either a decrease or increase in the rate of transcription. Studies of transgene methylation have shown that methylation patterns can be inherited in a parent-of-origin specific manner, suggesting that DNA methylation may play a role in genomic imprinting (or programming) [9]. DNA methylation can be effected by the availability of methyl groups and by changes in one-carbon metabolism by dietary and vitamin modifications. In this context, Lillycrop et al. [10] observed that dietary protein restriction of pregnant rats resulted in lower methylation and higher expression of PPARα, acyl-CoA carboxylase and glucocorticoid receptor genes in the livers of the offspring after weaning. Of interest, supplementation with folic acid prevented these epigenetic modifications. These studies are particularly relevant when interpreting the data of nutrition–gene interactions and other epidemiological correlations, particularly from societies with nutrient deficiencies [11]. Methionine, along with homocysteine and folate, are key components of the one-carbon metabolism [12]. Perturbations in the methionine cycle and secondarily DNA methylation could cause metabolic programming in the fetus and neonate that lead to morbidity in adult life. On the other hand, in the developed organism, perturbations in the methionine metabolism due to endocrine and metabolic changes in the tissue and organism could make it more prone to injury and thus propagation of the disease.

In the present review the alterations in the metabolism of methionine induced by normal human pregnancy, dietary protein restriction and with ectopic fat accumulation in nonalcoholic fatty liver disease (NAFLD) are discussed. The changes during development are speculated to result in the patterns of expression of certain genes in the fetus, while the perturbations in NAFLD are suggested to cause injury and propagation of the disease.

Metabolism of Methionine

Methionine, an essential amino acid required for protein synthesis, is an important source of methyl groups for a number of important methylation reactions such as transmethylation of nucleic acids (methylation of DNA in gene expression), protein, biogenic amines and phospholipids, etc. [12, 13]. Methionine is metabolized first by the ubiquitous transmethylation (or methionine) cycle wherein the methyl groups from methionine or from the folate-dependent one-carbon pool participate in various methyltransferase reactions (fig. 1). During transmethylation, methionine is converted to its active form S-adenosylmethionine (SAM), which is the major substrate for the methylation reactions. Following SAM-dependent transmethylation, the product S-adenosylhomocysteine (SAH) is metabolized to adenosine and homocysteine. Homocysteine is either converted to cysteine via transulfuration pathway, or remethylated back to methionine. The methyl group required for remethylation is obtained from either the folate-dependent one-carbon pool (5-methyltetrahydrofolate) or from betaine (in the liver). SAM is also converted to SAH by glycine N-methyltransferase (GNMT), an enzyme abundant in the liver where it makes up a very large component (~1%) of soluble proteins in the cytosol. It transfers a methyl group from SAM to glycine, resulting in the formation of N-methylglycine (sarcosine) and SAH. The function of GNMT is believed to serve as an alternate pathway for the conversion of SAM to SAH in order to maintain a normal SAM/SAH ratio [13, 14]. SAH is a potent inhibitor of most methyltransferases, and therefore the ratio of SAM/SAH is an index of methylation potential. SAM is also an allosteric inhibitor of 5,10-methylenetetrahydrofolate reductase (MTHFR), the enzyme that catalyzes the irreversible reduction of 5,10-methylenetetrahydrofolate to 5-methyltetrahydrofolate and an allosteric activator of cystathionine β-synthase (CβS). On the other hand, 5-methyltetrahydrofolate is an inhibitor of GNMT. Finally, tetrahydrofolate also plays an important role in the catabolism of histidine in the conversion of N-formimino glutamate (Figlu) to glutamate. The synthesis of SAM by SAM synthase is regulated by hypoxia [15], glutathione [16], availability of methionine [17], and modified by oxidant injury [18] and redox state [19] of the cell.

The transmethylation cycle does not result in catabolism of methionine. While methionine provides the carbon carrier for the cycle, the majority of the methyl groups for the methyltransferase reactions are provided by glycine and serine via the folate-dependent one-carbon pool. As shown in figure 2, the methionine transmethylation cycle is interdependent upon the folate cycle as the source of methyl groups for the conversion of

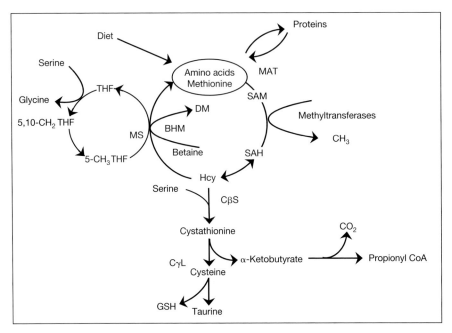

Fig. 1. Pathways of metabolism of methionine and its relation to the folate cycle are displayed (details in text).

homocysteine to methionine catabolized by methionine synthase (tetrahydrofolate methyltransferase).

As discussed by Brosnan and Brosnan [13], methionine metabolism requires a number of vitamins as cofactors, so that nutrient deficiencies can easily impact methionine metabolism (table 1). The key vitamins required for methionine metabolism are B_{12} for methionine synthase, folic acid for one-carbon pool, riboflavin for MTHFR, and pyridoxine for the transsulfuration pathway – CBS and CGL. In addition, the oxidative decarboxylation of the α-ketobutyrate catalyzed by pyruvate dehydrogenase requires niacin/thiamine and pentothenic acid (coenzyme A). Thus it is not surprising that deficiencies of these vitamins can impact methionine metabolism and may be associated with elevated plasma levels of homocysteine and other metabolic intermediates.

Human Pregnancy

There are very few data on methionine metabolism in human pregnancy. With the increased interest in the relationship between perturbations in one-carbon metabolism and its role in epigenetics and the developmental origin

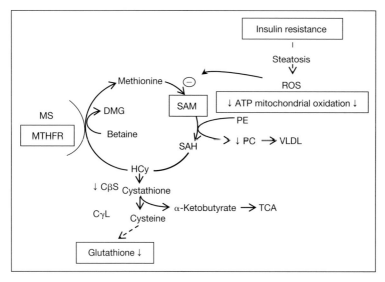

Fig. 2. Potential mechanism of propagation of hepatocellular injury in fatty liver disease (see text for details).

of adult health and disease, some new data have been published. However, human data are often confounded by the interactions between nutrient intake, nutrient status and other regional/societal interactions, and hence require careful interpretation. This is particularly important when evaluating data from societies with nutritional (vitamin) insufficiency. The data from studies in humans have been further confounded by the recent fortification of flour with folic acid in many countries.

The primary source of plasma methionine during fasting is that released from protein breakdown. Since the rate of breakdown of proteins has been shown to decrease during normal human pregnancy, there is a decrease in the concentrations of all amino acids in the plasma compartment [20]. Thus the plasma concentrations of all essential amino acids, including methionine, are lower during pregnancy when compared with non-pregnant women. Recent data from several studies show that the concentration of total homocysteine in the plasma is lower in normal healthy women in the 3rd trimester [21–23]. In fact, a progressive decrease in homocysteine concentration is evident starting early in pregnancy. This is associated with a progressive increase in plasma choline concentration. Of interest, the circulating levels of folate and vitamin B$_{12}$, respectively, increase and decrease with advancing gestation. The increase in plasma levels of choline have been interpreted as a mechanism to provide the increasing demands for choline by the fetus. In studies in the rat, the increase in plasma choline is associated with a decrease in the content of choline in the liver with advancing gestation. A decrease in

Table 1. Vitamins and methionine metabolism

Cobalamine (B_{12})	Methionine synthase
Folic acid	1-Carbon pool
Riboflavin (FAD)	MTHFR
Pyridoxine	CβS, CγL
Niacin (NAD)	Pyruvate dehydrogenase
Thiamine (thiamine pyrophosphate)	
Pantothenic acid (coenzyme A)	

hepatic choline content would impact the remethylation of homocysteine by lowering the availability of betaine. Although a number of significant statistical correlations have been observed for these metabolites, the mechanism of these changes and their physiological significance remains to be elucidated. Examination of the maternal–fetal gradients for these metabolites show that homocysteine is transported across the placenta along a concentration gradient so that the umbilical venous concentrations of tHcy are lower than in the simultaneously obtained maternal venous blood. In addition, the umbilical arterial concentrations of tHcy are lower than that in the umbilical vein, suggesting fetal utilization of homocysteine. Finally, the umbilical venous concentrations of methionine, choline, betaine and dimethylarginine were higher when compared with those in maternal venous blood [21].

Data from studies by Sturman et al. [24] and Gaull et al. [25], and recent studies of Levonen et al. [26], have shown the absence of transsulfuration activity in the human fetal liver and thus the inability of the fetus to synthesize cysteine. This is because of the low activity of CβS and the absence of cystathionine γ-lyase (CγL; protein) in the fetal liver. The fetal utilization of homocysteine and the umbilical uptake of betaine could be interpreted to support the transmethylation of methionine and homocysteine, and methylation demands in the fetus. These data would also suggest that any perturbations in the maternal methionine metabolism as a result of nutritional/environmental perturbations could have a significant impact on the fetal one-carbon metabolism.

Dietary Protein Restriction and IUGR

The dietary protein restriction during pregnancy model of IUGR has been used by a number of investigators to study the consequences of fetal growth retardation. These data show that protein restriction in pregnancy causes IUGR, selective changes in organ growth and permanent growth retardation, impaired insulin secretion, alterations in hepatic glucokinase expression and hepatic glucose output, and hypertension in the offspring [2–4]. These changes have been associated with changes in the hypothalamic-pituitary adrenal axis, changes in the reactivity of the vasculature, changes in the renin-angiotensin system and alterations in the catecholamine levels and adrenoreceptors in various tissues. Data from our studies suggest a higher rate of protein synthesis in the maternal liver and a lower rate of protein synthesis in the fetal liver in response to protein restriction [27]. In relation to methionine metabolism, dietary protein restriction in non-pregnant rats resulted in a marked increase in plasma, hepatic and skeletal muscle concentrations of serine and glycine, a significant change in hepatic SAM:SAH ratio, and downregulation of the hepatic transsulfuration pathway. These changes were associated with a change in the arterial-protein vein gradient for glycine and serine, resulting in a significant release of serine and a lower uptake of glycine by the gut [28]. Gene array analysis showed a marked upregulation of genes involved in serine and taurine biosynthesis (unpublished data). The biological significance of the changes in relation to whole body metabolism and to fetal growth remain to be determined.

Methionine and Nonalcoholic Fatty Liver Disease

NAFLD constitutes a wide spectrum ranging from the benign accumulation of triglycerides in the hepatocytes (hepatic steatosis) to steatohepatitis with inflammation, fibrosis and cirrhosis. Insulin resistance, obesity and ectopic fat (in the liver) are the hallmarks of the disorder [29]. It has been proposed that as a result of insulin resistance, there is an increase in the rate of lipolysis, which is not suppressed by infusion of glucose and insulin (clamp), resulting in a high rate of delivery to and uptake by the liver of free fatty acids. The accumulation of triglycerides in the liver (steatosis) has been attributed to the high uptake, high de novo lipogenesis, and to a decreased export of the lipids [30]. Hepatic steatosis results in hepatic insulin resistance, altered peroxisomal and microsomal lipid metabolism, lipid peroxidation and in increased production of reactive oxygen species (ROS), which can disrupt the mitochondrial membrane potential and cause a decline in the generation of hepatic ATP and lower ATP levels.

The changes in methionine metabolism are related to the insulin resistance and to the changes in hepatic metabolism as a result of ectopic fat accumulation. The data from human studies are confounded by the associated disorders, e.g. change in renal function, in addition to the possible differences in micronutrients, especially vitamin intake. Although the effects of insulin and insulin resistance on the metabolism of methionine have not been examined in humans, certain inferences can be drawn from the published data of studies in humans and animals. Studies in the rat show that a lack of insulin induced by streptozotocin results in lower plasma homocysteine levels and an increase in the activity of hepatic CβS and CγL [31]. The activities of enzymes involved in the transmethylation of methionine (MS, betaine:homocysteine methyltransferase, MTHFR) were not impacted by a lack of insulin [31, 32]. Insulin treatment reversed these changes. Similar changes in enzyme activity have been reported by the longitudinal studies of ZDF (fa/fa, type 2) diabetic rats [33]. Studies in patient with type 1 diabetes show that insulin deprivation results in a lower rate of transmethylation and a higher rate of transsulfuration, and that both effects could be reversed by insulin administration [34]. Somewhat variable effects have been observed by other investigators in studies in healthy subjects and in those with type 2 diabetes [35, 36]. Other data from humans in the insulin resistance state have shown that hyperhomocysteinemia is associated with hyperinsulinemia and insulin resistance [37].

In contrast to the repressive effect of insulin on transsulfuration and therefore decreased synthesis of cysteine, both insulin and hydrocortisone have been shown to increase the levels of glutathione in cultured hepatocytes. The increase in glutathione was related to the increase in the activity of γ-glutamylcysteine synthase (GCS), the key enzyme in the synthesis of glutathione [38]. A similar effect of insulin on glutathione metabolism was seen in vivo in streptozotocin-induced diabetes in the rat and in the plasma and red blood cell glutathione levels of human diabetic subjects.

In addition to insulin resistance, alterations in mitochondrial function resulting in lower mitochondrial oxidation, decreased synthesis of ATP, and increased peroxisomal production of ROS could also impair methionine metabolism in NAFLD. The high rate of ROS production may impact methionine metabolism by increasing glutathione consumption and thus change the hepatic redox state and impact the activity of methionine adenosyltransferase and the transmethylation of methionine. Finally, altered transmethylation of methionine may impact the hepatic VLDL export by altering the synthesis of phosphatidylcholine from phosphatidylethanolamine [39], and thus further contribute to the development of steatosis and steatohepatitis.

Preliminary data from our studies on subjects with biopsy-proven hepatic steatosis and nonalcoholic steatohepatitis (NASH) show that subjects with NASH, and without diabetes, are insulin-resistant, have lower plasma levels of glutathione and higher plasma concentrations of homocysteine and cysteine. A significant association of MTHFR 677C$\rightarrow$T homozygosity and NASH was also observed. Insulin resistance (HOMA) was negatively correlated with plasma glutathione ($r = 0.42$, $p < 0.001$) and positively correlated with plasma cysteine levels ($r = 0.25$, $p < 0.05$).

Based on these data, we propose the following hypothesis for the propagation of hepatic injury in NAFLD and the role of methionine in this process (fig. 2). Hepatic insulin resistance associated with obesity, type 2 diabetes or metabolic syndrome, results in an increased flux of fatty acid to the liver and in hepatic steatosis. As a consequence of lipid accumulation and increased fatty acid oxidation, there is a high rate of production of ROS, leading to decreased activity of methionine adenosyltransferase, disruption of mitochondrial membrane potential and cellular ATP level. A lower activity of methionine adenosyltransferase and a decreased rate of production of ATP leads to a lower rate of production of SAM. The lower concentration and the lower production of SAM then causes changes in the methionine transmethyl-ation and transsulfuration pathway. In addition, insulin resistance or the lack of insulin action may also cause the downregulation of glutathione synthesis. Decreased cellular glutathione levels lead to an unbalanced ROS and propagate these events. Decreased availability of SAM could impact the methylation of phosphatidylethanolamine to phosphatidylcholine, required for VLDL export, and thus interfering with fat mobilization.

In conclusion, metabolism of methionine, with all its interactions with folic acids, SAM-dependent methylation and one-carbon metabolism, is profoundly impacted by nutrient, hormone and environmental influences. During development, perturbations in methionine metabolism can result in long-term changes in the metabolism of the organism, possibly by causing changes in gene expression. In contrast, in mature organisms changes in methionine metabolism by impacting the physiological function may contribute to the propagation of injury.

Acknowledgment

The secretarial assistance of Mrs. Joyce Nolan is gratefully appreciated.

References

1 Dadhich JP, Paul V (eds): Newborn Health Issues in State of India's Newborn. New Delhi, National Neonatology Forum/Washington, Save the Children/US, 2004, pp 43–63.
2 Langley-Evans SC, Langley-Evans AJ, Marchand MC: Nutritional programming of blood pressure and renal morphology. Arch Physiol Biochem 2003;111:8–16.
3 Seckl JR, Meaney MJ: Glucocorticoid programming. Ann NY Acad Sci 2004;1032:63–84.
4 Brawley L, Poston L, Hanson MA: Mechanisms underlying the programming of small artery dysfunction: review of the model using low protein diet in pregnancy in the rat. Arch Physiol Biochem 2003;111:23–35.
5 Simmons RA: Developmental origins of diabetes: the role of epigenetic mechanisms. Curr Opin Endocrinol Diabetes Obes 2007;14:13–16.
6 Rees WD, Hay SM, Brown DS, et al: Maternal protein deficiency causes hypermethylation of DNA in the livers of rat fetuses. J Nutr 2000;130:1821–1826.
7 Waterland RA, Michels KB: Epigenetic epidemiology of the developmental origins hypothesis. Annu Rev Nutr 2007;27:363–388.
8 Jones PA, Takai D: The role of DNA methylation in mammalian epigenetics. Science 2001;293:1068–1070.
9 Cooney CA, Dave AA, Wolff GL: Maternal methyl supplements in mice affect epigenetic variation and DNA methylation of offspring. J Nutr 2002;132:2393S–2400S.
10 Lillycrop KA, Phillips ES, Jackson AA, et al: Dietary protein restriction of pregnant rats induces ad folic acid supplementation prevents epigenetic modification of hepatic gene expression in the offspring. J Nutr 2005;135:1382–1386.

11 Yajnik CS, Deshpande SS, Jackson AA, et al: Vitamin B_{12} and folate concentrations during pregnancy and insulin resistance in the offspring: the Pune Maternal Nutrition Study. Diabetologia 2008;51:29–38.
12 Finkelstein JD: Methionine metabolism in mammals. J Nutr Biochem 1990;1:228–237.
13 Brosnan JT, Brosnan ME: The sulfur-containing amino acids: an overview. J Nutr 2006;136:1636S–1640S.
14 Rowling MJ, McMullen MH, Chipman DC, Shalinske KL: Hepatic glycine N-methyltransferase is up-regulated by excess dietary methionine in rats. J Nutr 2002;132:2545–2550.
15 Avila MA, Carretero MV, Rodriguez EN, Mato JM: Regulation by hypoxia of methionine adenosyltransferase activity and gene expression in rat hepatocytes. Gastroenterology 1998;114:364–371.
16 Pajares MA, Durán C, Corrales F, et al: Modulation of rat liver S-adenosylmethionine synthetase activity by glutathione. J Biol Chem 1992;267:17698–17605.
17 Martínez-Chantar ML, Latasa MU, Varela-Rey M, et al: L-Methionine availability regulates expression of the methionine adenosyltransferase 2A gene in human hepatocarcinoma cells. J Biol Chem 2003;278:19885–19890.
18 Sánchez-Góngora E, Pastorino JG, Alvarez L, et al: Increased sensitivity to oxidative injury in Chinese hamster ovary cells stably transfected with rat S-adenosylmethionine synthetase cDNA. Biochem J 1996;319:767–773.
19 Lu SC, Huang Z-Z, Yang H, et al: Changes in methionine adenosyltransferase and S-adenosylmethionine homeostasis in alcoholic rat liver. Am J Physiol Gastrointest Liver Physiol 2000;729:G178–G185.
20 Kalhan SC: Protein metabolism in pregnancy. Am J Clin Nutr 2000;71:1249S–1255S.
21 Friesen RW, Novak EM, Hasman D, Innis SM: Relationship of dimethylglycine, choline, and betaine with oxoproline in plasma of pregnant women and their newborn infants. J Nutr 2007;137:2641–2646.
22 Molloy AM, Mills JL, Cox C, et al: Choline and homocysteine interrelations in umbilical cord and maternal plasma at delivery. Am J Clin Nutr 2005;82:836–842.
23 Molloy AM, Mills JL, McPartlin J, et al: Maternal and fetal plasma homocysteine concentrations at birth: the influence of folate, vitamin B_{12}, and the 5,10-methylenetetrahydrofolate reductase 677C→T variant. Am J Obstet Gynecol 2002;186:499–503.
24 Sturman JA, Gaull G, Raiha NCR: Absence of cystathionase in human fetal liver: is cystine essential? Science 1970;169:74–76.
25 Gaull G, Sturman JA, Raiha NCR: Development of mammalian sulfur metabolism: absence of cystathionase in human fetal tissues. Pediatr Res 1972;6:538–547.
26 Levonen A-L, Lapatto R, Saksela M, Raivio KO: Human cystathionine γ-lase: developmental and in vitro expression of two isoforms. Biochem J 2000;347:291–295.
27 Parimi PS, Cripe-Mamie C, Kalhan SC: Metabolic responses to protein restriction during pregnancy in rat and translation initiation factors in the mother and fetus. Pediatr Res 2004;56:423–431.
28 Kalhan SC, Parimi PS, Hanson RW: Impact of dietary protein restriction on one carbon metabolism in the rat. Pediatric Academic Societies Annual Meeting, 2006.
29 Utzschneider KM, Kahn SE: The role of insulin resistance in nonalcoholic fatty liver disease. J Clin Endocrinol Metab 2006;91:4753–4761.
30 Donnelly KL, Smith CI, Schwarzenberg SJ, et al: Sources of fatty acids stored in liver and secreted via lipoproteins in patients with nonalcoholic fatty liver disease. J Clin Invest 2005;115:1343–1351.
31 Jacobs RL, House JD, Brosnan ME, Brosnan JT: Effects of streptozotocin-induced diabetes and of insulin treatment of homocysteine metabolism in the rat. Diabetes 1998;47:1967–1970.
32 Ratnam S, Wijekoon EP, Hall B, et al: Effects of diabetes and insulin on betaine-homocysteine S-methyltransferase expression in rat liver. Am J Physiol Endocrinol Metab 2006;290:E933–E939.
33 Wijekoon EP, Hall B, Ratnam S, et al: Homocysteine metabolism in ZDF (type 2) diabetic rats. Diabetes 2005;54:3245–3251.
34 Abu-Lebdeh HS, Barazzoni R, Meek SE, et al: Effects of insulin deprivation and treatment on homocysteine metabolism in people with type 1 diabetes. J Clin Endocrinol Metab 2006;91:3344–3348.

35 Tessari P, Coracina A, Kiwanuka E, et al: Effects of insulin on methionine and homocysteine kinetics in type 2 diabetes with nephropathy. Diabetes 2005;54:2968–2976.
36 Tessari P, Kiwanuka E, Coracina A, et al: Insulin in methionine and homocysteine kinetics in healthy humans: plasma vs. intracellular models. Am J Physiol Endocrinol Metab 2005;288:E1270–E1276.
37 Meigs JB, Jacques PF, Selhub J, et al: Fasting plasma homocysteine levels in the insulin resistance syndrome. The Framingham Offspring Study. Diabetes Care 2001;24:1403–1410.
38 Mosharov E, Cranford MR, Banerjee R: The quantitatively important relationship between homocysteine metabolism and glutathione synthesis by the transsulfuration pathway and its regulation by redox changes. Biochemistry 2000;39:13005–13011.
39 Vance DE, Li Z, Jacobs RL: Hepatic phosphatidylethanolamine N-methyltransferase, unexpected roles in animal biochemistry and physiology. J Biol Chem 2007;282:33237–33241.

Discussion

Dr. Bohles: I would like you to speculate on two extremes. On one hand, what is the implication of a soy diet, soy protein being basically free of methionine? And, on the other hand, the other extreme, if homocysteinuria patients are treated with betaine they get tremendously high methionine concentrations as a result of the remethylation, and this is a constant phenomenon. What is the intellectual basis of handling these two extreme situations?

Dr. Kalhan: All soy formulas for infants are supplemented with methionine; it is a regulatory requirement; so you will not see a methionine-deficient state in babies. I would imagine that you will not want to eat protein alone without added methionine. In India they always eat dhal with bread and native American Indians mix corn with another source of protein. Soy protein by itself is an incomplete protein without methionine, it requires an additional source of methionine. I am not sure where exactly you are leading with this question because I don't think there is anybody on exclusively soy protein diet.

Dr. Bohles: My question refers to the constant effect on epigenetic phenomenon, like methylation, and possibly it is better viewed from the point of betaine therapy for homocysteinuria.

Dr. Kalhan: I will come back to homocysteinuria later. The source of methyl carbon is important for the maintenance of all these methyl reactions and there are some pilot data to suggest that if the source of methyl carbons is decreased in the diet, the methylation pattern of the genome can change. What are the implications of this in relation to the expression of physiological functions; to my knowledge this has not been studied and obviously needs to be examined in carefully done experiments. Yes, there is no question about it, we do need a constant source of methyl carbons in our diet and that is why, for example, when an animal is put on a choline betaine-deficient diet, it develops fatty liver disease and the whole phenomenon related to it. My impression is that, in vulnerable patients with homocysteinuria, when they are treated with betaine i.e. source of methyl groups, there is a tremendous transient increase in methionine which then gradually falls and returns to more reasonable levels. I have never managed a patient with homocysteinuria, so I can't tell you more than that.

Dr. Lafeber: Since we are both neonatologists, it would be interesting for us to speculate whether it is possible to create an intervention in order to influence this methylation process. For instance, if we observe the process of intrauterine growth retardation which occurred during the last trimester of gestation in the so-called Dutch hunger winter in Holland in 1944–1945, it is a process that is very similar to that observed in preterm infants at the neonatal intensive care unit. If we try to treat these infants optimally with oral and parenteral feeding, we still observe a growth deficit at the time of corrected term gestational age. At this time their weight is usually about 1 SD below that of normal term infants. We can then make our intervention by giving them a special diet. I just finished a study in which these preterm infants were provided with extra protein, but no extra calories. After 6 months we found that they were less fat and had lower insulin sensitivity [1]. We hope that this extra protein diet contributes to less metabolic syndrome in these preterm infants. Could you speculate on the total amount of protein and the quality of amino acids around the term age in preterm infants? I am sure you cannot say much about which specific amino acid is most important, although you have performed a trial similar to ours [2, 3] adding taurine or glutamine, for instance.

Dr. Kalhan: This is a very complex question. In spite of our best efforts, across the world when premature babies of less than 28–29 weeks gestation leave the neonatal intensive care units, their weight for the chronological gestation age is 1 or 2 SD below the fetal growth curve. The question whether this is permanent or can be reversed has always arisen. What Dr. Lafeber is referring to is that by changing the protein diet of these babies he has seen some remarkable changes at 6 and 8 months. Is this a reversable phenomenon? Time will tell. Actually we don't even know how these premature babies do in adulthood; this is a new population, it is a new cohort. There is some evidence to suggest that low birthweight babies have metabolic syndrome as adults, but remember the low birthweight babies are not the premature babies we are talking about right now. Low birthweight babies in the Delhi cohort or Dr. Yajnik's cohort are a very different population from the population we have in the west. The question of intervention is obviously very important. As was recently discussed at a meeting recently, the organism changes tremendously at birth, from fetus to newborn. It is probably the most dramatic event in life; the baby has to start breathing, has to maintain temperature, all sorts of things have to occur. But now we are feeding these babies for 15–16 weeks with all kinds of nutrients and we don't know the implications of doing these things. We know quite a bit, but still we don't know a whole lot about it. Have we destined this person to staying permanently small, we don't know that yet, and we are just about to start studying these phenomena. As Dr. Whitelaw, I also want to give caution that collecting DNA and measuring on the lymphocytes is not going to work when we talk about epigenetics or this permanent change in methylation. These are going to be tissue-specific changes and we will have to do studies on the tissues and not collect DNA in the cord blood lymphocytes. That is the best answer I can give today it is a rapidly evolving field.

Dr. Agarwal: Some 20 years back we started doing studies on the brain and neurotransmitters. The methionine-deficient diet showed a dissociation. Normally on a protein-deficient diet, it is the 9th to the 10th generation that ends up with a reduced brain size, but with the methionine diet it happens in the first generation. Therefore methionine is very important and this dissociation is something which could just be carried on.

Dr. Kalhan: I also want to point out that protein restriction is not the only one associated with methionine metabolism. Another commonly used model which has a human counterpart is hypoxia. The Chinese people who move up to Tibet or Peru have low birthweight babies, and it will take generations before that will change because they are recent migrants to the Tibetan altitude. Some beautiful studies have been done. The first generations have small babies compared to the local inhabitant Tibetans who have what we call the normal growth curve for that, which is very comparable to our population.

Dr. Agarwal: Latent iron deficiency without hypoxia reduces the size of the baby and changes the brain and neurotransmitters irreversibly; latent iron deficiency, not hypoxia.

Dr. Kalhan: Yes, hypoxia has been demonstrated to be associated with changes in methylation patterns in the fetus, in the brain and liver. Lane et al. [4] did those studies. There is also evidence without intervention. Iron deficiency also causes growth retardation, not severe iron deficiency, just restricting iron and there is probably a lot of those which ultimately have a common denominator to programming.

References

1   Amesz E, Schaafsma A, Lafeber HN: Similar growth but altered body composition in preterm infants fed enriched 'postdischarge' formula without extra calories, standard formula or human milk, from term until 6 months corrected age. J Pediatr Gastroenterol Nutr 2009, in press.
2   van den Berg A, van Elburg RM, Teerlink T, et al: A randomized controlled trial of enteral glutamine supplementation in very low birth weight infants: plasma amino acid concentrations. J Pediatr Gastroenterol Nutr 2005;41:66–71.
3   Kalhan SC, Parimi PS, Gruca LL, Hanson RW: Glutamine supplement with parenteral nutrition decreases whole body proteolysis in low birth weight infants. J Pediatr 2005;146:642–647.
4   Lane RH, Ramirez RJ, Tsirka AE, et al: Uteroplacental insufficiency lowers the threshold towards hypoxia-induced cerebral apoptosis in growth-retarded fetal rats. Brain Res 2001;895:186–193.

Kalhan SC, Prentice AM, Yajnik CS (eds): Emerging Societies – Coexistence of Childhood Malnutrition
and Obesity.
Nestlé Nutr Inst Workshop Ser Pediatr Program, vol 63, pp 135–150,
Nestec Ltd., Vevey/S. Karger AG, Basel, © 2009.

Adiposity and Comorbidities: Favorable Impact of Caloric Restriction

Eric Ravussin, Leanne M. Redman

Pennington Biomedical Research Center, Baton Rouge, LA, USA

Abstract

The focus here is on research involving long-term calorie restriction (CR) to prevent or delay the incidence of the metabolic syndrome with age. The current societal
environment is marked by overabundant accessibility of food coupled with a strong
trend to reduced physical activity, both leading to the development of a constellation of disorders including central obesity, insulin resistance, dyslipidemia and hypertension (metabolic syndrome). Prolonged CR has been shown to extend median and
maximal lifespan in a variety of lower species (yeast, worms, fish, rats, and mice).
Mechanisms of this lifespan extension by CR are not fully elucidated, but possibly
involve alterations in energy metabolism, oxidative damage, insulin sensitivity, and
functional changes in neuroendocrine systems. Ongoing studies of CR in humans now
makes it possible to identify changes in 'biomarkers of aging' to unravel some of the
mechanisms of its anti-aging phenomenon. Analyses from controlled human trials
involving long-term CR will allow investigators to link observed alterations from body
composition down to changes in molecular pathways and gene expression, with their
possible effects on the metabolic syndrome and aging.

Introduction

Anti-aging research by modern scientists continues to echo the quest of
the Spanish explorer Ponce de Leon, who searched for the 'Fountain of Youth'
on the shores of Florida in the early 1500s. Humans are no longer satisfied
with simply living longer; they want increased quality of life and prolonged
health during their senior years. Basic and clinical research is therefore conducted to understand the physiological and molecular mechanisms of aging
with the intent to postpone and possibly alleviate many of the illnesses associated with the aging process.

Ironically, as researchers aim to unravel the mysteries of delaying the biological aging process, the current societal environment is marked by overabundant accessibility of food coupled with a strong trend to reduced physical activity. As obesity rates have risen to over 30% among Americans [1], so have the prevalence of obesity-related chronic diseases such as diabetes mellitus, heart disease and stroke. This alarming increase in obesity is further coupled with a lower age at onset for the emergence of obesity-related comorbidities. It is now understood that obesity may cause up to 300,000 deaths per year in the USA [2]. Alarmingly, it now seems that babies born at the beginning of the 21st century will have shorter life expectancies than their parents [3].

Before the development of frank obesity, cardiovascular disease (CVD) and diabetes, individuals develop a constellation of disorders including central obesity, insulin resistance, dyslipidemia and hypertension, often termed the metabolic syndrome. Individuals with three or more of these key disorders have a 2–3 times greater risk of dying or being struck by heart attack or stroke and a 3–5 times greater risk of developing diabetes mellitus [4, 5]. It is estimated that worldwide 1 in 3 or 4 adults has the metabolic syndrome [6]. The first line of treatment is to adopt a healthy lifestyle [5]. However, the large individual variability in response to diet and exercise represents a huge challenge in clinical practice. A better understanding of the genetic and environmental influences in the physiopathology of the metabolic syndrome could ultimately deliver a customized treatment to those individuals who do not respond to intensive lifestyle changes and some medications.

Etiology of Obesity

Weight gain results from a sustained imbalance between energy intake and energy expenditure favoring positive energy balance. However, this simple statement belies the complex, multifactorial nature of obesity and the numerous biological and behavioral factors that can affect both sides of the energy balance equation. Figure 1a shows the major paths involved in obesity grouped according to behavioral, metabolic, and biological influences. These pathways and factors have been reviewed elsewhere [7, 8]. Figure 1b summarizes the major factors and the central integrators controlling energy balance.

Longitudinal studies of the same individuals over time have indicated that relative to body size, low metabolic rate, high respiratory quotient, insulin sensitivity, low sympathetic nervous system activity and low plasma leptin concentrations predict weight gain over time [9]. Upon gaining weight, the original 'abnormal' metabolic state becomes 'normalized'. Such 'normalization' with weight gain explains why cross-sectional studies have not led to the identification of metabolic risk factors for obesity. Weight gain thus causes an increase in metabolic rate, a decrease in respiratory quotient, a decrease in insulin sensitivity, an increase in sympathetic nervous activity and an increase

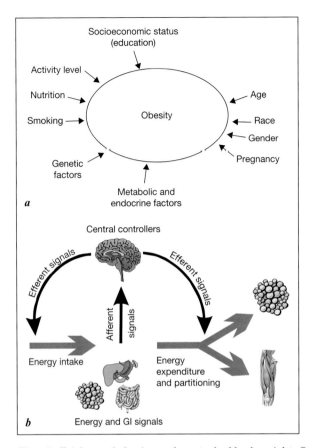

Fig. 1. Etiology of obesity and control of bodyweight. Several factors are known to predispose an individual to obesity (***a***), these include: behavioral factors (activity level, nutrition, smoking status, socioeconomic status); metabolic factors (physiological, metabolic, endocrine factors), and biological factors (genetic, racial, gender, age, pregnancy status). Bodyweight is regulated by an intricate balance between energy intake and energy expenditure (***b***). The figure depicts a negative feedback model for the regulation of bodyweight. Peripheral signals from energy stores (adipose tissue, muscle, and liver) as well as hormonal and gastrointestinal signals provide information to the central controllers in the brain, indicating the state of the external and internal environment as they relate to food, metabolic rates, and activity behavior. The central controllers in turn integrate all the information and transduce messages into efferent signals governing the behavioral search for the acquisition of food as well as modulating its subsequent deposition into energy storage compartments such as adipose tissue, liver, and muscle by modulating energy expenditure.

in plasma leptin concentrations, all of which serve to counteract further weight gain. Therefore it is not surprising that weight loss plateaus after a few months of therapy.

Aging and Obesity

Aging is associated with increased risk of metabolic disorders including overweight, obesity, insulin resistance, type 2 diabetes, atherosclerosis and cancer. Cross-sectional and longitudinal studies suggest that over-consumption of energy-dense foods and lack of physical activity are the leading causes of weight gain, obesity and the related health issues [10]. Recently researchers have learned that while increased adipose tissue per se is a health concern, the storage and distribution of fat within the body also has important implications for health. In particular, adipose tissues stored centrally in the visceral compartment of the abdomen and in non-adipose tissues, such as liver, heart, pancreas and skeletal muscle, are considered to be metabolic abnormalities that precede the development of impaired glucose tolerance, hyperlipidemia and insulin resistance. As individuals age, body weight even if maintained, is composed of increased fat mass, decreased fat-free mass [11] and increased ectopic fat stores in the abdominal visceral compartment [12], the liver and the skeletal muscle [13] associated with an increased incidence and prevalence of glucose intolerance and diabetes in older persons [14, 15]. It therefore seems that the link between aging and chronic disease may be inevitable in our current obesogenic environment. Interventions therefore that can attenuate the age-associated changes in body composition could delay (even prevent) the onset of metabolic disturbances of aging and result in extended lifespan.

Caloric Restriction and Lifespan

Since the 1930s calorie restriction (CR) has been shown by McCay et al. [16] to retard the aging process, extending the median and maximal lifespan in various models [17]. While the exact mechanisms through which CR is able to extend the lifespan have yet to be fully elucidated, CR reduces metabolic rate and oxidative damage, improves markers of age-related diseases including diabetes such as insulin resistance, and has been shown to alter neuroendocrine activities in animals [18] (fig. 2). Results from studies on rhesus monkeys suggest that prolonged CR can also oppose many age-associated pathophysiological changes including learning and behavior changes, body temperature, plasma insulin concentrations and resting energy expenditure. Since many changes associated with prolonged CR are important to the health and survival of humans, and excessive caloric intake is associated

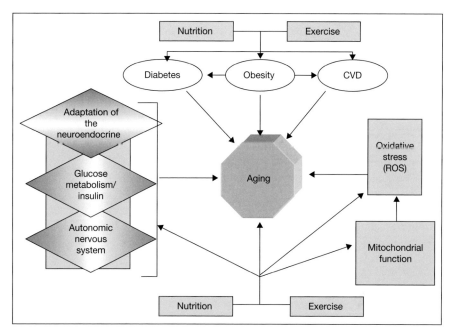

Fig. 2. Impact of calorie restriction (CR) on factors related to aging. Non-mutually exclusive candidate mechanisms of CR include: improved mitochondrial function; decreased oxidative damage due to reduced ROS generation and increased ROS removal; altered neuroendocrine function including growth axis, thyroid axis, hypothalamic pituitary axis, autonomic nervous system, and carbohydrate metabolism; decreased incidence of chronic diseases such as obesity, diabetes and cardiovascular disease, and delayed onset of aging-related markers (i.e. glucose, insulin, DHEAS, and body temperature).

with morbidity and the development of chronic diseases, it has become an important research objective to assess the feasibility, safety and efficiency of prolonged CR in well-controlled human trials.

CR May Alter the 'Rate of Living' and 'Oxidative Stress'

The aging process may be influenced by energy restriction through a reduction in the metabolic 'rate of living' [19], leading ultimately to reduced oxidative damage (fig. 2). An ongoing controversy among investigators appears to be whether chronic CR leads to 'metabolic adaptation', a reduction in the metabolic rate which is out of proportion to the diminished metabolic mass of the organism [18]. Results from rats and monkeys suggest that most of the collected data should be reevaluated using appropriate methods of normalizing the metabolic rate for changes in metabolic size [20]. For example, Blanc et al. [21] recently calculated a 13% reduction in resting energy expenditure after adjusting for fat-free mass in an 11-year-long study of energy-restricted monkeys. Recently, however, Selman et al. [22], using doubly labeled water to measure total energy expenditure, reported that calorie-restricted rats expended 30–50% more energy than expected.

The 'free radical theory of aging' or 'oxidative stress' hypotheses are well-supported theories of aging. It is widely accepted that the metabolic rate of an organism is a major factor in the rate of aging, and is inversely related to its lifespan [23]. Additionally, since 1–3% of consumed oxygen is associated with the production of reactive oxygen species (ROS), namely superoxide ($O_2^{\bullet-}$), hydrogen peroxide (H_2O_2), and the hydroxyl ion ($OH^{\bullet}$) [24], the production of these highly reactive molecules from normal aerobic metabolism is also in direct proportion to an organism's metabolic rate. Many investigators have shown that modulation of the oxidative stress of an organism through prolonged CR is able to retard the aging process in various species, including mammals [25, 26]. As a result of increased oxygen consumption, aerobic exercise is associated with increased production of ROS in muscle tissues [27]. However, exercise training boosts up the antioxidant capacity of skeletal muscle probably resulting in decreased overall oxidative stress [28].

CR, CVD, Insulin Resistance, Type 2 Diabetes Mellitus

Elevated levels of oxidized LDL, excessive ROS generation, hypertension and diabetes are all potential causes for the development of endothelial dysfunction, a precipitating event in the progression of atherosclerosis. These factors are believed to initiate an inflammatory response in the injured endothelial tissue. Long-term CR is associated with sustained reductions in factors related to endothelial dysfunction in humans, such as decreased blood pressure [29], reduced levels of total plasma cholesterol and triglycerides [30], and reduced markers of inflammation such as C-reactive protein, interleukin-6 and plasminogen activator inhibitor type-1 [31–33]. A recent long-term CR study in humans supports the feasibility of using CR as a protective effect against atherosclerosis by showing a 40% reduction in carotid artery intima-media thickness in CR participants relative to a control group [34].

Strong evidence shows that long-term energy restriction in lean and obese subjects improves insulin sensitivity, a mechanism by which CR may act to extend lifespan [30, 35]. Additionally, prolonged CR reduces fasting glucose and insulin concentrations, two factors believed to contribute to the aging process due to protein glycation [36] and mitogenic action [37], respectively. This compelling evidence suggests that weight loss due to CR may be the most effective means of improving insulin sensitivity, thereby decreasing the risk of the development of diabetes mellitus.

What Is Known from Humans?

Probably the most intriguing epidemiological evidence supporting the role of CR in lifespan extension in humans comes from the Okinawans [38]. Compared to most industrialized countries, Okinawa, Japan, has 4–5 times the average number of centenarians with an estimated 50 in every 100,000 people [39]. What is interesting about this population is that a low caloric intake was reported in schoolchildren on the island more than 40 years ago and later studies confirmed a 20% CR in adults residing on Okinawa compared to mainland Japan [40]. However the diets were typically rich in green leafy vegetables, soy and some fish providing adequate amounts of nutrients, essential vitamins and minerals [41].

To our knowledge there is only one other study that tested the effects of CR without malnutrition in non-obese humans [42]. This was a study of alternate day feeding in 60 male participants (1,500 kcal/day; 35% CR vs. controls) for 3 years, whereas the other 60 were ad libitum. While the initial report was brief, post-hoc analyses conducted several years later [43] indicated that the death rate tended to be lower in the CR group and hospital admissions were reduced in these individuals by approximately 50%.

The unexpected low availability of food during the 2-year Biosphere 2 experiment provided a unique opportunity to observe the effects of CR in non-obese humans. Eight individuals were completely isolated within this 3.15-acre 'mini-world' (ecological laboratory), where 100% of the air and water was recycled and all food was grown inside [44]. Due to unforeseen problems with agriculture early on, food supply was much lower than expected going rapidly from a projected ~2,500 to ~750 kcal/day during the first 6 months. The resulting $17 \pm 5\%$ weight loss was associated with many physiological, hematological, biochemical and metabolic alterations [44, 45] consistent with calorie-restricted primates including reductions in insulin, core temperature and metabolic rate. Furthermore CVD risk factors were improved, such as reductions in systolic/diastolic blood pressure and a 30% lowering of cholesterol [30].

Randomized Controlled Trials of Prolonged CR in Humans

As for randomized controlled trials, results from a 2-year study of CR in humans is only a few years away since the recruitment of volunteers began in March 2007. The National Institute on Aging (NIA) is sponsoring a trial called CALERIE (Comprehensive Assessment of the Long-term Effect of Reducing Intake of Energy) which for the first time is scientifically testing (randomized trial) the effects of 25% CR in ~150 non-obese (BMI 22–28) healthy men and women aged 25–45 years compared to 75 matched volunteers. Three clinical sites are involved in the trial: Washington University in St. Louis, Mo.; Tufts University in Boston, Mass., and Pennington Biomedical Research Center in Baton Rouge, La.

The Phase 1 CALERIE study conducted at Pennington involved 46 men and women randomized to 1 of 4 treatment groups for 6 months. For the CR group, the level of restriction imposed was a 25% reduction from the daily energy requirement for weight maintenance [46]. The other groups were: (1) CR plus exercise group where the calorie deficit was also set at 25% from weight maintenance with half (12.5%) achieved by CR and half (12.5%) by increased energy expenditure via structured aerobic exercise; (2) a low calorie diet group where participants consumed 890 kcal/day to achieve a 15% weight loss and thereafter followed a weight maintenance diet, and (3) a healthy diet control group that followed a weight-maintaining diet based on the American Heart Association Diet, Step 1.

Six months of CR induced favorable outcomes in terms of physiological, hormonal and biochemical parameters. The 12 participants assigned to this treatment group completed the study and reported no development of eating disorder symptoms [47] or reductions in quality of life indices [48]. After 6 months of 25% CR, the group lost 10.4 ± 0.9% of their body mass attributed to both a loss in fat mass (CR –24 ± 3%) and fat-free mass (CR –4 ± 1%). Central adiposity was reduced by 27% in both visceral (women –24 ± 4%, men –32 ± 6%) and subcutaneous fat depots (women –25 ± 2%, men –28 ± 7%). Interestingly the distribution of whole body fat, specifically within the abdomen was not altered by CR [49]. Abdominal fat cell size was reduced by ~20% and the deposition of lipid in the liver was lowered by ~37% but no change was noted in the lipid content within skeletal muscle [50]. Importantly the reduction in weight, visceral fat and abdominal fat cell size was associated with a 40% improvement in insulin sensitivity and reduced acute insulin response to glucose [50].

We also observed favorable changes in the lipoprotein profile. Triacyl-glycerol was reduced by 21%, HDL cholesterol increased by 9%, and factor VIIc reduced by 10%. No changes were observed in fibrinogen, homocysteine or endothelial function. Based on combined changes in lipid and blood pressure values, the estimated 10-year CVD risk declined by 29% in the CR group but as expected remained unchanged in the control group. Based on combined favorable changes in lipid and blood pressure levels, CR favorably reduces the risk of CVD [51].

With regard to longevity, 2 of 3 biomarkers of longevity [52] were improved in the CR group after 6 months [46]. Specifically, we observed significant reductions in both fasting insulin and core body temperature. Interestingly, in parallel with the decrease in core temperature, we observed a metabolic adaptation – lowering of metabolic rate larger than expected on the basis of weight loss – associated with reduced DNA damage probably due to lower production of ROS [46]. These findings of course echo results previously reported in nonhuman primates and rodents on CR and long-lived men in the Baltimore Longitudinal Study of Aging [52]. Importantly, CR was associated with an increase in the muscle expression of genes involved in mitochondrial biogenesis and mitochondrial fusion including PGC1-α, mitochondrial transcription factor A, endothelial nitric oxide, SIRT1 and PSARL [53]. In parallel, mitochondrial content increased by $35 \pm 5\%$ in the CR group with no change in the control group ($2 \pm 2\%$). However, the activity of key mitochondrial enzyme of the TCA cycle (citrate synthase), β-oxidation (β-HAD) and electron transport chain (COX II) were all unchanged. This suggests that 6 months of CR in non-obese humans was sufficient to improve biomarkers of aging and supports the theory that energy expenditure is reduced beyond expectation. Whether the observed metabolic adaptation translates into long-term overall reduced oxidative damage remains to be determined. The increased mitochondrial content in parallel with a decrease in DNA damage is, however, an important indication that CR improves mitochondrial function in skeletal muscle, a factor which may decrease cellular senescence.

Taken together the preliminary findings from the Phase I of CALERIE indicate promising benefits of CR for 6–12 months on body composition whereby total fat mass, visceral fat and ectopic fat stores are reduced. These body composition changes are associated with improvements in plasma lipids and reductions in cardiovascular and type 2 diabetes risk. Due to the pluripotent nature of energy restriction, the exact mechanisms by which CR extends lifespan are still being investigated, and will likely remain a challenge. However, controlled human trials such as the multicenter CALERIE study, are transforming this challenging investigation into a modern scientific reality.

Could CR Increase Longevity in Humans?

The wealth of CR literature in rodents, however, allows us to address some important questions relating to the practicality and feasibility of CR in humans. Relevant and practical questions are: (1) how much CR do we need to improve age-related health and possibly longevity, and (2) how long do we need to sustain CR in order to obtain these benefits? Analysis of 24 published studies of CR in mice or rats indicated a strong negative relationship between survival and energy intake [54] with more CR (up to 55%) associated with longer maximal lifespan.

The rodent data indicate that CR has greater benefits when more extreme and sustained over a longer period of time. Using the prediction equations derived from the rodent data above, we and others estimated that a 5-year life extension could be induced by 20% CR starting at age 25 and sustained for another 52 years, i.e. the life expectancy of a male in the US. However, if a 30% CR was initiated at age 55 for the next 22 years, the gain would only be 2 months.

Certainly there are individuals who self-impose CR with the CRON (Calorie Restriction with Optimal Nutrition) diet for health and longevity. A group of 18 CRONIES (only 3 women) have recently been studied after 3–15 years of CR [34]. Dietary analysis indicated an energy intake ~50% less than age-matched controls. In terms of body composition, the mean BMI of the males was 19.6 ± 1.9 with an extremely low percent body fat of ~7%. Atherosclerosis risk factors including total cholesterol, LDL cholesterol, HDL cholesterol and triglycerides fell within the 50th percentile of values for people in their age group. This report provides further evidence that longer term CR is highly effective in lowering the risk of developing coronary heart disease and other age-related comorbidities [34]. It remains to be seen if the CRONIES live longer than their age- and sex-matched counterparts.

Conclusion

The enormous public health burden resulting from obesity and its related morbidities compel researchers to challenge some of the existing classical clinical interventions. Despite recent pharmacological advances, development of insulin sensitizers, antihypertensive and hypolipidemic drugs the clinician has limited options to offer to the obese patient in terms of safe and efficacious alternative therapies. Intensive changes in lifestyle seem to benefit very few individuals suffering from obesity and its comorbidities. Only intensive public health messages, population-wide lifestyle interventions and major remodeling of our obesogenic environment may start to reverse the increasing incidence of common disorders such as obesity, CVD and diabetes.

Facing an 'obesogenic' environment, it seems very unlikely that a public health message be launched towards reducing the amount of ingested calories. Understanding the mechanisms leading to retarded senescence at the molecular and physiological levels is therefore important for the successful development of CR mimetics. Such natural compounds or botanical extracts would mimic the effect of CR without depriving people of their usual energy intake. Biotechnology and pharmaceutical companies are eager to search for small molecules mimicking the effect of CR and representing the 'Fountain of Youth'.

References

1 Flegal KM, Carroll MD, Ogden CL, Johnson CL: Prevalence and trends in obesity among US adults, 1999–2000. JAMA 2002;288:1723–1727.
2 Allison DB, Fontaine KR, Manson JE, et al: Annual deaths attributable to obesity in the United States. JAMA 1999;282:1530–1538.
3 Olshansky SJ, Passaro DJ, Hershow RC, et al: A potential decline in life expectancy in the United States in the 21st century. N Engl J Med 2005;352:1138–1145.
4 Grundy SM, Cleeman JI, Daniels SR, et al: Diagnosis and management of the metabolic syndrome. An American Heart Association/National Heart, Lung, and Blood Institute Scientific Statement. Executive summary. Cardiol Rev 2005;13:322–327.

5 Lorenzo C, Williams K, Hunt KJ, Haffner SM: The National Cholesterol Education Program – Adult Treatment Panel III, International Diabetes Federation, and World Health Organization definitions of the metabolic syndrome as predictors of incident cardiovascular disease and diabetes. Diabetes Care 2007;30:8–13.

6 Nieman DC, Brock DW, Butterworth D, et al: Reducing diet and/or exercise training decreases the lipid and lipoprotein risk factors of moderately obese women. J Am Coll Nutr 2002;21:344–350.

7 Ravussin E, Swinburn BA: Metabolic predictors of obesity: cross-sectional versus longitudinal data. Int J Obes Relat Metab Disord 1993;17(suppl 3):S28–S42.

8 Rosenbaum M, Leibel RL, Hirsch J: Obesity. N Engl J Med 1997;337:396–407.

9 Ravussin E, Bogardus C: A brief overview of human energy metabolism and its relationship to essential obesity. Am J Clin Nutr 1992;55(suppl):242S–245S.

10 Calle EE, Teras LR, Thun MJ: Adiposity and physical activity as predictors of mortality. N Engl J Med 2005;352:1381–1384.

11 Zamboni M, Zoico E, Scartezzini T, et al: Body composition changes in stable-weight elderly subjects: the effect of sex. Aging Clin Exp Res 2003;15:321–327.

12 Stanforth PR, Jackson AS, Green JS, et al: Generalized abdominal visceral fat prediction models for black and white adults aged 17–65 y: the HERITAGE Family Study. Int J Obes Relat Metab Disord 2004;28:925–932.

13 Cree MG, Newcomer BR, Katsanos CS, et al: Intramuscular and liver triglycerides are increased in the elderly. J Clin Endocrinol Metab 2004;89:3864–3871.

14 Folsom AR, Kushi LH, Anderson KE, et al: Associations of general and abdominal obesity with multiple health outcomes in older women: the Iowa Women's Health Study. Arch Intern Med 2000;160:2117–2128.

15 Reaven GM: Banting lecture 1988. Role of insulin resistance in human disease. Diabetes 1988;37:1595–1607.

16 McCay CM, Crowell MF, Maynard LA: The effect of retarded growth upon the length of life span and upon the ultimate body size. 1935. Nutrition 1989;5:155–172.

17 Walford RL, Harris SB, Weindruch R: Dietary restriction and aging: historical phases, mechanisms and current directions. J Nutr 1987;117:1650–1654.

18 Heilbronn LK, Ravussin E: Calorie restriction and aging: review of the literature and implications for studies in humans. Am J Clin Nutr 2003;78:361–369.

19 Sacher GA, Duffy PH: Genetic relation of life span to metabolic rate for inbred mouse strains and their hybrids. Fed Proc 1979;38:184–188.

20 Ravussin E, Bogardus C: Relationship of genetics, age, and physical fitness to daily energy expenditure and fuel utilization. Am J Clin Nutr 1989;49(suppl):968–975.

21 Blanc S, Schoeller D, Kemnitz J, et al: Energy expenditure of rhesus monkeys subjected to 11 years of dietary restriction. J Clin Endocrinol Metab 2003;88:16–23.

22 Selman C, Phillips T, Staib JL, et al: Energy expenditure of calorically restricted rats is higher than predicted from their altered body composition. Mech Ageing Dev 2005;126:783–793.

23 Sohal RS, Allen RG: Relationship between metabolic rate, free radicals, differentiation and aging: a unified theory. Basic Life Sci 1985;35:75–104.

24 Alexeyev MF, Ledoux SP, Wilson GL: Mitochondrial DNA and aging. Clin Sci (Lond) 2004;107:355–364.

25 Weindruch R, Walford RL, Fligiel S, Guthrie D: The retardation of aging in mice by dietary restriction: longevity, cancer, immunity and lifetime energy intake. J Nutr 1986;116:641–654.

26 Sohal RS, Weindruch R: Oxidative stress, caloric restriction, and aging. Science 1996;273:59–63.

27 Fulle S, Protasi F, Di Tano G, et al: The contribution of reactive oxygen species to sarcopenia and muscle ageing. Exp Gerontol 2004;39:17–24.

28 Sachdev S, Davies KJ: Production, detection, and adaptive responses to free radicals in exercise. Free Radic Biol Med 2008;44:215–223.

29 Velthuis-te Wierik EJ, van den Berg H, Schaafsma G, et al: Energy restriction, a useful intervention to retard human ageing? Results of a feasibility study. Eur J Clin Nutr 1994;48:138–148.

30 Walford RL, Mock D, Verdery R, MacCallum T: Calorie restriction in biosphere 2:alterations in physiologic, hematologic, hormonal, and biochemical parameters in humans restricted for a 2-year period. J Gerontol A Biol Sci Med Sci 2002;57:B211–B224.

31 Heilbronn LK, Noakes M, Clifton PM: Energy restriction and weight loss on very-low-fat diets reduce C-reactive protein concentrations in obese, healthy women. Arterioscler Thromb Vasc Biol 2001;21:968–970.

32 Bastard JP, Jardel C, Bruckert E, et al: Elevated levels of interleukin 6 are reduced in serum and subcutaneous adipose tissue of obese women after weight loss. J Clin Endocrinol Metab 2000;85:3338–3342.

33 Mavri A, Alessi MC, Bastelica D, et al: Subcutaneous abdominal, but not femoral fat expression of plasminogen activator inhibitor-1 (PAI-1) is related to plasma PAI-1 levels and insulin resistance and decreases after weight loss. Diabetologia 2001;44:2025–2031.

34 Fontana L, Meyer TE, Klein S, Holloszy JO: Long-term calorie restriction is highly effective in reducing the risk for atherosclerosis in humans. Proc Natl Acad Sci USA 2004;101:6659–6663.

35 Walford RL, Mock D, MacCallum T, Laseter JL: Physiologic changes in humans subjected to severe, selective calorie restriction for two years in biosphere 2: health, aging, and toxicological perspectives. Toxicol Sci 1999;52(suppl):61–65.

36 Robertson RP: Chronic oxidative stress as a central mechanism for glucose toxicity in pancreatic islet beta cells in diabetes. J Biol Chem 2004;279:42351–42354.

37 Stenkula KG, Said L, Karlsson M, et al: Expression of a mutant IRS inhibits metabolic and mitogenic signalling of insulin in human adipocytes. Mol Cell Endocrinol 2004;221:1–8.

38 Kagawa Y: Impact of Westernization on the nutrition of Japanese: changes in physique, cancer, longevity and centenarians. Prev Med 1978;7:205–217.

39 Japan Ministry of Health Law: Journal of Health and Welfare Statistics. Tokyo, Health and Welfare Statistics Association, 2005.

40 Suzuki M, Wilcox BJ, Wilcox CD: Implications from and for food cultures for cardiovascular disease: longevity. Asia Pac J Clin Nutr 2001;10:165–171.

41 Willcox DC, Willcox BJ, Todoriki H, et al: Caloric restriction and human longevity: what can we learn from the Okinawans? Biogerontology 2006;7:173–177.

42 Vallejo EA: Hunger diet on alternate days in the nutrition of the aged (in Spanish). Prensa Med Argent 1957;44:119–120.

43 Stunkard AJ: Nutrition, longevity and obesity; in Rockstein M, Sussman ML (eds): Nutrition, Aging and Obesity. New York, Academic Press, 1976, pp 253–284.

44 Walford RL, Harris SB, Gunion MW: The calorically restricted low-fat nutrient-dense diet in Biosphere 2 significantly lowers blood glucose, total leukocyte count, cholesterol, and blood pressure in humans. Proc Natl Acad Sci USA 1992;89:11533–11537.

45 Weyer C, Walford RL, Harper IT, et al: Energy metabolism after 2 y of energy restriction: the biosphere 2 experiment. Am J Clin Nutr 2000;72:946–953.

46 Heilbronn LK, de Jonge L, Frisard MI, et al: Effect of 6-month calorie restriction on biomarkers of longevity, metabolic adaptation, and oxidative stress in overweight individuals: a randomized controlled trial. JAMA 2006;295:1539–1548.

47 Williamson DA, Martin CK, Anton SD, et al: Is caloric restriction associated with development of eating disorder syndrome? Results from the CALERIE trial. Health Psychol 2008;27(suppl):S32–S42.

48 Martin CK, Anton SD, Han H, et al: Examination of cognitive function during six-months calorie restriction: results of a randomized controlled trial. Rejuvenation Res 2007;10:179–189.

49 Redman LM, Heilbronn LK, Martin CK, et al: Effect of calorie restriction with or without exercise on body composition and fat distribution. J Clin Endocrinol Metab 2007;92:865–872.

50 Larson-Meyer DE, Heilbronn LK, Redman LM, et al: Effect of calorie restriction with or without exercise on insulin sensitivity, beta-cell function, fat cell size, and ectopic lipid in overweight subjects. Diabetes Care 2006;29:1337–1344.

51 Lefevre M, Redman LM, Heilbronn LK, et al: Caloric restriction alone and with exercise improves CVD risk in healthy non-obese individuals. Atherosclerosis 2008 July 3 (Epub ahead of print).

52 Roth GS, Lane MA, Ingram DK, et al: Biomarkers of caloric restriction may predict longevity in humans. Science 2002;297:811.

53 Civitarese AE, Carling S, Heilbronn LK, et al: Calorie restriction increases muscle mitochondrial biogenesis in healthy humans. PLoS Med 2007;4:e76.

54 Merry BJ: Calorie restriction and age-related oxidative stress. Ann NY Acad Sci 2000;908:180–198.

Discussion

Dr. M. Chatterjee: You have talked much about caloric restriction. What role do bioflavanoids play, especially the very colorful ones, prunes, colored cabbages and berries?

Dr. Ravussin: Nutrition companies have a real interest in what is called calorie restriction mimetics. In other words if you know the mechanisms of how calorie restriction expands lifespan, you can mimic this by giving blueberries as a natural way. It is true that the redder and bluer the fruits the more resveratrol and flavonoids they have, and the better for life extension. We don't know enough about what the mechanisms are. In studies on resveratrol in rats, for example, it was the equivalent of about 16 liters of wine a day. If you extrapolate that to humans it probably would not be very good for health. But yes, nutrition companies do have an interest, and I am sure Nestlé is in the business of calorie restriction mimetics.

Dr. Prentice: I was very interested in both your survival plots for the rats and your final statement when you had recalculated the advantage of 30% caloric restriction on your own potential lifespan. It did seem from those initial survival curves that actually the differential mortality was happening very early and that they were probably parallel after about 700 days or so in the rats, and that would presumably tie in with the calculation when you said you could only get the 2 months advantage. So the question in terms of this conference is: would you care to speculate much further back in earlier life as to what we could achieve by modulating feeding patterns? I am rather confused by some of Barker's data at the moment which sometimes gives evidence that a high weight at 1 year is beneficial and other times it is the reverse.

Dr. Ravussin: That is a very good point. As I said, the earlier the better. You are absolutely right, in all the survival curves there is a gap very early, and then it does not increase very much anymore. One thing we have to be absolutely clear about is that people, who call themselves CRONies (Caloric Restriction Optimal Nutrition) and practice caloric restriction, are very well educated, they know nutrition, have no deficiency in any micronutrients, and know exactly what they are eating. I think there is a lot to be learned from these people, some of whom started very young, but of course what is the control group and what is the effect? There is no reason to doubt that caloric restriction with optimal nutrition can really expand lifespan by decreasing what is called secondary aging, which is basically chronic diseases of aging, obesity, diabetes, cardiovascular disease, and also by decreasing primary aging, which is at the cellular level, why do we have senescence in the cells. I think it would be very interesting to learn more about the mechanism of primary aging.

Dr. Ajayi: Due to the appreciation evolving regarding the understanding of nutritional science, I think we need to begin looking at the normal standards that have been set for BMI and caloric intake. It seems obvious from these results that we needn't eat as much as we do, so caloric intake could be less, and if we select our food very well, we will still benefit. So perhaps we need now to review the BMI standards and caloric intakes set for every age group. Particularly after puberty, we need to look strictly at these and then begin to make some fresh recommendations for the populations.

Dr. Ravussin: Should there be a potential reappraisal of these BMI curves versus mortality? Looking at these curves, it is always a J curve, and there are people with a low BMI of around 18 like the CRONies. There is a lot of confusion about this J curve with regard to smoking: should smoking be deleted and so on. Again I would not speculate on the mortality curve, which of course is very likely to be different in different populations. In Pima Indians, for example, there is no way that the best BMI for them is 22.5 or 23, because it is really a higher BMI which is good for Pima

Indians, and in India it is also true that this BMI and the mortality curve may be displaced.

Dr. Klassen: I have a question related to the exercise part. In your very early slides you showed that running already had a small effect, but it seems that, with additional exercise, caloric restriction does not make an impact. I was wondering if you could elaborate on the extent of physical activity? Would for example a triathlon runner or marathon runner experience an inverse effect, i.e. would you expect them to produce more ROS and thus can there be a limit to the benefit of exercise?

Dr. Ravussin: There is a lot of controversy about oxidative stress and exercise. At the mitochondrial level about 1–2% of the oxygen escapes ATP production and therefore produces ROS. But on the other hand we know that exercisers have better defense; the antioxidants are upregulated. Of course we know that epidemiologically exercisers are more likely to live longer, at least the average lifespan. But once again in all the studies, the paradox is that the maximum lifespan is not extended by exercise. Exercisers have a lot of lipid in their muscle but they are not insulin-resistant. There are a few paradoxes with exercise.

Dr. Haschke: What would happen if you apply the same caloric restriction (15%) to people with a BMI of >30 without metabolic syndrome. What would be the effect of exercise? Probably these studies have been done.

Dr. Ravussin: There are a lot of weight loss studies in obese people, and we know the results of these studies. People can drop their weight, there is no problem with that, but the maintenance of that weight 5 years after stopping the active intervention is less than 5%. I don't know about those without metabolic syndrome. It has been claimed that it doesn't matter how fat you are, as long as you are metabolically fit. I have a hard time with the dissection of those epidemiological data because there are very few people who are fat and fit. I think the benefit would be much less in people who do not have the metabolic syndrome than in people who have the metabolic syndrome.

Dr. Haschke: In your phase 2 study, are you looking at test parameters that are indicative for cognitive function?

Dr. Ravussin: I teamed up with a psychologist and in phase 1 we made a lot of cognitive measurements and there was no detrimental effect. But this was too short. Now over 2 years, the concerns are bone health, immune function, and also cognitive function. What has been done, and this has not been published but I am aware of the data, is a comparison with basically calorie-restricted CRONies versus marathon runners who have the same BMI, 19–20, or very close. One group, the marathon runners, had a high energy flux, and the other group had very little, and no difference was found in cognitive function. That is all that I can say.

Dr. Popkin: The issue of resveratrol raises the question of how we can extrapolate from animal studies to human studies and this is very complex. We do not find effects in humans, so one has to be very careful on all these anti-aging issues because all the work has been done on animals, and when we pull it forward it gets very complex in humans. Although I love red wine I would not want to oversell it. I do not think we can replicate your research in infants. Can you see a way that we can go after Dr. Prentice's question, because you are talking about a well-balanced diet plus caloric restriction and I don't think under any human circumstances we will ever be able to find that. All the Barker and fetal origins studies do not replicate those two combinations.

Dr. Ravussin: The first point is well taken, except that there are no randomized clinical trials with resveratrol, they are all epidemiology. The secondly, and I kind of escaped Dr. Prentice's question, at the fetal age once again all the nutrients and proteins are needed for the development of this fetus. I think first of all, these are not experiments which are going to be done. I don't know the answer.

Dr. Haschke: There are data in infants showing that feeding influences the metabolic outcome from the first day of life. It has clearly been shown that the differences between breastfed infants and infants fed formulas with a high protein content are that they have much lower insulin secretion. We have much less data on growth hormone and IGF1; so there is something from early life onwards. I am not saying that this can be extrapolated clinically. It is not caloric restriction, but it is protein restriction to a certain extent. Growth of the breastfed infant is very much modulated by the protein content. We consider this healthy growth, but growth can be accelerated in an infant if more protein is given.

Dr. Giovannini: About caloric restriction, do we mean a low carbohydrate intake or a low fat intake, or does a low protein intake play a role? A European project is assessing the correlation between obesity and protein intake in the first year of life.

Dr. Ravussin: That is a good question. These people were interested in longevity and tested all that in rodents, and it is mostly the calories which count. Of course if protein intake is too low then there is a problem, but it doesn't make any difference if it is carbohydrate or fat. The alternate-day fast in rodents is very interesting. When a rat is starved and given food ad libitum every other day for a long time, there is no difference in weight but there are all the advantages of caloric restriction. There is a lot of interest in that now. There are some mechanisms that we don't understand: cells are needed, a stressor is needed, and is that an alternative stress or just eating less calories? We don't know.

Dr. Arora: As prolonged caloric restriction may not be possible, what is the impact of intermittent caloric restriction? Are there some studies on that?

Dr. Ravussin: There are no studies in humans. I am embarking on a study of people with impaired glucose intolerance. Every other day they are put on 25% of the energy requirement, and then we look at insulin sensitivity. All that with the hope that we could have an intervention which is basically easier than caloric restriction, because it is tough to start counting all your calories and this kind of thing.

Dr. Ganapathy: Since the discussion is about red wine I thought why not touch upon probiotics. There was a beautiful article in *Nature* [1] in which two sets of mice, obese and thin, were compared. It was found that there definitely is a difference in the gut flora constitution, more saccharolytic and less proteolytic in the thin rats, and it was the other way round in the obese rats. The second thing that I want to talk about is the accelerator hypothesis of caloric restriction in diabetes, that type 1 and type 2 belong to the same spectrum but different ends, that if as a child you are exposed to a high caloric diet and you develop insulin resistance very early in life, it upregulates your pancreas and makes it more prone to an immune response. There are a lot of studies being done on that by Wilkin [2]. The last thing that I want to talk about is about sleep. A good night's sleep just makes you save about 120 cal.

Dr. Ravussin: Let me start with the last one. First of all we did not measure the duration of sleep in our subjects. This was when the subjects were in a chamber, in an artificial environment. In phase 2 we have a questionnaire about sleep. Now your second point is about malnutrition and b-cell growth or immune resistance? We simply do not have the answers.

Dr. Ganapathy: No, the upregulation of the islet cells secondary to increased calorie exposure and hyperinsulinism. This is a new hypothesis that has come from Barker, now it is the accelerator hypothesis. We were talking about longevity and aging, but I am more interested in the probiotic part.

Dr. Ravussin: I am aware of some data in South Africa on malnutrition and basically decreased b-cell mass, but I am not familiar with the data that you are talking about.

Dr. Whitelaw: I was interested in your significant change in the DNA damage. Do you want to talk more about comet assay and what you think it means? Also was that done on blood or what tissues?

Dr. Ravussin: It was done on mononucleated blood cells. We looked at this because a reviewer asked whether it is the same if we take CD8 versus CD4, etc., and we had exactly the same answer on whole blood DNA versus sorting the T cells. There are two assays, one which is basically an electrical field and the DNA migrates. The more damage there is the more DNA is left behind and it makes a comet. For a positive control the DNA is then also treated with hydrogen peroxide, and then mostly the comet remains but there is no nucleus anymore.

Dr. Whitelaw: So chromatin might be involved in contributing to those kinds of assays, I am not sure if anybody has look at that. Telomeres come to mind if you have got damaged DNA and aging effects. So I wonder if your telomeres are getting shorter or longer?

Dr. Ravussin: That is a very interesting question because one of the theories of aging is also shortening of the telomeres and therefore more potential mutations at these genes towards the end of the chromosome. First of all if you take epidemiological data and with age you have a reduction in telomere length. I am now doing a study comparing some less mitotic tissue, like skeletal muscle versus blood cell or sperm, and it seems that the length of the telomere at birth is very variable between people. If mitotic tissue is normal, the birth telomere length is normal, and then after a turnover of skin cells or mononucleotide blood cells, and attrition can be seen, the difference being the attrition. If you have the misfortune of being born with short telomeres and have a very rapid rate of attrition, it will be the worst scenario. But this is one of these 25–100 theories of aging, and I don't know if anyone has ever put everything together.

References

1 Turnbaugh PJ, Ley RE, Mahowald MA, et al: An obesity-associated gut microbiome with increased capacity for energy harvest. Nature 2006;444:1027–1031.
2 Wilkin TJ: Diabetes: 1 and 2, or one and the same? Progress with the accelerator hypothesis. Pediatr Diabetes 2008;9:23–32.

Kalhan SC, Prentice AM, Yajnik CS (eds): Emerging Societies – Coexistence of Childhood Malnutrition and Obesity.
Nestlé Nutr Inst Workshop Ser Pediatr Program, vol 63, pp 151–162,
Nestec Ltd., Vevey/S. Karger AG, Basel, © 2009.

Obesity, Inflammation, and Macrophages

Vidya Subramanian[a], Anthony W. Ferrante, Jr.[a,b]

[a]Department of Medicine and [b]Naomi Berrie Diabetes Center, Columbia University, New York, NY, USA

Abstract

The World Health Organization estimates that since 1980 the prevalence of obesity has increased more than threefold throughout much of the world, and this increase is not limited to developed nations. Indeed, the incidence of obesity is increasing most rapidly among rapidly industrializing countries raising the specter of a burgeoning epidemic in obesity-associated diseases, including diabetes, dyslipidemia, nonalcoholic fatty liver disease and atherosclerosis. Reducing the rates of obesity and its attendant complications will require both coordinated public health policy and a better understanding of the pathophysiology of obesity. Obesity is associated with low grade chronic inflammation, a common feature of many complications of obesity that appears to emanate in part from adipose tissue. In obese individuals and rodents adipose tissue macrophage accumulation is a critical component in the development of obesity-induced inflammation. The macrophages in adipose tissue are bone marrow-derived and their number is strongly correlated with bodyweight, body mass index and total body fat. The recruited macrophages in adipose tissue express high levels of inflammatory factors that contribute to systemic inflammation and insulin resistance. Interventions aimed at either reducing macrophage numbers or decreasing their inflammatory characteristics improves insulin sensitivity and decreases inflammation. Macrophage accumulation and adipose tissue inflammation are dynamic processes under the control of multiple mechanisms. Investigating the role of macrophages in adipose tissue biology and the mechanisms involved in their recruitment and activation in obesity will provide useful insights for developing therapeutic approaches to treating obesity-induced complications.

Introduction

Obesity is caused by a chronic imbalance between caloric intake and energy expenditure, leading to the storage of excess calories as body fat. The incidence of obesity has dramatically increased worldwide in the last quarter century. Once considered a disease of the affluent countries, obesity is now on the rise in developing nations. The World Health Organization estimates that approximately 1.6 billion adults worldwide are overweight and about 400 million adults are obese [1, 2]. This increased prevalence has translated to a disturbing increase in the incidence of obesity-related diseases and an associated increase in morbidity and mortality. Obesity contributes significantly to the development of insulin resistance and type 2 diabetes mellitus, dyslipidemia, atherosclerosis, hypertension, osteoarthritis, non-alcoholic fatty liver disease, and certain forms of cancer [2]. The increase in prevalence of obesity is not restricted to adults, but is increasing rapidly among children and adolescents as well [3]. Worldwide, approximately 20 million children are overweight [1]. This increased prevalence of obesity has lead to a disturbing rate of obesity-associated complications in children that predicts future morbidity not seen in previous generations [3]. If the challenge of obesity is unmet by the scientific and clinical community, the human and economic toll on the world will continue to grow exponentially.

Obesity-Induced Inflammation

Over that last dozen years, research has revealed that a chronic state of low-grade systemic inflammation is a common feature of obesity and that this inflammatory state mechanistically links obesity to many of its complications [4]. Originally recognized as the response to invading pathogens, inflammation is now broadly recognized as the complex biological response to noxious stimuli such as infectious agents, damaged cells or foreign bodies. Inflammation can either be acute or chronic in nature [5]. Acute inflammation is a short-term response, usually lasting a few days, in which the body rapidly removes the eliciting stimulus. Chronic inflammation occurs when there is no resolution and the stimulus is not removed. Classically, acute inflammation is characterized by swelling, redness, heat, and pain at the site of the insult [5]. Most acute inflammatory responses are characterized by resolution, which is critical for repair, regeneration and ultimately survival of the organism. Acute inflammation that does not resolve can either escalate to a lethal state typified by sepsis or can develop into a chronic state. While the signs and symptoms of acute inflammation are often apparent, the effects of chronic inflammation are often, at least initially, more subtle. However, with time the effects of chronic inflammation are often manifested with deterioration of one or more specific tissues or systems. Obesity induces a state of chronic low-grade inflammation as measured by activation of inflammatory signaling pathways, production of increased cytokines and alterations in immune cell function.

Epidemiological and clinical studies, some dating from the 1960s, revealed an association of inflammatory markers, e.g. circulating concentration of fibronectin, with both obesity and diabetes. In the mid-1990s Hotamisligil et al. [6] observed that adipose tissue expression of tumor necrosis factor-α (TNF-α), the prototypical inflammatory cytokine, is increased by obesity and argued it to be responsible for obesity-induced diabetes in some rodent models. They showed that the expression and secretion of the classic inflammatory cytokine TNF-α from adipose tissue was significantly increased in rodent models of obesity [6]. In some studies, neutralizing TNF-α in obese mice with antibodies improved insulin sensitivity [7]. In humans, a similar correlation of TNF-α expression with adiposity was observed, although attempts to improve insulin sensitivity by neutralizing TNF-α have not been successful [8, 9]. Nonetheless, these initial studies of TNF-α revealed that the production of an inflammatory molecule can play a significant role in the development of obesity-induced complications. Since this initial observation, many studies have shown that obesity increases adipose tissue expression and secretion of other inflammatory markers including, interleukin-6 (IL-6), C-reactive protein (CRP), resistin, monocyte chemoattractant protein-1 (MCP-1), and plasminogen activator inhibitor-1 (PAI-1) [4]. Studies in animal models demonstrated that genetic deletion of individual inflammatory factors can modestly improve insulin sensitivity in mice on a high fat diet suggesting a role for inflammation in the development of obesity-induced insulin resistance. Furthermore, an increased concentration of circulating proinflammatory proteins, e.g. IL-6, predicts the development of insulin resistance, type 2 diabetes, and cardiovascular disease in humans. That no single inflammatory factor fully explains the inflammatory changes associated with obesity suggests that there is a complex interplay between multiple pathways and systems.

Adipose Tissue Macrophages

Hotamisligil et al. [6] originally postulated that adipose tissue production of TNF-α and other inflammatory molecules is derived from adipocytes. However, adipose tissue is a heterogeneous organ that in addition to adipocytes contains pre-adipocytes, fibroblasts, endothelial cells, and immune cells including macrophages and lymphocytes. Fain et al. [10, 11] separated adipose tissue into adipocytes and non-adipocyte populations and found that while adipocytes express some of the inflammatory cytokines induced by obesity, the majority of these cytokines are derived from the stromal vascular fraction. This observation was initially puzzling and some suggested an artifact of isolation and in vitro culture. However, two recent reports demonstrated that in obesity, adipose tissue is infiltrated by macrophages and that these cells indeed express a substantial portion of inflammatory factors that are linked to obesity-related complications [12, 13].

Macrophages belong to the mononuclear phagocyte system and are derived largely from circulating monocytes. Macrophages are present in most tissues

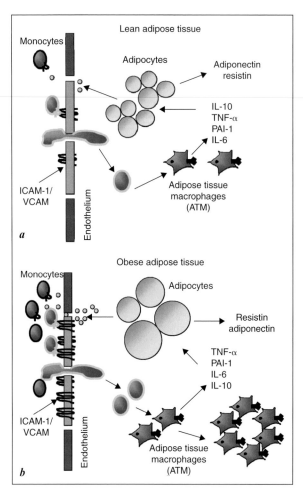

Fig. 1. Adipose tissue macrophages in obesity-induced inflammation. *a* In lean
animals the macrophage content is low in adipose tissue. These macrophages express
low amounts of inflammatory factors including tumor necrosis factor-α(TNF-α),
interleukin-6 (IL-6), and plasminogen activator inhibitor-1 (PAI-1) and high levels
of anti-inflammatory factors including interleukin-10 (IL-10). *b* Obesity increases
monocyte adhesion and recruitment to adipose tissue, consequently increasing
macrophage number in adipose tissue. The macrophages in obese adipose tissue
express increased amounts of inflammatory factors including TNF-α, IL-6, and PAI-1
and decreased amounts of IL-10. The inflammatory molecules act locally in a paracrine
fashion to alter adipocyte function and adipokine production.

and have distinct phenotypes and functions specific to their local microenvironment. They are the primary effectors of the innate immune system, and therefore, form a first line of defense against foreign pathogens. Resident tissue macrophages also are critical for maintaining normal tissue function by clearing apoptotic and dead cells and cellular debris especially following tissue injuries [5], and in response to injury play a central role in coordinating the reparative response.

Studies of adipose tissue macrophages (ATMs) in both humans and rodents demonstrate that increases in adiposity are closely associated with increases in the macrophage content of adipose tissue. Consistent with ATMs being authentic macrophages, bone marrow transplant studies in rodents demonstrate that almost all of the macrophages in adipose tissue are bone marrow-derived and are dependent upon the key regulator of macrophage differentiation and development, macrophage colony-stimulating factor (M-CSF or CSF-1) [12].

In obesity, the initial instigator of adipose tissue inflammation is not clear. Data suggest that dying cells, hypoxia and excess local concentrations of free fatty acids can contribute to the inflammatory signal that attract and sustain ATMs. However, once initiated it is clear that ATMs play a critical role in the inflammatory response seen in obesity. In humans and rodents, the number of macrophages in fat depots correlates positively with adipocyte size, body mass index, and percent body fat [12]. In obese mice [12] and severely obese individuals [14], visceral adipose tissue, which is strongly correlated with the development of insulin resistance and metabolic syndrome, contains higher numbers of macrophages than subcutaneous adipose tissue. The higher macrophage content of visceral adipose tissue depots is also reflected in the high expression of inflammatory molecules from these depots compared to subcutaneous ones. Defining the mechanisms that lead to differences in ATM content between visceral and subcutaneous depots will likely provide insights into the functional differences between these depots.

Recruitment of Monocytes to Adipose Tissue

The recruitment of bone marrow-derived circulating monocytes to tissues is a complex process under the control of numerous chemokines, cytokines, and other local factors [15]. Under homeostatic conditions peripheral monocytes cross the endothelium into the tissue and replenish any loss of resident macrophages, thus maintaining the resident tissue macrophage populations. However, the presence of local inflammation causes activation of endothelial cells and production of chemoattractant proteins. A necessary step in the accumulation of macrophages is the adhesion of circulating monocytes to activated endothelial cells and transmigration into the tissue. Cytokines like TNF-α secreted from adipose tissue are capable of activating endothelial cells.

In obesity, adipose tissue expression of adhesion molecules including inter-cellular adhesion molecule-1 (ICAM-1) and vascular cell adhesion molecule-1 (VCAM-1) is increased [12]. However, there are conflicting data as to the met-abolic effects of ICAM-1 deficiency [16, 17]. An initial analysis of macrophage content in the adipose tissue of ICAM-1-deficient mice did not reveal a sig-nificant effect. Further studies are therefore required to identify the adhesion molecules critical for recruitment of monocytes to adipose tissue in obesity.

Chemokines are a large, structurally related family of proteins that regu-late immune cell trafficking and activation. Profiling of adipose tissue expres-sion has revealed that obesity increases expression of MCPs, members of the C-C chemokine ligand family. MCP-1 (CCL2) is the prototypical MCP and its expression is increased in obesity. Studies in mice have demonstrated that overexpression of MCP-1 within adipocytes induces macrophage accumula-tion and inflammation in adipose tissue, and reduces insulin sensitivity [18, 19]. There are conflicting data as to whether a genetic deficiency of MCP-1 is sufficient to reduce macrophage accumulation in adipose tissue and improve glucose homeostasis in obese rodents [19, 20]. This may in part be due to the redundancy of ligands that can bind a key MCP-1 receptor, C-C chemokine receptor 2 (CCR2). Obesity increases adipose tissue expression of MCP-1, MCP-3, MCP-5, all of which bind the CCR2. Genetic deletion or pharmacologi-cal antagonism of CCR2 reduces macrophage accumulation in adipose tissue of high fat fed mice by ~30%. This reduction is accompanied by decreased adi-pose tissue inflammation, increased systemic insulin sensitivity, and reduced hepatic steatosis [21]. These studies suggest that MCPs through CCR2 are important for the recruitment of monocytes to adipose tissue and the devel-opment of obesity-induced inflammation and metabolic syndrome. However, CCR2 alone does not account for obesity-induced accumulation of ATMs.

Once recruited to the tissue, monocyte differentiation to macrophages is governed by local signals. CSF-1 is the primary regulator of macrophage differentiation, survival and proliferation. This is supported by the observa-tion that mice deficient in either CSF-1 (Csf1[op/op]) or the CSF-1 receptor have markedly reduced macrophage content in almost all tissues [22, 23]. Consistent with a role for CSF-1 in ATM function, adipose tissue from mice lacking CSF-1 has significantly reduced the number of macrophages com-pared to those from control mice [12].

The population of macrophages in adipose tissue is diverse. Broadly, macrophage populations in most tissues can be divided into resident and recruited macrophages. Resident macrophages are a stable population of cellular sentries that reside in tissue under non-pathological states. By con-trast, recruited macrophages hone to tissues in response to pathological or immunological stimuli [24]. The stable populations of resident macrophages in various tissues have distinct phenotypes and functions specific to the local microenvironment in the tissue. In the lean state resident macrophages in adipose tissue produce low levels of classic inflammatory molecules (alternately activated macrophages). In contrast, macrophages actively recruited to sites of injury or infection express high levels of inflammatory molecules [24]. The majority of macrophages in adipose tissue from obese individuals has a distinctly inflammatory character typical of classically activated macrophages, and thus, expresses high levels of inflammatory molecules, including TNF-α, MCP-1 and inducible nitric oxide synthase [12]. Alternative activation of macrophages is the typical response seen to some parasitic infections and important in the resolution of inflammation. Peroxisome proliferator-activated receptor-γ (PPAR-γ) is an important regulator of macrophage alternative activation, and deletion of PPAR-γ impairs alternative activation. In high fat diet-induced obesity, deletion of PPAR-γ specifically in myeloid cells increases adipose tissue inflammation and further impairs glucose homeostasis [25, 26].

Role of Macrophages in Metabolic Diseases

Adipose tissue inflammation and macrophage content are dynamic, regulated by weight changes and correlated with insulin resistance. Intervention studies aimed at either reducing macrophage numbers or manipulating their inflammatory state in murine models have improved insulin sensitivity and decreased overall adipose tissue inflammation. In humans, weight loss following gastric bypass is associated with a significant decrease in macrophage number in subcutaneous adipose tissue [27]. Concomitantly, there was also a significant decrease in circulating levels of proinflammatory factors. Thiazolidinediones are potent insulin-sensitizing compounds that also exhibit powerful anti-inflammatory effects [28]. Treating obese mice [13] and humans [29, 30] with thiazolidinediones reduces ATM content and improves insulin sensitivity.

Conclusion

Obesity is associated with a state of chronic low grade inflammation. Adipose tissue is an important source of systemic inflammation. The macrophage population within adipose tissue and their activation state are increased in obesity, contributing to the systemic low grade inflammation associated with weight gain. Furthermore, these immune cells have been implicated in the development of obesity-associated complications, including insulin resistance, cardiovascular disease and nonalcoholic fatty liver disease. However, there are still numerous questions that will likely be answered in the coming years as to the role of ATMs in systemic and local inflammation. The understanding of the interaction between immune cells and adipocytes is still incomplete. Understanding the role of immune cells in adipose tissue

Subramanian/Ferrante, Jr.

physiology, and the molecular signals needed and the kinetics of recruitment, survival, and activation of these cells in obesity will help identify new therapeutic candidates for treating obesity-related complications.

References

1 World Health Organization: The World Health Report 2002 – Reducing Risks, Promoting Healthy Life. Geneva, World Health Organization, 2002.
2 World Health Organization: Obesity and Overweight; in Fact Sheet No. 311. Geneva, World Health Organization, 2006.
3 Bibbins-Domingo K, Coxson P, Pletcher MJ, et al: Adolescent overweight and future adult coronary heart disease. N Engl J Med 2007;357:2371–2379.
4 Wellen KE, Hotamisligil GS: Inflammation, stress, and diabetes. J Clin Invest 2005;115:1111–1119.
5 Janeway CA, Walport M, Shlomchik M: Immunobiology, ed 6. New York, Garland, 2004.
6 Hotamisligil GS, Shargill NS, Spiegelman BM: Adipose expression of tumor necrosis factor-alpha: direct role in obesity-linked insulin resistance. Science 1993;259:87–91.
7 Hotamisligil GS, Spiegelman BM: Tumor necrosis factor alpha: a key component of the obesity-diabetes link. Diabetes 1994;43:1271–1278.
8 Ofei F, Hurel S, Newkirk J, et al: Effects of an engineered human anti-TNF-alpha antibody (CDP571) on insulin sensitivity and glycemic control in patients with NIDDM. Diabetes 1996;45:881–885.
9 Paquot N, Castillo MJ, Lefèbvre PJ, Scheen AJ: No increased insulin sensitivity after a single intravenous administration of a recombinant human tumor necrosis factor receptor: Fc fusion protein in obese insulin-resistant patients. J Clin Endocrinol Metab 2000;85:1316–1319.
10 Fain JN, Cheema PS, Bahouth SW, Lloyd Hiler M: Resistin release by human adipose tissue explants in primary culture. Biochem Biophys Res Commun 2003;300:674–678.
11 Fain JN, Madan AK, Hiler ML, et al: Comparison of the release of adipokines by adipose tissue, adipose tissue matrix, and adipocytes from visceral and subcutaneous abdominal adipose tissues of obese humans. Endocrinology 2004;145:2273–2282.
12 Weisberg S, McCann D, Desai M, et al: Obesity is associated with macrophage accumulation in adipose tissue. J Clin Invest 2003;112:1796–1808.
13 Xu H, Barnes GT, Yang Q, et al: Chronic inflammation in fat plays a crucial role in the development of obesity-related insulin resistance. J Clin Invest 2003;112:1821–1830.
14 Cancello R, Tordjman J, Poitou C, et al: Increased infiltration of macrophages in omental adipose tissue is associated with marked hepatic lesions in morbid human obesity. Diabetes 2006;55:1554–1561.
15 Charo IF, Ransohoff RM: The many roles of chemokines and chemokine receptors in inflammation. N Engl J Med 2006;354:610–621.
16 Dong ZM, Gutierrez-Ramos JC, Coxon A, et al: A new class of obesity genes encodes leukocyte adhesion receptors. Proc Natl Acad Sci USA 1997;94:7526–7530.
17 Gregoire FM, Zhang Q, Smith SJ, et al: Diet-induced obesity and hepatic gene expression alterations in C57BL/6J and ICAM-1-deficient mice. Am J Physiol Endocrinol Metab 2002;282:E703–E713.
18 Kamei N, Tobe K, Suzuki R, et al: Overexpression of monocyte chemoattractant protein-1 in adipose tissues causes macrophage recruitment and insulin resistance. J Biol Chem 2006;281:26602–26614.
19 Kanda H, Tateya S, Tamori Y, et al: MCP-1 contributes to macrophage infiltration into adipose tissue, insulin resistance, and hepatic steatosis in obesity. J Clin Invest 2006;116:1494–1505.
20 Inouye KE, Shi H, Howard JK, et al: Absence of CC chemokine ligand 2 does not limit obesity-associated infiltration of macrophages into adipose tissue. Diabetes 2007;56:2242–2250.
21 Weisberg SP, Hunter D, Huber R, et al: CCR2 modulates inflammatory and metabolic effects of high-fat feeding. J Clin Invest 2006;116:115–124.

158

22 Cecchini MG, Dominguez MG, Mocci S, et al: Role of colony stimulating factor-1 in the establishment and regulation of tissue macrophages during postnatal development of the mouse. Development 1994;120:1357–1372.
23 Dai XM, Ryan GR, Hapel AJ, et al: Targeted disruption of the mouse colony-stimulating factor 1 receptor gene results in osteopetrosis, mononuclear phagocyte deficiency, increased primitive progenitor cell frequencies, and reproductive defects. Blood 2002;99:111–120.
24 Gordon S: Alternative activation of macrophages. Nat Rev Immunol 2003;3:23–35.
25 Hevener AL, Olefsky JM, Reichart D, et al: Macrophage PPAR gamma is required for normal skeletal muscle and hepatic insulin sensitivity and full antidiabetic effects of thiazolidinediones. J Clin Invest 2007;117:1658–1669.
26 Odegaard JI, et al: Macrophage-specific PPARgamma controls alternative activation and improves insulin resistance. Nature 2007;447(7148):1116–1120.
27 Cancello R, Henegar C, Viguerie N, et al: Reduction of macrophage infiltration and chemoattractant gene expression changes in white adipose tissue of morbidly obese subjects after surgery-induced weight loss. Diabetes 2005;54:2277–2286.
28 Ricote M, Li AC, Willson TM, et al: The peroxisome proliferator-activated receptor-gamma is a negative regulator of macrophage activation. Nature 1998;391:79–82.
29 Di Gregorio GB, Yao-Borengasser A, Rasouli N, et al: Expression of CD68 and macrophage chemoattractant protein-1 genes in human adipose and muscle tissues: association with cytokine expression, insulin resistance, and reduction by pioglitazone. Diabetes 2005;54:2305–2313.
30 Mohanty P, Aljada A, Ghanim H, et al: Evidence for a potent antiinflammatory effect of rosiglitazone. J Clin Endocrinol Metab 2004;89:2728–2735.

Discussion

Dr. Chowdhury: What is the role of n-3 fatty acids in manipulating obesity-induced inflammation? In particular have you found in your laboratory or in any other report that it can reduce the hepatic expression of MCP-1?

Dr. Subramanian: Actually there is a lot of work on the type of fatty acids in n-3 versus n-6, saturated versus unsaturated. At least in in vitro models it seems that saturated fatty acids activate the macrophages and result in more proinflammatory states whereas n-3 fatty acids actually do not induce inflammation. So the type of fatty acid seems to play an important role in the extent of the inflammatory process. I don't know if anybody has actually measured MCP-1 in the liver, but I think MCP-1 automatically decreases as inflammation and macrophages decrease. So yes, the various types of fatty acids have different inflammatory effects. We have looked at the various fats in rodents: visceral, subcutaneous, and mesenteric fat which surrounds the intestine. So as I showed before, in all depots there is accumulation of macrophages and it correlates with the degree of adiposity or the adipocyte site, but there is a difference in absolute numbers of macrophages. So it seems in rodents that the perigonadal adipose tissue has more macrophages than subcutaneous. You are very right, the secretion of cytokines is completely different in the various adipose tissues. So there are differences in terms of accumulation. But all the macrophage depots that are accumulating are proinflammatory. In humans with weight loss, subcutaneous adipose tissue could actually be sampled and a decrease in macrophages and in the expression of the proinflammatory cytokines could be seen. But I don't think anybody has actually very clearly or very thoroughly dissected the different adipose tissues. We know that the adipose tissues are different so there are going to be differences in terms of accumulation of macrophages and the extent of inflammation just by the fact that is the depots are different, but the macrophages of all depots are inflammatory.

Dr. Mathur: What are your views on some papers available on incriminating infective etiology in triggering the inflammatory processes for obesity [1, 2]? In addition, How well does your hypothesis apply to the immune-compromised state of obesity?

Dr. Subramanian: Let me answer the second question first. In the immune-compromised state the processes are different. In obesity there is no immune compromise. The immune system is activated but it is fully functional and capable of mounting an immune response. It is very difficult to compare the inflammatory process in obesity to immunosuppressor or other states because in those conditions you have the complication that the immune system is actually not primed or cannot handle whatever the underlying disease condition is. Regarding your first question, I actually don't know the literature you are talking about in terms of viruses causing inflammatory processes. I am sure any infective agent can cause an inflammatory response, but in obesity we think that this whole process is triggered by the adipose tissue or the adipocytes that are expanding. I know that, at least in the last year, literature has been published on gut microflora and their role in obesity and inflammation. It is a very new topic, but for most part we think that this inflammatory process is not started by a pathogen but it is the response of the body to the expanding adipocytes.

Dr. Prentice: You suggested that the initial driver of this process is a metabolic perturbation without any detail to that, probably because we don't know about it. I just wanted to try the possibility that there could be a physical perturbation because adipose tissue obviously has to be perfused. There is a large growth of the capillary bed, I would imagine. Intuitively to me it seems that if there is a big mass of adipose tissue there may be problems in perfusing that bed. Is there any evidence as to whether that is part of the story or not?

Dr. Subramanian: Metabolic perturbation is again only part of the story. There is a hypothesis out there that the dimension, the expanding adipose tissue, is very hard to study because a lot of neovascularization is needed to get blood flow to this expanding adipose tissue, and hypoxia is another big factor in the recruitment of macrophages to adipose tissue. Actually there is some evidence showing that it is actually the inability of the fat cell to expand continuously to recruit these macrophages, and if you were able to just keep on expanding the fat cell you probably would not have this accumulation or some of the complications of obesity because the fat would be where it should be. So yes, in addition to metabolic factors the physical expansion of the adipocyte and hypoxia induced by it play a role in recruiting macrophages to the tissue.

Dr. Ganapathy: You just mentioned inflammatory markers and obesity. One of the mechanisms of macrophage activation is TNF-a endotoxin and macrophages have now been subdivided into three categories: one for TH1, one for TH2, and one for the immune complex. Could it be that the inflammatory markers themselves are activating the macrophage system, and have we done anything on the inducible NOS system because that could go a long way to control the inflammatory side effects of obesity?

Dr. Subramanian: The inflammatory cytokines actually do feed back and activate the macrophages and these macrophages that you see in obese adipose tissue are proinflammatory type 1, the TH1 response macrophages. About the iNOS, we see increases in iNOS expression in obese adipose tissue and I think that mice lacking iNOS are actually protected from obesity-induced macrophages as well as systemic insulin resistance. We haven't specifically looked at iNOS, but we are looking at all of the mixtures of these proinflammatory cytokines.

Dr. Ganapathy: You told us a little bit about the PPAR system. Could you add something more about PPAR and its role? Are you trying to produce drugs through the TNF-b receptors? You mentioned a slide about the PPAR ligand and it was also mentioned in the first talk about the inheritance and genetic basis for PPAR. Does it play a role?

Dr. Subramanian: I don't know about the genetic basis of PPAR, I definitely can't answer. But PPAR seems to play a role because knocking out the PPAR-g actually primes the macrophage to be more proinflammatory and these macrophages actually secrete more inflammatory proteins compared to wild-type macrophages that have PPAR-g, and this is also true for the other isoforms as well PPAR-d. So these PPARs seem to play a role in priming the macrophages or in controlling the activation of macrophages type 1 versus the TH2 macrophages. So at this point the data are very preliminary, but we think that the normal function of the PPARs at macrophages is to clamp down on the proinflammatory state.

Dr. Ganapathy: Could it also be possible that if there is a parasitic infection and macrophages of the TH2 type that this is an anti-inflammatory state, just as in inflammatory bowel disease? We have tried to use hepatocytes to get the TH2 changed since we are talking about inflammation.

Dr. Subramanian: I don't know about bowel disease but there is evidence showing that in obesity the resident macrophages in the adipose tissue are actually TH2, they are more anti-inflammatory. As weight is gained and macrophages are recruited, these macrophages are more TH1, so they are more proinflammatory.

Dr. Ravussin: You have shown the infiltration of macrophages in the adipose tissue and then in the liver. Systemic insulin resistance, in humans at least, as measured by clamp is in the muscle. Do you have data showing that there would be some infiltration by macrophages in the muscle, or is the increase in cytokines, TNF-a, IL-6 enough to explain the decrease in glucose disposal into the muscle?

Dr. Subramanian: With regard to the muscle, in obesity there is intramyocellular fat and there is macrophage accumulation in intramyocellular fat, but the role of those macrophages in muscle insulin resistance is really not known. It could be that those macrophages locally produce inflammatory cytokines that play a role in impairing myocyte, glucose uptake, and systemically it could be TNF, IL-6. So it could be both, macrophages in the fat within muscle as well as systemic inflammatory markers could both contribute to muscle insulin resistance.

Dr. Jaigirdar: You mentioned the CCR2 receptor protein. Is there any way, any drug or any physiological way to decrease it?

Dr. Subramanian: No, we really don't want to mess with immune systems without really understanding what is going on in obesity-induced inflammation. But there is a company in the US that has a small antagonist for CCR2 and I think they are looking at it in terms of using it in arthritis and multiple sclerosis. Actually I did not present the data but if the CCR2 antagonist is given to rodents, a fairly similar effect is seen; there is decreased macrophage accumulation in adipose tissue and increased insulin sensitivity. But to advocate the use of that drug in large scale human studies, more data and more research are needed to actually see what other systems are being perturbed by knocking out CCR2.

Dr. Jatana: Did you look at calorie restriction diets or increased activity in these rodents to decrease macrophages, or do we only need to reduce the amount of adipose tissue in order to reduce the macrophages?

Dr. Subramanian: The studies about caloric restriction are actually currently underway in the laboratory, and the results are actually not that clear-cut. In terms of physical activity I don't think we have looked at it. We have looked at physical activity in terms of a genetically obese model, the agouti and the obese strain, but I cannot recall the data in terms of macrophage accumulation and inflammation.

Dr. Arora: In severe malnutrition there is a lot of fat in the liver and there is no fat elsewhere. What is the inflammatory status in the fatty liver of the severely malnourished individual? Are there situations in which there is adipose tissue and obesity without evidence of ongoing inflammation? In other words I am asking whether inflammation triggers adiposity or adiposity triggers inflammation?

Dr. Subramanian: To answer your first question on malnutrition, fatty liver and inflammatory state; this is just a speculation I actually have no data or expertise in that area. The inflammation or the immune response in malnutrition is again slightly different from that in obesity because in malnutrition and undernutrition the immune system is immunocompromised, it is not able to function normally, while in obesity the functions are very normal. So the immune response or the inflammation in malnutrition and obesity may be completely different. To answer to your second question, we really don't know whether adiposity triggers macrophage accumulation or macrophage accumulation triggers adiposity.

Dr. Giovannini: Is the inflammatory process in obesity linked to the development of atherosclerosis?

Dr. Subramanian: There is some evidence in rodents but I cannot recall the exact data. Obesity-induced inflammation results in an inflammatory cascade in the endothelial cells which play a major role in atherosclerosis plaque formation, so we think that obesity-induced inflammation plays a major role in atherosclerosis, but I can't recall the exact data.

Dr. Jatana: Is there a difference between childhood obesity and age-onset obesity and the number of years a person was obese, and whether it was reversible? Are there any studies?

Dr. Subramanian: The accumulation of macrophages in adipose tissue was actually first reported in 2003 from our laboratory. There have not been a lot of studies looking at childhood obesity versus age-onset obesity and how much this reversal occurs during weight loss. These are studies that are probably ongoing right now, but there are no results so far.

References

1   Kalliomäki M, Collado MC, Salminen S, Isolauri E: Early differences in fecal microbiota composition in children may predict overweight. Am J Clin Nutr 2008;87:534–538.
2   Atkinson RL: Viruses as an etiology of obesity. Mayo Clin Proc 2007;82:1192–1198.

Kalhan SC, Prentice AM, Yajnik CS (eds): Emerging Societies – Coexistence of Childhood Malnutrition
and Obesity.
Nestlé Nutr Inst Workshop Ser Pediatr Program, vol 63, pp 163–176,
Nestec Ltd., Vevey/S. Karger AG, Basel, © 2009.

Obesity, Hepatic Metabolism and Disease

John M. Edmison, Satish C. Kalhan, Arthur J. McCullough

Department of Gastroenterology and Hepatology, Cleveland Clinic, Cleveland, OH, USA

Abstract

Nonalcoholic steatohepatitis (NASH), which is the most severe histological form of
nonalcoholic fatty liver disease, is emerging as the most common clinically important
form of liver disease in developed countries. Although its prevalence is 3% in the general population, this increases to 20–40% in obese patients. Since NASH is associated
with obesity, its prevalence has been predicted to increase along with the growing
epidemic of obesity and type 2 diabetes mellitus. The importance of this observation
comes from the fact that NASH is a progressive fibrotic disease in which cirrhosis
and liver-related death occur in 25 and 10% in these patients, respectively, over a
10-year period. This is of particular concern given the increasing recognition of NASH
in the developing world. Treatment consists of treating obesity and its comorbidities:
diabetes and hyperlipidemia. Nascent studies suggest that a number of pharmacological therapies may be effective, but all remain unproven at present. Histological and
laboratory improvement occurs with a 10% decrease in bodyweight. Bariatric surgery
is indicated in selected patients. A greater understanding of the pathophysiological
progression of NASH in obese patients must be obtained in order to develop more
focused and improved therapy.

Introduction

In the United States, over the last quarter century, there has been an obesity epidemic which has yet to plateau. Dietary modification and sedentary
lifestyle have been identified as key perpetuates. The prevalence of the metabolic (insulin resistance) syndrome and its sequelae (e.g. type 2 diabetes mellitus, cardiovascular disease, nonalcoholic fatty liver disease) have increased
in parallel fashion [1–3]. Similar trends are now being discovered worldwide
in populations which have undergone migration and urbanization. We are
just now beginning to realize the devastating effect these trends may have in
terms of future health risk.

Obesity

From 1960 to 2000 in the United States the prevalence of obesity (BMI ≥30) for adults aged 20–74 years has increased from 13.4 to 30.9% [4] (table 1). The prevalence of obesity was relatively constant from 1960 to 1980, then increased by 8.3% from 1980 to 1990 and 7.6% from 1990 to 2000. Likewise, the prevalence of overweight (BMI for age ≥95th percentile) among children in the United States increased in similar fashion from 1960 to 2000, culminating in a prevalence of 10% for 2- to 5-year-olds and 15% for 6- to 19-year-olds [5] (table 2).

Similar trends have been seen in migrant populations which are likely due to the adoption of 'Westernized' dietary and lifestyle habits. The prevalence of overweight Mexican-Americans increased 30.9–39.1% in men and 41.5–48.1% in women from approximately 1984 to 1990 [6]. A cross-sectional study in people of African origin showed a stepwise increase in the prevalence of obesity from Nigeria (5.4%) to Jamaica (23.2%) to the United States (39.0%), following the approximate path of migration [7]. Likewise, migrant Asian Indians tend to have higher BMI than those of urban- or rural-based sedentees in India [8]. Furthermore, Tokelauans who migrated to New Zealand because of a natural disaster increased their BMI levels from 24.1 to 28.7 between 1968 and 1982, while BMI levels in non-migrants only increased from 24.8 to 26.1 [9].

Urbanization of developing countries has shown trends in obesity similar to that of the United States. The prevalence of obesity from 1975 to 2003 among adult Brazilian men aged ≥20 years increased from 2.7 to 8.8%, and in Brazilian women it increased from 7.4 to 13%, reflecting a prevalence rate which almost doubled in both genders over a 28-year period [10]. Likewise, the prevalence of overweight and obesity increased 2.0–5.2% from 1992 to 2002 among Vietnamese adults, affecting urban residents more than their rural counterparts [11]. These trends hold true for adolescents as well as adults. The prevalence of overweight in young persons aged 6–18 years increased 4.1–13.9% in Brazil (from 1975 to 1997), 6.4–7.7% in China (from 1991 to 1997), and 15.4–25.6% in the United States (from 1974 to 1994) [12].

Using Western Criteria for Defining Obesity

Using Western criteria for defining obesity (BMI >30), less than 5% of South Asians and Asian Pacific populations will be defined as obese. However, obesity-related metabolic disorders occur at lower BMI levels in Asians. Data from South Asia, Singapore and Hong Kong demonstrate that in those native populations, the clustering of metabolic risk factors begins to increase at BMI of approximately 23. Therefore the recommended BMI cutoff values for

Table 1. Trends in age-adjusted and age-specific prevalence of obesity for adults aged 20–74 years, 1960–2000 [4]

Sex	Age years[1]	Prevalence, %					Change, % (95% CI)[2]	
		NHES 1960–1962 (n = 6,126)	NHANES I 1971–1974 (n = 12,911)	NHANES II 1976–1980 (n = 11,765)	NHANES III 1988–1994 (n = 14,468)	NHANES continuous 1999–2000 (n = 3,601)	NHANES II to NHANES III	NHANES III to NHANES 1999–2000
Both sexes	20–74	13.4	14.5	15.0	23.3	30.9	8.3 (6.6–10.0)	7.6 (4.2–11.0)
Men	20–74	10.7	12.1	12.7	20.6	27.7	7.9 (6.0–9.8)	7.1 (3.4–10.8)
	20–39	9.8	10.2	9.8	14.9	23.7	5.1 (2.9–7.2)	8.8 (4.8–12.8)
	40–59	12.6	14.7	15.4	25.4	28.8	10.0 (6.9–13.0)	3.4 (–2.8–9.6)
	60–74	8.4	10.5	13.5	23.8	35.8	10.3 (6.3–14.3)	12.0 (5.0–19.0)
Women	20–74	15.8	16.6	17.0	25.9	34.0	8.9 (6.5–11.3)	8.1 (3.7–12.5)
	20–39	9.3	11.2	12.3	20.6	28.4	8.3 (5.2–11.4)	7.8 (2.5–13.1)
	40–59	18.5	19.7	20.4	30.4	37.8	10.0 (6.1–13.9)	7.4 (0.5–14.3)
	60–74	26.2	23.4	21.3	28.6	39.6	7.3 (3.9–10.6)	11.0 (4.6–17.4)

NHES = National Health Examination Survey; NHANES = National l Health and Nutrition Examination Survey; CI = confidence interval.
[1] Estimated prevalences for ages 20–74 years were age-standardized by the direct method to the 2000 census population using age groups 20–39, 40–59 and 60–74 years.
[2] Overall and within each age-sex group, the changes between 1988–1994 and 1999–2000 are not significantly different from the changes between 1976–1980 and 1988–1994.

Table 2. Trends in overweight for children birth through 19 years by sex and age group [5]

Age		NHES 2 1963–1965	NHES 3 1966–1970	NHANES I 1971–1974	NHANES II 1976–1980	NHANES III 1988–1994	NHANES 1999–2000	p values NHANES III vs. NHANES 1999–2000
6–23 months[1]	Total					08.9 (0.7)	11.6 (1.9)	0.09
	Male					09.9 (0.8)	09.8 (2.2)	0.48
	Female					07.9 (1.0)	14.3 (3.5)	0.04
2–5 years[2]	Total			5.0 (0.6)	5.0 (0.6)	07.2 (0.7)	10.4 (1.7)	0.04
	Boys			5.0 (0.9)	4.7 (0.6)	06.1 (0.8)	09.9 (2.2)	0.06
	Girls			4.9 (0.8)	5.3 (1.0)	08.2 (1.1)	11.0 (2.5)	0.16
6–11 years[2]	Total	4.2 (0.4)		4.0 (0.5)	6.5 (0.6)	11.3 (1.0)	15.3 (1.7)	0.02
	Boys	4.0 (0.4)		4.3 (0.8)	6.6 (0.8)	11.6 (1.3)	16.0 (2.3)	0.05
	Girls	4.5 (0.6)		3.6 (0.6)	6.4 (1.0)	11.0 (1.4)	14.5 (2.5)	0.11
12–19 years[2]	Total		4.6 (0.3)	6.1 (0.6)	5.0 (0.5)	10.5 (0.9)	15.5 (1.2)	<0.001
	Adolescent boys		4.5 (0.4)	6.1 (0.8)	4.8 (0.5)	11.3 (1.3)	15.5 (1.6)	0.02
	Adolescent girls		4.7 (0.3)	6.2 (0.8)	5.3 (0.8)	09.7 (1.1)	15.5 (1.6)	0.002

Values are expressed as percentages with standard error in parentheses.
[1] Weight for length at the 95th percentile or higher is considered overweight.
[2] Body mass index for age at the 95th percentile or higher is considered overweight.

Table 3. Prevalence (%) of obesity in Asia using WHO criteria for Asians

Country	Men	Women
China	12	14
Japan	24	20
Malaysia	24	18
Philippines	13	15
Taiwan	18	16
Thailand	17	20

overweight for Asians are from 23–25 and for obesity more than 25, according to the new WHO guidelines.

Applying these new criteria, the prevalence of obesity in Asian populations is significant (table 3). There are also emerging data that the numbers will worsen with the increasing adoption of a Western lifestyle.

Metabolic (Insulin Resistance) Syndrome

Components of the metabolic syndrome include central obesity (waist circumference $\geq$102 cm in men, $\geq$88 cm in women), hypertriglyceridemia (serum triglycerides $\geq$150 mg•dl^{-1}), low HDL cholesterol (<40 mg•dl^{-1} in men, <50 mg•dl^{-1} in women), hypertension (blood pressure $\geq$130/85 mm Hg), and hyperglycemia (fasting glucose $\geq$100 mg•dl^{-1}) [13, 14]. At least three of the above criteria are necessary to be labeled as having metabolic syndrome [13].

The prevalence of the metabolic syndrome among US adults aged $\geq$20 years increased from 28% (or ~50 million people) in 1990 to 31.9% (or ~64 million people) in 2000, a relative change of 13.8% [15] (table 4). The prevalence of the metabolic syndrome in US adolescents aged 12–19 years in 2000 was 9.4% (or 2.9 million people); the prevalence in obese adolescents was 44.2% (table 5), which underscores the importance of adiposity in the development of insulin resistance and the metabolic syndrome [16].

Of particular interest is South Asia where abdominal obesity is common and evident even in non-obese people. The prevalence of the metabolic syndrome in South Asian populations ranges from 11 to 41% depending on the region of India, and South Asians have an unusually high tendency to develop type 2 diabetes mellitus and coronary heart disease [17–19]. Even though the prevalence of the metabolic syndrome in Asian Indian adolescents is low, the prevalence of insulin resistance remains high (27%) [20, 21].

Table 4. Unadjusted and age-adjusted prevalence (%) of the metabolic syndrome among U.S. adults aged ≥ 20 years [2]

	n		Original NCEP/ATP III definition					Revised NCEP/ATP II definition				
	NHANES III	NHANES 1999–2000	NHANES III	NHANES 1999–2000	relative change %	absolute difference %	p	NHANES III	NHANES 1999–2000	relative change %	absolute difference %	p
Total												
Unadjusted	6,436	1,677	23.1 (0.9)	26.7 (1.5)	15.7	3.6	0.043	28.0 (1.1)	31.9 (1.5)	13.8	3.9	0.041
Age adjusted	6,436	1,677	24.1 (0.8)	27.0 (1.5)	12.1	2.9	0.088	29.2 (0.9)	32.3 (1.5)	10.9	3.2	0.072
Men												
Total												
Unadjusted	3,069	0,841	22.9 (1.4)	24.1 (2.1)	5.4	1.2	0.625	29.3 (1.6)	30.6 (2.1)	04.2	1.2	0.648
Age adjusted	3,069	0,841	24.6 (1.4)	25.2 (2.1)	2.2	0.5	0.831	31.4 (1.4)	31.8 (2.2)	01.4	0.4	0.866
20–39 years	1,218	1,283	10.2 (1.7)	10.7 (1.9)	4.4	0.4	0.858	15.7 (2.1)	16.5 (2.5)	04.9	0.8	0.815
40–59 years	1,841	1,234	29.3 (2.4)	33.0 (3.8)	12.9	3.8	0.399	36.3 (2.3)	40.3 (4.4)	10.9	4.0	0.426
≥60 years	1,010	1,324	42.6 (2.4)	39.7 (4.3)	–6.8	–2.9	0.560	50.5 (2.3)	46.4 (4.3)	–8.2	–4.1	0.404
Women												
Total												
Unadjusted	3,367	1,836	23.3 (1.3)	29.3 (2.0)	25.8	6.0	0.016	26.8 (1.4)	33.2 (1.9)	24.0	6.4	0.010
Age adjusted	3,367	3,836	23.5 (1.1)	29.0 (2.0)	23.5	5.5	0.021	27.0 (1.2)	32.9 (2.0)	21.8	5.9	0.014
20–39 years	1,250	1,430	09.7 (1.6)	18.0 (2.8)	86.1	8.3	0.013	10.8 (1.7)	19.1 (2.9)	76.7	8.3	0.018
40–59 years	1,281	1,949	26.0 (2.3)	30.6 (3.8)	17.8	4.6	0.303	30.5 (2.3)	33.8 (3.8)	10.9	3.3	0.459
≥60 years	1,305	1,988	43.9 (2.0)	46.1 (3.7)	05.0	2.2	0.601	50.3 (2.2)	56.0 (4.0)	11.3	5.7	0.214

Values are presented as percentages with standard errors in parentheses.

Table 5. Prevalence of the metabolic syndrome in US adolescents using various definitions, NHANES 1999–2002 [16]

	Cook/Ford % (SE)	Cruz % (SE)	Caprio % (SE)	Adult % (SE)
Overall	9.2 (1.2)	2.0 (0.4)	2.4 (0.4)	5.8 (0.9)
	2.9 million	600,000	700,000	1.8 million
Sex				
Male	13.2 (2.0)	3.0 (0.8)	3.8 (0.8)	7.0 (1.4)
Female	05.3 (1.2)	1.0 (0.4)	0.6 (0.3)	4.5 (1.2)
Race/ethnicity				
White	10.7 (1.9)	2.2 (0.5)	2.5 (0.6)	6.0 (1.4)
Black	05.2 (1.1)	1.6 (0.5)	1.9 (0.7)	4.7 (1.1)
Mexican-American/ Hispanic	11.1 (1.2)	2.6 (0.6)	3.1 (0.7)	6.0 (0.9)
BMI status				
Normal	01.6 (0.7)	12.0 (0)	12.0 (0)	01.1 (0.5)
At risk	47.8 (3.6)	12.0 (0)	12.0 (0)	05.8 (2.8)
Overweight	44.2 (2.9)	12.4 (2.5)	14.1 (2.6)	26.2 (3.6)

Nonalcoholic Fatty Liver Disease

Nonalcoholic fatty liver disease (NAFLD) is a spectrum of disease ranging from simple steatosis to nonalcoholic steatohepatitis (NASH), which carries a risk of progression to cirrhosis and end-stage liver disease [22, 23]. NAFLD is considered the hepatic manifestation of the metabolic (insulin resistance) syndrome and its prevalence has paralleled the rise in obesity such that NAFLD is currently the most common chronic liver disease in the United States [24–26].

The prevalence of hepatic steatosis in a probability-based population from Dallas, Tex., was 31%; the prevalences per ethnic group were: Whites (33%), Blacks (24%), and Hispanics (45%) [25]. The prevalence of the metabolic syndrome in an unselected cohort of subjects with NASH was found to be 87%; when NASH subjects with type 2 diabetes mellitus were excluded, the prevalence remained higher than the general population at 38% [27, 28].

Nearly 25% of the urban population of India has NAFLD [19] and therefore may be at risk of developing the same clinical sequelae that has been described in other populations. It should be emphasized that NASH should be considered as the most severe form of a larger spectrum of NAFLD with histologic findings ranging from fat alone, to fat plus inflammation, to fat plus hepatocyte injury (ballooning degeneration) with or without fibrosis, polymorphonuclear cells or Mallory hyaline. Only fat plus hepatocyte injury with

Table 6. Pathophysiological based treatment of nonalcoholic fatty liver disease

Pathological mechanisms	Treatment
Nonhepatic causes	
Obesity	Moderate weight loss[1]
	Bariatric surgery[2]
	Orlistat[2]
Western diet	Vitamins, fiber, type of diet
Abnormal cytokines/adipokines	Anticytokine therapy
	Inhibitors
	Blockade
	Replacement[3]
Increased visceral fat	Weight loss
	Omental resection[3]
Bacterial overgrowth	Nonabsorbable antibiotics[3]
	Probiotics[3]
Insulin resistance	Thiazolidinedione[2]
	Metformin[2]
	Exercise
Hypertriglyceridemia	Hypolipidemics
	Clofibrate[2,4]
	Gemfibrozil[2]
	Probucol[2]
Hepatic causes	
Oxidative stress	Antioxidant[1,2]
Lipid peroxidation	PPAR-α[3]
Iron	Phlebotomy
Cytoprotection	Ursodeoxycholic acid[1,4]
Glutathione deficiency	Betaine[b]/SAMe[3]
Apoptosis	Caspase inhibition
	A-adrenergic agonists[3]

[1] At least one controlled trial in humans has been performed.

[2] Uncontrolled trial in humans has been performed.

[3] Used only in animal models thus far.

[4] Not effective. The only controlled trials (vitamin E, vitamin C, or ursodeoxycholic diet) were no better than controls.

or without fibrosis should be considered NASH. The significance of these histologic categories rests not only on the fact that the prevalence varies by histology, with steatosis alone with or without inflammation being more common than NASH, but that clinical outcomes also vary by histologic category. Therefore, it is important to reliably distinguish NASH from other histologic types of NAFLD.

Cirrhosis develops in 15–25% of NASH patients [29], and once developed, 40% of these patients may experience a liver-related death over a 10-year period, with mortality rates similar to or worse than cirrhosis associated with hepatitis C. NASH is also now considered the major cause of cryptogenic cirrhosis. NASH-associated cirrhosis can also decompensate into acute liver failure, progress to hepatocellular carcinoma, and recur after transplantation.

In contrast, steatosis alone is reported to have a more benign clinical course, although progression of fibrosis in cirrhosis has occurred in 3% of those patients with steatosis alone.

Pathophysiological Treatment

There are many potential pathophysiological factors that, either alone or in combination, may provide the basis for effective therapy that has yet to be established. Table 6 lists each of the proposed pathophysiologic factors and the potential therapies. Further proof-of-principle studies are required to determine the optimal therapeutic strategies for NAFLD that may vary among different populations.

References

1 Wilson PW, D'Agostino RB, Parise H, et al: Metabolic syndrome as a precursor of cardiovascular disease and type 2 diabetes mellitus. Circulation 2005;112:3066–3072.
2 Ford ES: The metabolic syndrome and mortality from cardiovascular disease and all-causes: findings from the National Health and Nutrition Examination Survey II Mortality Study. Atherosclerosis 2004;173:309–314.
3 Lakka HM, Laaksonen DE, Lakka TA, et al: The metabolic syndrome and total and cardiovascular disease mortality in middle-aged men. JAMA 2002;288:2709–2716.
4 Flegal KM, Carroll MD, Ogden CL, Johnson CL: Prevalence and trends in obesity among US adults, 1999–2000. JAMA 2002;288:1723–1727.
5 Ogden CL, Flegal KM, Carroll MD, Johnson CL: Prevalence and trends in overweight among US children and adolescents, 1999–2000. JAMA 2002;288:1728–1732.
6 Kuczmarski RJ, Flegal KM, Campbell SM, Johnson CL: Increasing prevalence of overweight among US adults. The National Health and Nutrition Examination Surveys, 1960 to 1991. JAMA 1994;272:205–211.
7 Luke A, Guo X, Adeyemo AA, et al: Heritability of obesity-related traits among Nigerians, Jamaicans and US black people. Int J Obes Relat Metab Disord 2001;25:1034–1041.
8 Misra A, Vikram NK: Insulin resistance syndrome (metabolic syndrome) and obesity in Asian Indians: evidence and implications. Nutrition 2004;20:482–491.
9 Salmond CE, Prior IA, Wessen AF: Blood pressure patterns and migration: a 14-year cohort study of adult Tokelauans. Am J Epidemiol 1989;130:37–52.
10 Monteiro CA, Conde WL, Popkin BM: Income-specific trends in obesity in Brazil: 1975–2003. Am J Public Health 2007;97:1808–1812.
11 Tuan NT, Tuong PD, Popkin BM: Body mass index (BMI) dynamics in Vietnam. Eur J Clin Nutr 2008;62:78–86.
12 Wang Y, Monteiro C, Popkin BM: Trends of obesity and underweight in older children and adolescents in the United States, Brazil, China, and Russia. Am J Clin Nutr 2002;75:971–977.
13 Executive Summary of the Third Report of the National Cholesterol Education Program (NCEP) Expert Panel on Detection, Evaluation, and Treatment of High Blood Cholesterol In Adults (Adult Treatment Panel III). JAMA 2001;285:2486–2497.
14 Genuth S, Alberti KG, Bennett P, et al: Follow-up report on the diagnosis of diabetes mellitus. Diabetes Care 2003;26:3160–3167.
15 Ford ES, Giles WH, Mokdad AH: Increasing prevalence of the metabolic syndrome among US Adults. Diabetes Care 2004;27:2444–2449.

16 Cook S, Auinger P, Li C, Ford ES: Metabolic syndrome rates in United States adolescents, from the National Health and Nutrition Examination Survey, 1999–2002. J Pediatr 2008;152:165–170.
17 King H, Aubert RE, Herman WH: Global burden of diabetes, 1995–2025:prevalence, numerical estimates, and projections. Diabetes Care 1998;21:1414–1431.
18 Reddy KS, Yusuf S: Emerging epidemic of cardiovascular disease in developing countries. Circulation 1998;97:596–601.
19 Misra A, Misra R, Wijesuriya M, Banerjee D: The metabolic syndrome in South Asians: continuing escalation & possible solutions. Indian J Med Res 2007;125:345–354.
20 Vikram NK, Misra A, Pandey RM, et al: Heterogeneous phenotypes of insulin resistance and its implications for defining metabolic syndrome in Asian Indian adolescents. Atherosclerosis 2006;186:193–199.
21 Misra A, Vikram NK, Arya S, et al: High prevalence of insulin resistance in postpubertal Asian Indian children is associated with adverse truncal body fat patterning, abdominal adiposity and excess body fat. Int J Obes Relat Metab Disord 2004;28:1217–1226.
22 Matteoni CA, Younossi ZM, Gramlich T, et al: Nonalcoholic fatty liver disease: a spectrum of clinical and pathological severity. Gastroenterology 1999;116:1413–1419.
23 Younossi ZM, Gramlich T, Liu YC, et al: Nonalcoholic fatty liver disease: assessment of variability in pathologic interpretations. Mod Pathol 1998;11:560–565.
24 McCullough AJ: The epidemiology and risk factors of NASH; in Farrell G, George J, Hall P, McCullough AJ (eds): Fatty Liver Disease: NASH and Related Disorders. Oxford, Blackwell, 2005, pp 23–37.
25 Browning JD, Szczepaniak LS, Dobbins R, et al: Prevalence of hepatic steatosis in an urban population in the United States: impact of ethnicity. Hepatology 2004;40:1387–1395.
26 Marchesini G, Forlani G: NASH: from liver diseases to metabolic disorders and back to clinical hepatology. Hepatology 2002;35:497–499.
27 Marchesini G, Bugianesi E, Forlani G, et al: Nonalcoholic fatty liver, steatohepatitis, and the metabolic syndrome. Hepatology 2003;37:917–923.
28 Chitturi S, Abeygunasekera S, Farrell GC, et al: NASH and insulin resistance: Insulin hypersecretion and specific association with the insulin resistance syndrome. Hepatology 2002;35:373–379.
29 McCullough AJ: The epidemiology and risk factors of NASH; in Farrell G, George J, Hall P, McCullough AJ (eds): Fatty Liver Disease: NASH and Related Disorders. Oxford, Blackwell, 2005, pp 23–37.

Discussion

Dr. Mathur: Could you enlighten us more on lean NASH and how does it develop [1]? Secondly, as a hepatologist, what clinical and public health advice would you give for tackling simple steatosis?

Dr. McCullough: The majority of people with lean NASH or fatty liver are really not lean; there is increased visceral fat in the majority of those patients. As opposed to the US, in the majority of cases the appropriate BMI in developing countries is much less. There are clear cases of high triglycerides by themselves increasing fatty liver. On the second question regarding the impact on healthcare of simple steatosis, I think this only pertains to very selective groups of patients. We are now increasingly using liver donors, and because 30% of America is fat, if the donors have steatosis, those livers can't be used. Fatty liver disease also adversely affects the progression of hepatitis C, and people with fatty liver disease have a much higher progression to cirrhosis. The 3rd point is that, although this is not as clear as the first two that I just mentioned, it is likely that these livers are more sensitive to drugs and it is also becoming with a little more certain that they are more sensitive to anesthesia. But steatosis itself in the progression of cirrhosis is not a bad thing (2%), but what it does to chronic inflammation, I don't know.

Dr. Giovannini: Alcoholism is very interesting because there is a big difference when we speak only about beer, but if we speak about wine types it must be remembered that there is a difference between red and white wine. Are obese people protected from NAFLD? To what extent may hepatic metabolism influence brain activity?

Dr. McCullough: The association with red wine is probably the strongest. Pinot noir has the highest concentration of resorbitol. I really don't know what effect it has on the brain. We know that the canabinoid receptors are activated in the brain, but obesity and the brain is not my field of expertise. I really don't know if obese people are protected from NAFLD. Actually some of the best data have come from Northern Italy. It is the same as in the United States, only 30% of people have increased fat. But those studies were done with ultrasounds. About 30% of the liver must be replaced by fat tissue. Mass spectroscopy can pick up 5%, and 5% of fat is normal if metabolic processes are being studied. I really don't know the answer to that question.

Dr. Giovannini: The problem in Asian and African countries is alcohol dehydrogenase deficiency. Perhaps Caucasians have more alcohol dehydrogenase enzymatic activity, and some problems have arisen with a lower alcohol dehydrogenase activity.

Dr. McCullough: That is somewhat different. If everyone here drank 60 g alcohol/day, we would all get fatty liver; that's not a question, that's a dose effect. The pathways of fat in the liver are completely different, and the enzyme pathway is something that probably has not been considered. The pathways that are activated in fatty liver disease are lysosomes, mitochondria and peroxisomes.

Dr. Kayal: In children with fatty liver, what would be the least invasive and least expensive way to monitor them for their fat content in the liver?

Dr. McCullough: In United States the prevalence is not as clear as in adults, but in pediatrics the best data come from San Diego. About 19% have fatty liver disease and there is a report of early cirrhosis developing in a 5-year-old from this disease. There is a statement, but without much data that I am aware of, that in the average United States high school about 2–3 children will have cirrhosis. Monitoring is a problem. People and parents in particular don't want to have their children biopsied. In the NASH study we had a pediatric population and a lot of trouble recruiting children because we only put children with NASH on a treatment protocol. So the answer to that also is not known, but I did not discuss alternate ways of diagnosing NASH other than apoptosis. Function tests are coming that will look at the activation of lysosomes and mitochondria perhaps. What we need are good noninvasive methods, if they are functional or static tests that give us a reliability of probably 85%, that will be acceptable. But this epidemic is coming to the pediatricians. I have a metabolic clinic and I am frequently seeing 20-year-olds with cirrhosis from this disease.

Dr. Sesikaran: M30 is a noninvasive marker and is expressed in many other apoptotic cells as well. We have studied intestinal epithelial cells, even when they undergo apoptosis they express M30. How could it be specific to liver cell apoptosis because when there is oxidative stress many other cells in the body also undergo apoptosis?

Dr. McCullough: I look forward to that data because this is specific for cytocarotene-18; so that is predominantly in the liver. Initially these were our own data, but they have been reproduced now by 2 other laboratories.

Dr. Sesikaran: We used M30 in the in situ tissue kit, and this was demonstrated in intestinal cells undergoing apoptosis [2].

Dr. Jaigirdar: In pediatrics, especially in enterology, we treated a fatty acid oxidation disorder with L-carnitine. I would like to ask about NASH and L-carnitine?

Dr. McCullough: The evidence shows that there is no trouble with mitochondrial oxidation in this disease.

Dr. Popkin: This is a slightly different but related issue. From my understanding we have fatty liver that may be benign not inflamed, not damaged, and then we have fatty liver disease, which is a tiny subset of everybody with fatty liver. Clearly in the US and in many countries we have enormous amounts of fatty liver. If we are studying the metabolic syndrome and find someone has 4 or 5 of the various symptoms at a high level, forgetting about whether there is a syndrome or not, do we need to study your ELISA and will it really add anything to what we know from a diagnostic side?

Dr. McCullough: I did not show these data, but it is clear that the more the components of the metabolic syndrome, the more likely that you have fatty liver disease. If you have 3, you have an about 45 or 50% chance of having fatty liver disease.

Dr. Popkin: So there is enough variability that one would gain in diagnostics by testing for fatty liver disease independently. The question is does your ELISA separate between fatty liver and fatty liver disease at enough specificity?

Dr. McCullough: This test has not yet been marketed and I am not suggesting that it be used as a diagnostic test; I was simply using it as an example of what we need to make the separation between good and bad fat in a noninvasive fashion. There are a number of different discriminative functions out there that I chose not to discuss because they are worse than that. What I am usually asked by hepatologists is, should we screen? The answer is probably not yet because we don't have a treatment. Once we have safe treatment then that question becomes somewhat moot because then we have to separate good fat from bad fat, and a noninvasive test with even an 85% predictability will probably be cost-effective.

Dr. Matthai: What is the effect of lipid-lowering agents on the progression of NAFLD? Do they play any role at all?

Dr. McCullough: That is a very good question. Clofibrate didn't work, but there are some data that gemfibrozil decreases ALT. The usual problem is that people say that it is not safe to use those drugs. But they are absolutely safe to use, there is no contraindication.

Dr. Kalhan: For a variety of reasons there is a large burden of background inflammation. What is the impact of this background inflammation on obesity, NAFLD and all the comorbidities?

Dr. McCullough: Inflammation is absolutely present in NAFLD. T cells are important. If the inflammation is suppressed by suppressing macrophage activity, just as in alcoholic liver disease, NAFLD in certain animal models gets better. So chronic inflammation is a very important component of liver disease.

Dr. Kalhan: My question was more in relation to other chronic inflammations in the body. In the organism or human being living in a developing country with a large burden of parasites or whatever, if you measure their circulating cytokines they are probably higher than in the Western societies. Does obesity have a different form in these people? Does liver disease worsen in these types of people? Are there any data?

Dr. McCullough: I am not aware of any data in terms of the ratio of good fat to bad fat in developing countries. The data I showed on prevalence are just based on ultrasounds.

Dr. Yajnik: We have a study, called the Coronary Risk of Insulin Sensitivity in Indians (CRISIS). We measured body fat by different techniques in 150 men from rural areas, 150 from urban slums, and 150 middle income patients. We found progressive increases in body adiposity, liver fat (measured by CT), and abdominal fat volume measured by MRI. We also measured a number of inflammatory markers. CRP levels were highest in the urban middle class, while total leukocyte count, IL-6 and TNF-a were highest in slum dwellers, suggesting a contribution from the infective environment. We found that hyperglycemia and insulin resistance in the urban middle class were substantially enhanced by their adiposity [3]. We are looking at other markers.

Obesity and Fatty Liver

Dr. McCullough: When I heard the presentations by Dr. Prentice and Dr. Popkin, in your world this does not have a high priority. There are many other diseases that you are more concerned about, and as society develops it is coming to you. It is just a matter of how soon.

Dr. Yajnik: Previously we did not call it NASH. Liver problems were there but fewer. Working in a diabetic clinic for 25 years I have seen an increasing number of people who develop liver cirrhosis. Is this part of the central visceral adiposity? You showed analyses where you compared NAFLD with controls. Did you adjust for total body adiposity or visceral fat in that analysis?

Dr. McCullough: Those studies did not look at visceral fat.

Dr. Yajnik: You have been calling it central obesity and this is a component of central obesity or adiposity, and part of it is ectopic adiposity.

Dr. Genuino: In the new food guide pyramid released by the National Institutes of Health, there is a recommendation on fats that you can go beyond the 30% limitation as long as these are polyunsaturated fats. What is your opinion?

Dr. McCullough: Depending on the type of fat I think it is probably fine; the oceanic societies eat a lot of n-3, and they do fine.

Dr. Arora: What is the difference in fat accumulation due to obesity and that due to severe malnutrition in the liver?

Dr. McCullough: With severe malnutrition you get fatty liver disease and the problem is you don't have enough export proteins of the triglycerides. Whether that is an inflammatory state or not, I don't know.

Dr. Sesikaran: We always believed that fatty liver with undernutrition never leads to cirrhosis unless it coexists with hepatitis B. Yet there is a situation in which a fatty liver could lead to cirrhosis. So the fat accumulation in the liver due to undernutrition and that associated with excess adiposity obviously seem to have a different etiopathologies.

Dr. McCullough: Did you say that malnutrition in fatty liver disease can progress to cirrhosis?

Dr. Sesikaran: It can, but it does not unless there is a coexistent hepatitis B.

Dr. McCullough: I am pretty sure that the mechanism for fatty liver disease in that condition is failure to export protein. I assume that it is not an inflammatory state, but I have never looked at liver tissue from that type of patient, so I don't know.

Dr. Ganapathy: I was just wondering whether, in a state of type 2 diabetes, by the time it is manifest the patient has already gone through a phase with an altered immune status. Gut-associated lymphoid tissue is the biggest system, and endotoxins, lipopolysaccharides, translocation of organisms, they all get into the liver. Kupffer cells can be altered with altered cytokine profile in the liver, and we have seen this in neonates who have sepsis with jaundice and negative blood cultures. So could this be a contributing factor to NASH and could we do something at the gut level to prevent this from happening?

Dr. McCullough: There are some very preliminary studies looking at probiotics that help to decrease endotoxin. The thought is that in obesity there is a leaky gut, and there is some information about that which would suggest measuring endotoxin, and then induce macrophages by TL4 or CD38 or those receptors, and I think it is a reasonable hypothesis to test. I myself am not a big probiotic fan because there have been some deaths described in the United States mostly in inflammatory bowel disease. I like prebiotics, fibers that type of thing, but I think it is a very reasonable hypothesis in this disease because a lot of this disease very closely mimics alcoholic liver disease, and that disease is largely mediated by endotoxin, gut endotoxin in active drinkers. I think you are probably right.

175

References

1   Angulo P: Nonalcoholic fatty liver disease. N Engl J Med 2002;346:1221–1231.
2   Vijayalakshmi B, Sesikeran B, Udaykumar P, et al: Chronic low vitamin intake potentiates cisplatin-induced intestinal epithelial cell apoptosis in WNIN rats. World J Gastroenterol 2006;12:1078–1085.
3   Yajnik CS, Joglekar CV, Lubree HG, et al: Adiposity, inflammation and hyperglycaemia in rural and urban Indian men: Coronary Risk of Insulin Sensitivity in Indian Subjects (CRISIS) Study. Diabetologia 2008;51:39–46.

Kalhan SC, Prentice AM, Yajnik CS (eds): Emerging Societies – Coexistence of Childhood Malnutrition
and Obesity.
Nestlé Nutr Inst Workshop Ser Pediatr Program, vol 63, pp 177–194,
Nestec Ltd., Vevey/S. Karger AG, Basel, © 2009.

Imperative of Preventive Measures Addressing the Life-Cycle

Chittaranjan S. Yajnik

Diabetes Unit, KEM Hospital, Pune, India

Abstract

The epidemiological characteristics of chronic non-communicable diseases (NCD) are fast changing. The prevalence has risen to unprecedented levels, and the young and the underprivileged are increasingly affected. The classic view of the etiology of NCD consists of a genetic susceptibility which is precipitated by aging and modern lifestyle. In a virtual absence of any methods to tackle genetic susceptibility, the preventive approach has so far been focused on the control of lifestyle factors in those at high risk (old, and those with positive family history and elevated risk factors). Such an approach might help high risk individuals, but is unlikely to curtail the burgeoning epidemic of obesity and diabetes. Recent research has suggested that susceptibility to NCD originates in early life through non-genetic mechanisms *(fetal programming)*. Tackling these may offer an exciting opportunity to control the NCD epidemic by influencing the susceptibility in a more durable manner than only controlling the lifestyle factors in adult life. The imperative is to address the life cycle rather than concentrate on the end stages.

Introduction

The world is facing an unprecedented epidemic of type 2 diabetes (T2D) and other chronic non-communicable diseases (NCDs). The rise in the prevalence of T2D in the last few decades has been phenomenal, perhaps unmatched by any other chronic condition. The pattern of affliction is rapidly changing; the poor and the young are increasingly affected. In 2007, there were an estimated 246 million diabetic patients in the world, of which 165 million (80%) were in the developing world [1, 2]. A substantial number are diagnosed before 40 years of age, and it is increasingly common to see T2D in children. Current trials of diabetes prevention have concentrated on

Yajnik

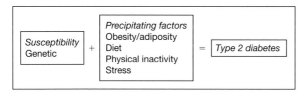

Fig. 1. The conventional model for the origin of type 2 diabetes. The current diabetes prevention trials are based on the conventional model.

modifying lifestyle in middle-aged people with advanced risk factors (obese and impaired glucose tolerant). Such attempts are unlikely to curtail the epidemic, fuelled by the increasing incidence in the young.

Over last three decades there has been growing recognition that early life factors have a major influence on the risk of T2D. Studies in Pima Indians showed that maternal hyperglycemia in pregnancy increased the risk of obesity and diabetes in the offspring [3]. On the other hand studies in the UK showed that low birthweight (LBW) was a risk factor for T2D diabetes in the offspring [4]. These studies focused attention on intrauterine environment as an important determinant of subsequent risk of T2D. Subsequent studies demonstrated that rapid childhood growth was also a strong risk factor for obesity and T2D. Thus, factors influencing intrauterine and childhood growth seem to affect the risk of T2D. These new developments have challenged the rather limited idea of controlling the diabetes epidemic by intervening in the middle-aged population with advanced risk factors.

Here we will review some of these new ideas and discuss the imperative for a life-course approach to the prevention of chronic NCD, with focus on T2D.

Conventional Model of Pathogenesis of Type 2 Diabetes and Prevention Strategies

The classic view of the etiology of T2D suggests that aging and modern-day lifestyle factors (dietary excess and physical inactivity) cause hyperglycemia in those genetically predisposed (fig. 1). The lifestyle factors act to promote obesity, which is an integral part of this process ('diabesity') and thought to act by causing insulin resistance (IR). The contribution of genetics is less clear. Recent genome-wide association studies have shown that variations in more than 10 regions in the human genome increase the risk of T2D, the majority of these seem to affect pancreatic β-cell function [5]. In the absence of any methods to tackle genetic susceptibility, the preventive approach has so far focused on the control of lifestyle factors in those at high risk (middle-aged, those with a family history of diabetes, obese and impaired glucose tolerance). A number of studies across the world demonstrated that dietary modifications

178

and promotion of physical activity (sometimes with a pharmacological agent) improved glycemia in individuals with impaired glucose tolerance (IGT) [6]. This has been interpreted to mean 'prevention' of diabetes, which may be a bit naïve. Obesity and IGT are both 'end-stage' conditions with arbitrary cutoff points (which have changed substantially over last 2 decades). Trying to treat only such 'high risk' individuals is unlikely to curtail the burgeoning epidemic of obesity and diabetes, which is rapidly spreading to involve the younger and the poorer. Controlling obesity and metabolism in post-reproductive years will not benefit the offspring, a major limitation to our efforts at curtailing the epidemic.

Changing Epidemiology of Obesity and Type 2 Diabetes

A few decades ago T2D was considered a disease of the affluent ('what gout was to the royalty in the UK'). However the scene has rapidly changed. There are more diabetic patients in developing countries than in developed countries. Moreover, in many developed countries and in some developing countries, the prevalence of obesity and diabetes is higher in the lower socio-economic groups compared to the affluent ('reversal' of the socioeconomic gradient). While part of this change could be ascribed to the healthy behavior of the affluent and the educated, other biological factors seem to operate.

Some striking features of diabetes epidemiology in developing countries (like India) include: (1) younger age at diagnosis; (2) lower body mass index; (3) higher adiposity (body fat percent) and central adiposity (waist–hip ratio and visceral fat, 'thin and fat'), and (4) higher IR [7]. Over the last few decades, age at diagnosis of T2D has fallen by many years in India. Children are increasingly affected with obesity and T2D, especially in the urban affluent. Clearly the diabetogenic influences are operating at a much younger age and at lower threshold of body size. We know that hyperglycemia is usually present for many years before clinical diagnosis [8] and that the risk factors are present for a long time before glucose concentrations start rising [9, 10]. It is increasingly clear that preventive strategies will have to start very early in life.

Early Life Factors and Risk of Diabetes

Maternal Diabetes and Offspring Obesity and Diabetes
Pettitt et al. [3] and Dabelea et al. [11] made a very interesting observation in Pima Indians. Taking advantage of a prospective serial database in the Pima Indian community, they analyzed the contribution of genetics and intrauterine environment to the risk of obesity and diabetes in the offspring. The risk of diabetes was many times higher if the mother had diabetes during pregnancy ('intrauterine exposure') compared to the risk in the children whose mothers developed diabetes after pregnancy ('genetic risk'). They

suggested that intrauterine hyperglycemia is more important in intergenerational propagation of diabetes compared to genetic factors. Diabetes in young girls is thus a major factor in the escalating epidemic of diabetes. A subsequent analysis showed that 70% of diabetes in young Pima Indians could be ascribed to maternal diabetes.

Maternal Nutrition and Offspring Diabetes

Barker [12] proposed a novel model for the etiology of T2D and cardiovascular disease (CVD) when they demonstrated that LBW was a risk factor for these conditions. In addition to LBW, other measures of small size at birth (length, ponderal index, etc.) also predicted future T2D or its two pathogenic mechanisms, i.e. IR and impaired β-cell function. It was proposed that intrauterine growth restriction (IUGR) consequent upon maternal undernutrition contributed to this association. In the original form this was called the 'thrifty phenotype' hypothesis and other terms like 'fetal origins' and 'small baby syndrome' were also used. Many studies across different populations confirmed the association between small size at birth and later diabetes [13].

Size at birth is only a surrogate for events during intrauterine life. It is useful to remember that it is an intermediate phenotype between the intrauterine exposures and the final outcome. It is also a nonspecific and insensitive marker for nutritional exposures, and does not provide a clue to the nutrient or the time of exposure. Another point of relevance is that the association between birthweight and T2D is U-shaped (as shown in Pima Indians [14]), thus both LBW and large birth weight (contributed by maternal diabetes) increase risk of T2D. Target for intervention is thus the intrauterine environment rather than birthweight.

Fetal Programming

The associations between size at birth and later disease have been explained by the concept of 'fetal programming'. It refers to a permanent change in the structure and function of a developing organism in response to an environmental factor [15]. The intrauterine environment thus assumes a great significance in determining the future prospects for the fetus. Programming is thought to be a 'predictive' adaptation [16]. The programmed fetus will do well in a similar postnatal environment, but if the environment is substantially different, the fetal 'programs' are unable to cope and result in disease.

I will review briefly some of the findings of the studies in Pune, which have helped the thinking in this field.

Pune Children's Study

In 1991 Prof. David Barker visited us and discussed the idea of 'intrauterine origins'. With his help we started a study of over 400 children whose birthweights were available from the labor room records at King Edward Memorial Hospital in Pune. We studied their anthropometry, glucose

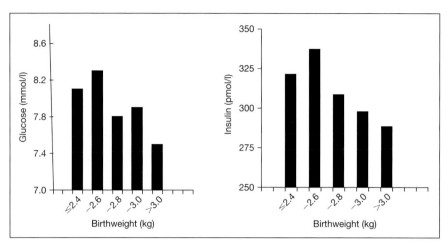

Fig. 2. Plasma glucose and insulin concentrations after an oral glucose load in 4-year-old Indian children. Significance of the trend is corrected for age, gender and current bodyweight. The results show that low birthweight is associated with higher glucose and insulin concentrations [17, 18a].

tolerance and circulating insulin concentrations. Plasma glucose and insulin concentrations 30 min after the glucose load were inversely related to birthweight (fig. 2). [17] This provided the first proof for Barker's hypothesis in a developing country. Given the fact that almost a third of the babies born India are small by international standards, this could have enormous implications for the diabetes epidemic.

We studied these children again at 8 years of age, and confirmed the association of LBW with higher IR [18]. In addition, we found that the levels of the risk factors for diabetes and CVD (glucose, IR, lipids, blood pressure, leptin concentrations, etc.) were highest in children who were born lightest but were heaviest by 8 years of age (fig. 3). This finding focused attention on rapid childhood growth as a risk factor for T2D. We also found that children born to short parents were more insulin resistant, and those who had grown taller in relation to parental height were the most insulin resistant, suggesting an intergenerational influence of poor parental growth on the metabolic risk of the offspring. A discordance in size (presumably due to nutritional factors) in one's lifetime (LBW and later overweight) as well as across generations (short parents and tall children) predicts a higher metabolic risk.

A study in Delhi provided further proof that rapid childhood growth predisposes to T2D [19]. Over 1,500 men and women, for whom growth data were available from birth, were studied at 28 years of age. The diabetic subjects were born lighter, grew more slowly during infancy but progressively faster from 3 years of age compared to those who were normal glucose tolerant (fig. 4). They had an earlier adiposity rebound.

181

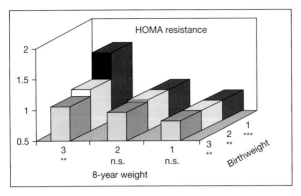

Fig. 3. The mean levels of insulin resistance (HOMA) in 8-year-old children by tertiles of birthweight and 8-year weight. Those born the lightest but having grown heaviest are the most insulin-resistant. The effect of the 'rapid transition' in one's lifetime is highlighted, and the effect of the double burden (early life undernutrition and subsequent overnutrition) in an individual is depicted. n.s. = Not significant. * p < 0.05; ** p < 0.01; *** p < 0.001 [18a, b].

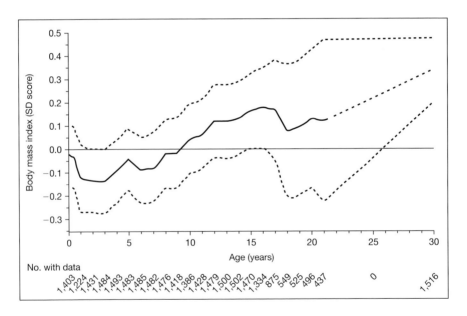

Fig. 4. Mean sex-specific unadjusted SD scores for body mass index, according to age, for subjects in whom impaired glucose tolerance or diabetes developed. The mean SD scores (solid lines) are obtained by linear interpolation of yearly means, with one additional observation at 6 months. The dotted lines represent 95% confidence intervals. The dashed portions of the lines indicate years in which there was no follow-up. The SD score for the cohort is set at zero (solid horizontal line). Printed with permission from [19].

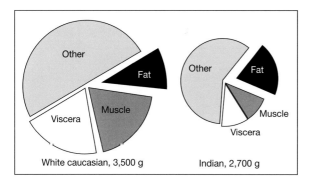

Fig. 5. A schematic diagram to compare the body composition of Indian and White Caucasian (UK) newborn babies. The Indian babies are approximately 800 g lighter, have less muscle but higher adiposity than the White babies.

In all these studies only size measurements were available at birth and later. The possible role of nutrition in these associations is speculative. We therefore set up a prospective, community-based study of maternal nutrition and fetal growth, with a view to follow the children until adult life for the risk of NCD.

Pune Maternal Nutrition Study

The Pune Maternal Nutrition Study (PMNS) was started in 1993 in 6 villages near Pune. Over 2,500 eligible nonpregnant women were followed up regularly, of whom over 800 women became pregnant during the study. We measured their nutrition, physical activity, biochemistry and fetal growth. Newborn babies were measured for size in detail at birth and every 6 months thereafter. Every 6 years we do a detailed assessment of body composition, IR and a range of other cardiovascular risk factors. Over 700 children are being followed up currently at 12 years of age.

We made an interesting observation that Indian babies, though small, short and thin, had comparable subscapular skin-fold-thickness measurements compared to White Caucasian babies born in the UK [20]. In other words they were 'thin but fat' very similar to our previous description of Indian adults. This suggests that body composition is established at birth (fig. 5). In a subsequent study we compared cord blood measurements, and showed that Indian babies have higher concentrations of insulin and leptin but lower concentrations of adiponectin, compared with those in White Caucasian babies in the UK, again suggesting that the high risk Indian phenotype for T2D is established at birth [21]. If we were to think of a real preventive intervention, it will have to start in utero, and improving the health of young girls will be a very important aspect of such an approach. This must represent a paradigm shift in thinking about the prevention of the T2D epidemic.

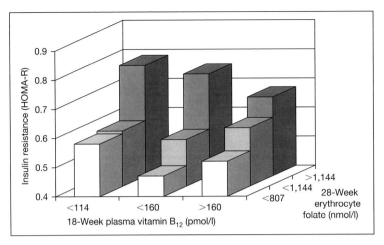

Fig. 6. Insulin resistance (HOMA-R) in children at 6 years in relation to maternal vitamin B_{12} (18 weeks) and erythrocyte folate (28 weeks). Printed with permission from [24].

Another important observation in the PMNS was that maternal micronutrient nutrition was an important determinant of fetal growth in this population. Maternal intake of calories, proteins and fats did not have a significant effect on fetal growth but the frequency of consumption of green leafy vegetables, milk and fruits had a major effect [22]. Additionally we found that higher maternal circulating concentrations of homocysteine predicted IUGR [23]. Over two thirds of mothers had low vitamin B_{12} concentrations, while only one woman had folate deficiency. Low vitamin B_{12} status in this population was ascribable to low dietary intake, predominantly due to vegetarianism. Even more interestingly, at 6 years of age the children's adiposity and IR were significantly related to maternal B_{12} and folate levels in pregnancy [24]. Children born to mothers with low B_{12} concentrations but high folate concentrations were the most insulin resistant (fig. 6). This is the first demonstration in a prospective study of a relationship between maternal nutrition in pregnancy and offspring risk of T2D.

Thus, a deficiency as well as an imbalance between these two related vitamins which affect one-carbon (methyl) metabolism may be responsible for structural and functional programming. Maternal nutritional disturbance of these two vitamins disturbs fetal growth and development, which may manifest as early abortions, congenital anomalies (neural tube defects and cardiovascular anomalies), IUGR or a change in neurocognitive function, body composition and metabolism. To include such a spectrum of effects we propose a new term, 'nutrient-mediated teratogenesis' analogous to Freinkel's [25] concept of 'fuel-mediated teratogenesis' in a diabetic pregnancy.

Experimental Models and the Concept of Epigenetics

Animal models of maternal undernutrition and fetal programming have provided crucial information on these phenomena. A review is outside the scope of this article and readers are referred to work from Hoet and Hanson [26] and Hales et al. [27].

Animal models have provided exciting information on the role of methyl groups in fetal programming. Waterland and Jirtle [28] fed genetically obese Agouti mice with a 'methylating cocktail' (B_{12}, folic acid, choline and beta-ine) and showed that the offspring had a different coat color and were less obese, despite inheriting the Agouti mutation. This was related to the methylation status of the promoter region of the Agouti gene. Lillycrop et al. [29] demonstrated that folate rescue in the rat model of mater-nal protein deficiency was related to methylation in some of the genetic sequences. Sinclair et al. [30] produced methionine deficiency in female sheep (by dietary restriction of methionine, B_{12} and folate). Ova from these sheep were fertilized in vitro, and the blastocysts were transferred to sur-rogate mothers with normal methionine status. The offspring were obese and insulin resistant, especially males. They demonstrated a differential methylation at number of sites in the genome of these animals. This model highlights the importance of periconceptional one-carbon (methyl) metabo-lism in fetal programming.

These phenomena are included under the concept of 'epigenetics' which refers to heritable modifications in the genome not associated with a change in the base sequence [31]. Periconceptional, embryonic and fetal life are con-sidered the most opportune times for epigenetic manipulation, though it may continue postnatally. Many of these changes are organ-specific and contribute to differentiation and development. Methylation of cytosine residues in the CpG dinucleotide regions of DNA and acetylation of lysine residues of the his-tones are two known mechanisms that affect gene expression and function.

Fetal Programming in Rapid Transition

In countries undergoing rapid transition there is a double burden of dis-ease: the rapidly emerging T2D and CVD along with the unconquered nutri-tional and infective disorders. This is evident in the morbidity and mortality statistics of rural and urban populations in India. The rural populations pre-dominantly suffer from undernutrition and infections while urban popula-tions are increasingly affected by overnutrition-related NCD (T2D and CVD). Often the two coexist, for example urban women have the double burden of micronutrient deficiencies and gestational diabetes with potentially grave consequences for fetal programming. Such a combination of factors could be at the heart of the rapidly escalating epidemic of T2D.

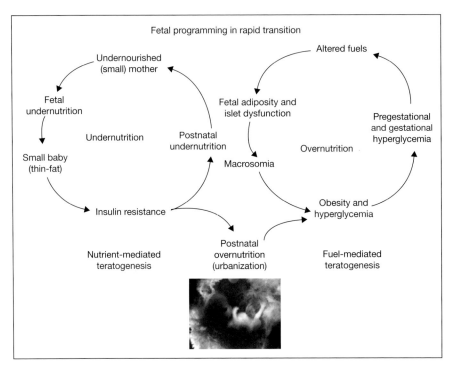

Fig. 7. The interrelationship of two major maternal factors (undernutrition and overnutrition) in fetal programming is shown. An undernourished mother produces a small (thin-fat) insulin-resistant baby. If this baby remains undernourished in postnatal life, the cycle is propagated. If the thin-fat insulin-resistant baby is overnourished, it becomes obese and hyperglycemic. An obese and hyperglycemic mother produces a 'macrosomic' baby at a higher risk of obesity and hyperglycemia. Thus the intergenerational insulin resistance–diabetes cycle is propagated through a girl child. Rapid transition shifts the balance from undernutrition to overnutrition, and contributes to escalation of the diabetes epidemic. Improving the health of a girl child is of paramount importance in controlling the diabetes epidemic [32].

We have conceptualized this complex interplay in a model based on data from our own and other research. It proposes that the two cycles of fetal programming (related to 'undernutrition' and obesity-diabetes related 'overnutrition') operate separately, overlap or combine to produce a spectrum of NCD that are influenced by postnatal nutrition. Thus, 'nutrient-mediated teratogenesis' and 'fuel-mediated teratogenesis' are two operational faces of the same coin (fig. 7) [32]. The undernutrition 'track' produces 'small, thin and fat' babies who are insulin resistant and remain so if postnatal nutrition is not excessive. They have low rates of NCD. When postnatal nutrition is relatively plentiful, it promotes obesity and hyperglycemia, many times without correction of the micronutrient imbalance. In a female such

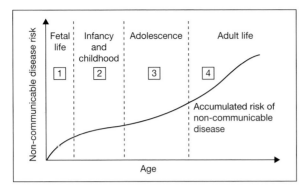

Fig. 8. The World Health Organization's life-course model of non-communicable disease. The model suggests that non-communicable diseases have their origins in early life. The risk progressively accumulates throughout the life course and the disease becomes manifest in later life [34].

a situation exposes her fetus to multiple adverse programming influences, resulting in a complex phenotype that includes exaggerated adiposity ('macrosomia') and pancreatic islet dysfunction with a tendency to develop diabetes, CVD and other disorders at a young age. The nutritional history of a population thus becomes an important determinant of the health of the present generation.

The Life-Course Model and DOHaD

Kuh and Ben-Shlomo [33] synthesized such ideas into a 'life-course' model for NCD which stresses that risk of these conditions is not attributable solely to either early life or adult experiences but instead they operate cumulatively throughout life. A WHO committee adopted these ideas to include many disorders (fig. 8) [34]. To accommodate the new evidence since the coining of the original term 'fetal origins of adult disease', the international council of 'early life origins' also adopted a new term 'developmental origins of health and disease' (DOHaD) [35]. All these terms represent the growing recognition of the importance of environmental factors acting on the genotype throughout the life cycle of an individual to progressively modify its phenotype (fig. 9). Clearly there are 'windows' of time in the lifecycle when the susceptibility of the genome to such an influence is very high. The periconceptional and intrauterine period seems to be the most crucial time, when a small change in environment could have a large effect on the phenotype. The need is to define these periods and the environmental exposures of importance. Research in this area has a lot to contribute to our understanding of the determinants of health and disease in populations.

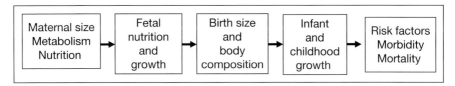

Fig. 9. Current concept of the Developmental Origins of Health and Disease (DOHaD). The influence of early life factors (including maternal factors and childhood growth) on the burden of type 2 diabetes and other non-communicable disease is shown.

The Imperative of Life-Cycle Prevention

I hope, the above discussion has highlighted the need to start early in life to prevent NCD. Current teaching and medical practice revolve around the idea of 'fixing' the end-stage conditions, which is difficult, expensive and unaffordable for the majority. The lack of appreciation of the life-course evolution of these conditions has resulted in prevention trials that concentrate on high-risk adults. Such an approach leaves the larger and more important issue of 'susceptibility' unanswered, and has no benefits for the offspring who are at an even higher risk. Recognition that intergenerational environmental influences ('epigenetic' rather than 'genetic') might be important has opened new avenues for research and intervention in NCD. Maternal nutrition and metabolism appear crucial to the risk of the offspring. Thus, improving early life environment may be more beneficial and cost-effective than only concentrating on the lifestyle factors in later life and devising newer treatments for the end-stage conditions. The health of young girls and women is of paramount importance, as highlighted in the Millennium Development Goals [36]. A recent meeting captured this well in its slogan: 'Woman's health is nation's wealth' [32]. It is time to capitalize on the new exciting ideas in this field and promote translation research.

References

1 International Diabetes Federation: Diabetes Atlas, ed 3. Brussels, IDF, 2006.
2 Wild S, Roglic G, Green A, et al: Global prevalence of diabetes: estimates for the year 2000 and estimates for year 2030. Diabetes Care 2004;27:1047–1053.
3 Pettitt DJ, Aleck KA, Baird HR, et al: Congenital susceptibility to NIDDM. Role of intrauterine environment. Diabetes 1988;37:622–628.
4 Hales CN, Barker DJP, Clark PMS, et al: Fetal and infant growth and impaired glucose tolerance at age 64. BMJ 1991;303:1019–1022.
5 Frayling TM: Genome-wide association studies provide new insights into type 2 diabetes aetiology. Nat Rev Genet 2007;8:657–662.
6 Gillies CL, Abrams KR, Lambert PC, et al: Pharmacological and lifestyle interventions to prevent or delay type 2 diabetes in people with impaired glucose tolerance: systematic review and meta-analysis. BMJ 2007;334:299.

7   Yajnik CS: The insulin resistance epidemic in India: fetal origins, later lifestyle, or both? Nutr Rev 2001;59:1–9.
8   Harris MI, Klein R, Welborn TA, Knuiman MW: Onset of NIDDM occurs at least 4–7 years before clinical diagnosis. Diabetes Care 1992;15:815–819.
9   Yudkin JS, Yajnik CS, Mohammed Ali V, Bulmer K: High levels of circulating proinflammatory cytokines and leptin in urban, but not rural, Asian Indians. Diabetes Care 1999;22:363–364.
10 QM, SR, JH, et al: Changes in risk variables of metabolic syndrome since childhood in prediabetic and type 2 diabetic subjects: the Bogalusa Heart Study. Diabetes Care 2008;31:2044–2049.
11 Dabelea D, Knowler WC, Pettitt DJ: Effect of diabetes in pregnancy on offspring: follow-up research in the Pima Indians. J Matern Fetal Med 2000;9:83–88.
12 Barker DJP: Fetal nutrition and cardiovascular disease in later life. Br Med Bull 1997,53.90–108.
13 Barker DJP: Mothers, Babies and Health in Later Life, ed 2. Edinburgh, Churchill Livingstone, 1998.
14 McCance DR, Pettitt DJ, Hanson RL, et al: Birth weight and non-insulin dependent diabetes: thrifty genotype, thrifty phenotype, or surviving small baby genotype? BMJ 1994;308:942–945.
15 Lucas A: Programming by early nutrition in man. Ciba Found Symp 1991;156:38–55.
16 Gluckman PD, Hanson MA: Living with the past: evolution, development, and patterns of disease. Science 2004;305:1733.
17 Yajnik CS, Fall CH, Vaidya U, et al: Fetal growth and glucose and insulin metabolism in four-year-old Indian children. Diabet Med 1995;12:330–336.
18a Yajnik CS: The lifecycle effects of nutrition and body size on adult adiposity, diabetes and cardiovascular disease. Obes Rev 2002;3:217–224.
18b Bavdekar A, Yajnik CS, Fall CH, et al: Insulin resistance syndrome in 8-year-old Indian children: small at birth, big at 8 years, or both? Diabetes 1999;48:2422–2429.
19 Bhargava SK, Sachdev HS, Fall CH, et al: Relation of serial changes in childhood body-mass index to impaired glucose tolerance in young adulthood. N Engl J Med 2004;350:865–875.
20 Yajnik CS, Fall CHD, Coyaji KJ, et al: Neonatal anthropometry: the thin-fat Indian baby: the Pune Maternal Nutrition Study. Int J Obes 2003;26:173–180.
21 Yajnik CS, Lubree HG, Rege SS, et al: Adiposity and hyperinsulinemia in Indians are present at birth. J Clin Endocrinol Metab 2002;87:5575–5580.
22 Rao S, Yajnik CS, Kanade A, et al: Intake of micronutrient-rich foods in rural Indian mothers is associated with the size of their babies at birth: Pune Maternal Nutrition Study. J Nutr 2001;131:1217–1224.
23 Yajnik CS, Deshpande SS, Panchanadikar AV, et al: Maternal total homocysteine concentration and neonatal size in India. Asia Pac J Clin Nutr 2005;14:179–181.
24 Yajnik CS, Deshpande SS, Jackson AA, et al: Vitamin B_{12} and folate concentrations during pregnancy and insulin resistance in the offspring: the Pune Maternal Nutri-tion Study. Diabetologia 2008;51:29–38.
25 Freinkel N: Banting Lecture 1980. Of pregnancy and progeny. Diabetes 1980;29:1023–1035.
26 Hoet JJ, Hanson MA: Intrauterine nutrition: its importance during critical periods for cardiovascular and endocrine development. J Physiol 1999;514:617–627.
27 Hales CN, Desai M, Ozanne SE, Crowther NJ: Fishing in the stream of diabetes: from measuring insulin to the control of fetal organogenesis. Biochem Soc Trans 1996;24:341–350.
28 Waterland RA, Jirtle RL: Transposable elements: targets for early nutritional effects on epigenetic gene regulation. Mol Cell Biol 2003;23:5293–5300.
29 Lillycrop KA, Phillips ES, Jackson AA, et al: Dietary protein restriction of pregnant rats induces and folic acid supplementation prevents epigenetic modification of hepatic gene expression in the offspring. J Nutr 2005;135:1382–1386.
30 Sinclair KD, Allegrucci C, Singh R, et al: DNA methylation, insulin resistance, and blood pressure in offspring determined by maternal periconceptional B vitamin and methionine status. Proc Natl Acad Sci USA 2007;104:19351–19356.
31 Robertson K: DNA methylation and human disease. Nat Rev Genet 2005;6:597–610.
32 Diabetes, Women, and Development. Meeting Summary, Expert Recommendations for Policy Action, Conclusions and Follow up Actions (2008). Expert meeting, UN headquarters. http://

www.gawh.org/programs/2008_04_08/Report-Final-Expert-Meeting-on-Diabetes-Women-and-Development.pdf?CAMEFROM = SYMPOSIA&id = 34. Accessed August 26, 2008.

33 Kuh D, Ben-Shlomo Y: A Life-Course Approach to Chronic Disease Epidemiology. Oxford, Oxford University Press, 1997.

34 Aboderin I, Kalache A, Ben-Shlomo Y: Life Course Perspectives on Coronary Heart Disease, Stroke and Diabetes: Key Issues and Implications for Policy and Research. Geneva, WHO, 2001.

35 International Society for Developmental Origins of Health and Disease: DOHaD. www.mrc.soton.ac.uk/dohad/. Accessed August 26, 2008.

36 United Nations Millennium Development Goals: http://www.undp.org/mdg/basics.shtml. Accessed August 26, 2008.

Discussion

Dr. Wharton: So far we have done a lot on the coexistence of these two conditions and I did hope that for the rest of the conference we could be discussing whether there was interaction. I think throughout there has been an underlying assumption, which we just heard about in detail very elegantly, that a period of malnutrition primes, programs or predisposes, whichever word you wish to use, to later obesity. We have heard quite a lot about secular changes in the amount of obesity and then we haven't heard anything about secular changes in birthweight in any of these countries, and I think we would need to do that if we were developing that theme; some on the reduction in childhood malnutrition; perhaps not very much on the growth patterns whether there is a secular change in growth patterns in the first few months of life to fit in with the fetal or early catch-up growth hypothesis, whichever one you support, we would need to know about. I just have a slightly uncomfortable feeling about taking on the idea that early undernutrition leads to later obesity because if we look at so many countries we find that childhood malnutrition is going down but adult obesity is going up. China is probably the best one to quote because of such extensive figures on this. Of course the cohort studies seem to leave no doubt, but they don't seem to account for the temporal changes we are seeing in societies because there is less childhood malnutrition in many but their obesity is going up. The same applies to other ideas about adult obesity. We are getting more breastfeeding in communities throughout the world but obesity is going up. The amount of protein that we give to the very young is going down mainly because we rely less on whole cow's milk and yet obesity is going up. So those overall population observations don't seem to fit in very well with the results that you conclude from the cohort studies. Now I can't fault the cohort studies but I do see a sort of mismatch of conclusions in the cohort studies, but does it explain these big population changes that we are seeing throughout the world?

Dr. Yajnik: Sachdev [1] wrote a systematic review a few years ago about birthweight in India and showed the magnitude of an increase in birthweight of about 52–126 g over a period of 25 years. Studies in Indian immigrants in the UK have not shown much change in birthweight [2, 3]. The question you ask is, 'Is the increasing obesity in adults matched by increasing birthweight?' The transfer of nutrients to the fetus is complex and if the fetus grew bigger compared to the mother's pelvis there would be a disaster. Christian and Osrin [4] analyzed the outcomes of maternal intervention in Nepal and Bangladesh where a multi-nutrient supplementation to the underweight women increased birthweight but also increased the perinatal and infant mortality.

Dr. Wharton: What I am saying is that there has been a 200-gram increase in birthweight, which is an amazing change in population terms on average birthweight. The conclusions we draw from cohort studies, shouldn't that increase in birthweight being accompanied by a reduction in obesity and yet you are seeing actually increases in obesity?

Dr. Yajnik: Birthweight is one aspect, ponderal index is the next complexity and body composition the next. Indian babies put on more fat when they put on weight. So increasing birthweight in Indian babies because of their adipose composition might increase the problem.

Dr. Shahkhalili: The increase in average birthweight is also due to a continuous increase in the number and weight of large babies, especially among obese/overweight mothers with gestational diabetes. Thus an increase in average birthweight does not reflect a birthweight improvement among small babies.

Dr. Popkin: I think we are completely mixing concepts related to averages vs. distributions. We are talking about the proportion of children with a certain ponderal index and a certain fetal environment and what comes later. Even in a country like China average birthweight is going up and low birthweight is going down, so we still have a subset of children who still suffer the kinds of problems that we have with the DOHAD group. You must be careful not to extrapolate too much from trends in cinome, etc., without studying the proportion poor.

Dr. Sawaya: I don't think birthweight is a good measurement or a good marker; I would say lean body mass. You need to know if lean body mass is increasing or not because just an increase in birthweight means an increase in body fat in many Western countries. I would like you to help me to understand your data in comparison to our data about the increase in height. You mentioned that in short parents there was an increase in the height of the baby and this was related to an increase in insulin resistance.

Dr. Yajnik: No, what I said was children who had grown more than what we would expect from the parental height had the highest insulin resistance. But this is an observational cross-sectional study.

Dr. Sawaya: As I showed you yesterday we had the normalization of height and in this case we had the normalization of insulin resistance as well. So that is not different to what you are showing.

Dr. Yajnik: It would be interesting to intervene and see if we are able to achieve this.

Dr. Sawaya: Among adults we showed that a BMI of <21.5 decreased productivity in Brazil in sugarcane workers. You are saying that a BMI of 18.1 is good enough in Indian terms to label capacity. I would like you to comment on these differences. Why do you think it is happening?

Dr. Yajnik: Basically we have described the average village woman. I am not saying that lower BMI does not compromise work activity because at a BMI of 20 she might have done better. But the WHO idea that at a BMI of <18.5 you are severely incapacitated is just not true because that one woman's activity in 1 day is more than my activity in a week.

Dr. Prentice: I have a question, but first I would quickly like to make a comment because the results of this discussion are going to appear in the book and I feel that there may be a misunderstanding. To my knowledge, and I have done quite a considerable amount of reading and analysis of this, there is actually no indication that low birthweight predisposes to obesity. We constantly quote the Ravelli study [5] in which there was in 19-year-olds a significant increase in a very small component of the population. The other Ravelli study [6] suggests that there is an association, but if you read it clearly there is no significant association. Meta-analyses have been done on this and in fact it is big babies that become obese, not small babies. There is a little bit of information to suggest that body fat pattern may be altered, a higher waist-hip

191

ratio in small babies but even there the effects are extremely small. So I think we need to be careful not to make any implication that small babies lead to obesity, there are different patterns that are going on and it is, as Dr. Yajnik has so elegantly shown, the disharmony of growth between what the child is programmed to do and what he actually does that causes the metabolic damage. If I could quickly ask a question, and again I congratulate you on your fantastic presentation and for leaving such novel thoughts in this field, the question is about extrapolatability. You have got a very heavily vegetarian population there, would you be able to extrapolate to African populations to some extent, and could you quickly comment on the conflicts and the paradoxes that your data reveal in relation to folate recommendations? And the final point is, what are the key markers? You have looked at homocysteine in terms of your pilot intervention but from your mechanistic model in your latest paper it may be that homocysteine is actually not the best thing to be measured.

Dr. Yajnik: The first question about extrapolation. When I started presenting these results, everyone told me that there is no B_{12} deficiency in India, so it took us 6 years to publish that. The reason was a paper from Vellore which was published 30 years ago and said that drinking 1.5 liters of water from a well provided enough B_{12} to the population. They were referring to microbial contamination. It was predicted that with better hygiene and a piped water supply, people will have B_{12} deficiency. We surveyed the literature from 1954, and a series of papers has been published about B_{12} deficiency in India, in migrant Indians in the UK, US and Singapore. We have analyzed samples from Delhi and South Indian and from Exeter in the UK. We found that Indians everywhere seem to have much lower B_{12} concentrations starting from cord blood to adult life [7]. Muthayya et al. [8] measured this in Bangalore and showed that low maternal B_{12} was a strong risk factor for intrauterine growth retardation. In Mysore and Exeter we have now found that low B_{12} is associated with obesity. So I think there is a basic biological association in this which needs investigation. Probably we should take Dr. Kalhan's advise on what we should measure, and probably use his help to do isotope studies to look at different pathways. In addition we plan to measure nonesterified fatty acids and 3-hydroxybutyrate. The ratio of 3-hydroxybutyrate to any fatty acid might give us an indication whether B_{12} deficiency blocks ketogenesis. This takes me back 25 years when my first few papers were actually on ketosis resistance in Indians. We seem to have one full circle. About folate supplementation there is a controversy. More than 50 countries have already introduced folic acid fortification in some form or other; in many countries it is mandatory; Australia has recently come on board; the UK I think is just now discussing the final stages, and there have been discussions in India on how to fortify flour with folic acid. My take on this is that both the vitamin B_{12} status of the population and the amount of folic acid need to be carefully considered. There is concern about an increase in dementia in the elderly and an increase in different forms of cancer. Smith et al. [9] wrote a review article on this subject. In India we should consider B_{12} supplementation along with folic acid. Otherwise we are likely to create a bigger imbalance and might open Pandora's box.

Dr. Haschke: My comment is also related to the potential imbalance between folic acid and vitamin B_{12} intake in the study population. The Nestlé Nutrition Institute recently conducted a survey among Indian obstetricians asking which supplements are important during pregnancy. Folic acid supplementation is generally accepted, but multivitamin supplements (including B_{12}) is seen by many obstetricians as a gimmick promoted by the industry. There seems to be a consensus during this discussion, however, that the vegetarian population in India has an increased risk of vitamin B_{12} deficiency.

Dr. Yajnik: There is another question of supplementing folic acid in already folate-replete populations because folic acid is different from folate. There are a number of chemical differences, a number of possible toxicities or unmetabolized folic acid. Smith et al. [9] have beautifully reviewed this, and recently there was a paper from Selhub et al. [10] showing that in B_{12}-deficient people increasing folate concentrations are associated with increasing homocysteine levels.

Dr. Kalhan: I just want to add that B_{12}–folate interaction is so important. If a large amount of folate is given to a B_{12}-deficient subject, folate is not going to work. We used to call that the folate trap and it should be kept in mind.

Dr. Vaidya: The presentation concerns clinical neonatology and pediatrics. All these data show the profound implications of rapid growth in later life. In neonatology today we are still making IUGR babies grow faster. We give them parenteral amino acids; we don't have the best formulas so we give them additional fortifications with fat. There is tremendous confusion as to what is the real benchmark for catch-up growth. How much should we make our babies grow? So far everybody is focusing on making IUGR babies grow and making them catch up faster. From these data we are very confused about the extent to which we make them catch up or do not make them catch up at all. What would you recommend; how should we neonatologists and pediatricians approach this problem in the community practice?

Dr. Yajnik: My first response is these are observational studies, not intervention studies. Our observation is that children who are born small but become big later tend to have trouble. This is not to say that you don't do anything, I just don't know what to do. Barker faced this criticism and therefore he went back to the Finnish cohort where many measurements were made in the first 2 years of life. What he showed is that poor growth in the first 2 years of life, what they call infant growth, predisposed to problems and it is the rapid growth after that period. We have now analyzed some of the data in the Pune Maternal Nutrition Study and found that insulin resistance at 6 years was associated with poor growth in the first 6 months, but after that they caught up. I think this needs to be investigated in very properly conducted trials.

Dr. Al Waili: In our country we have a program of folate supplementation and flour is fortified with folate. We rarely look at vitamin B_{12} although there is anemia, but we don't know if it is because of iron or vitamin B_{12} deficiency. Do you think the children in your studies have adiposity because the mothers consume more than 70% carbohydrates which convert to esterified fatty acid? What is the role of breastfeeding? We advise the mothers to exclusively breastfeed their children up to 6 months and we know that it will prevent adiposity, and it will also prevent diabetes later in life.

Dr. Yajnik: The micronutrient content of the diet did not relate to fetal growth in our study. That is not to say that it is not important; many people have suggested that a high carbohydrate content could be responsible for adiposity. I don't have a definite answer to that. We found an association between maternal intake of micronutrients and inflammatory markers (CRP) at 6 years. About breastfeeding in villages, almost every child was exclusively breastfed for a minimum of 6 months and yes, we advise breastfeeding.

Dr. Ajayi: As nutritionists we have been advising mothers to feed their children very well knowing that the intergenerational problems will not affect them. At what age does insulin resistance increase? In developing countries the majority of mothers give birth at home (70%), so we have no idea about the birthweight. What advise do we give the mothers, because the message has been feed your child to grow well? What role do fathers play in this life cycle? When you talk of the parents is the father included or is it only the mother?

Dr. Yajnik: About the role of the father, we were the first to include the father's measurements in the PMNS. The Exeter team has also written a number of papers

Yajnik

showing that maternal factors influence the soft tissues and adiposity in the baby, while paternal factors affect skeletal growth more. There are complexities within this scheme so that we are thinking of two things: one is the parent of origin effect and second the gender specificity because it seems that the effects may be different for boys and girls. We have discussed this issue in an editorial on fetal programming [11].

Dr. Singhal: The issue of promoting catch-up growth in small babies is very controversial but I think the important thing to remember is that the effect is different in various populations. Going back to the question about neonates, there is no doubt that promotion of growth in preterm babies or babies who are vulnerable is important for brain function and for the survival of the baby. In that population we would advocate that you should be promoting growth because of the favorable risk/benefit balance. I think the same applies to babies who are born in a vulnerable environment where it has been shown that promotion of growth helps survival. But I think faster growth promotion in small full-term babies from richer countries could have the opposite effect. There are roughly 27 studies showing that babies who grow faster in infancy are at increased risk of later obesity [12]. In the UK we don't advocate the promotion of growth in the healthy SGA baby [13]. So I think it is more complicated than applying a policy for all babies.

References

1 Sachdev HP: Low birth weight in south Asia: epidemiology and options for control. Int J Diab Dev Countries 2001;21:13–33.
2 Dhawan S: Birth weights of infants of first generation Asian women in Britain compared with second generation Asian women. BMJ 1995;311:86–88.
3 Margetts BM, Mohd Yusof S, Al Dallal Z, Jackson AA: Persistence of lower birth weight in second generation South Asian babies born in the United Kingdom. J Epidemiol Community Health 2002;56:684–687.
4 Christian P, Osrin D, Manandhar DS, et al: Antenatal micronutrient supplements in Nepal. Lancet 2005;366:711–712.
5 Ravelli GP, Stein ZA, Susser MW: Obesity in young men after famine exposure in utero and early infancy. N Engl J Med 1976;295:349–353.
6 Ravelli AC, van Der Meulen JH, Osmond C, et al: Obesity at the age of 50 y in men and women exposed to famine prenatally. Am J Clin Nutr 1999;70:811–816.
7 Yajnik CS, Deshpande SS, Lubree HG, et al: Vitamin B12 deficiency and hyperhomocysteinemia in rural and urban Indians. J Assoc Physicians India 2006;54:775–782.
8 Muthayya S, Kurpad AV, Duggan CP, et al: Low maternal vitamin B12 status is associated with intrauterine growth retardation in urban South Indians. Eur J Clin Nutr 2006;60:791–801.
9 Smith AD, Kim YI, Refsum H: Is folic acid good for everyone? Am J Clin Nutr 2008;87:517–533.
10 Selhub J, Morris MS, Jacques PF: In vitamin B_{12} deficiency, higher serum folate is associated with increased total homocysteine and methylmalonic acid concentrations. Proc Natl Acad Sci USA 2007;104:19995–20000.
11 Yajnik CS, Godbole K, Otiv SR, Lubree HG: Fetal programming of type 2 diabetes: is sex important? Diabetes Care 2007;30:2754–2755.
12 Ong KK, Ahmed ML, Emmett PM, et al: Association between postnatal catch-up growth and obesity in childhood: prospective cohort study. BMJ 2000;320:967–971.
13 Clayton PE, Cianfarani S, Czernichow P, et al: Management of the child born small for gestational age through to adulthood: a consensus statement of the International Societies of Pediatric Endocrinology and the Growth Hormone Research Society. J Clin Endocrinol Metab 2007;92:804–810.

Kalhan SC, Prentice AM, Yajnik CS (eds): Emerging Societies – Coexistence of Childhood Malnutrition and Obesity.
Nestlé Nutr Inst Workshop Ser Pediatr Program, vol 63, pp 195–208,
Nestec Ltd., Vevey/S. Karger AG, Basel, © 2009.

New Approaches to Optimizing Early Diets

Staffan Polberger

Neonatal Intensive Care Unit, Department of Paediatrics, University Hospital, Lund, Sweden

Abstract

Most extremely low birthweight (ELBW; <1,000 g) infants will survive if cared for at a tertiary neonatal intensive care unit, and should be given optimal nutrition for brain development. Human milk confers nutritional and non-nutritional advantages over infant formula, and is started during the first hours of life. In Sweden, most ELBW infants are fed individually with mother's own milk (preferred) and banked milk, with supplementary parenteral nutrition. There is an enormous variation particularly in the fat and protein content of milk between mothers, during the day and the course of lactation. Infrared macronutrient analyses on 24-hour collections of mother's milk are performed once a week allowing for optimal protein and energy intakes. All banked milk is analyzed, and the most protein-rich milk is given to a newborn ELBW infant. After 2 weeks, the milk may be fortified if the protein or energy intakes need to be further increased, and fortification is continued throughout the tube-feeding period. Parenteral nutrition is continued until the enteral intake constitutes 75–80% of the total volume intake. Protein markers, e.g. serum urea and transthyretin, are assessed, and growth is monitored by measurements of weight, crown–heel length and head circumference.

Introduction

The increasing number of extremely preterm infants who survive with gestational ages of 23 weeks and birthweights of 400 g is a new challenge to neonatology and neonatal nutrition. The vast majority of extremely low birthweight (ELBW) infants will survive if they are born and taken care of at a hospital with a tertiary neonatal intensive care unit. Nutrition is essential over several weeks consisting of periods of intermittent ventilator

Polberger

treatment, episodes of septicemia and persistent ductus arteriosus, which consistently lead to varying degrees of malnutrition upon discharge from hospital.

ELBW infants, particularly those born at 23–26 weeks of gestation, have an increased risk of school and cognitive problems and, to a limited extent, motor and vision problems [1]. There is also an epidemiologic association between low birthweight and cardiovascular disease later in life, particularly with rapid catch-up growth [2]. However, the general view is that preterm infants should be given optimal nutrition for brain growth and development [3]. Nutrition during the vulnerable preterm period, preferably based on human milk, should lead to adequate growth, at least corresponding to the intrauterine growth rate.

Feeding Systems

The best available method for nutrition of these infants during the preterm period is a combination of parenteral and enteral nutrition. Today, in Sweden most immature infants are fed according to the following scheme: (1) mother's own milk (preferred); (2) banked milk (if mother's own milk is not available); (3) preterm infant formula (only if human milk is not available), and (4) supplementary parenteral nutrition (starting at birth or immediately thereafter).

Parenteral Nutrition

There is a trend to a more 'aggressive' nutrition of preterm infants, i.e. initiating parenteral nutrition early after birth including starting administration of not only intravenous glucose but also amino acids and lipids immediately after birth or during the first day of life [4]. Enteral feeding with human milk is also started during the first few hours of life [5]. Parenteral nutrition is continued until the enteral intake constitutes 75–80% of the total volume intake. It has been shown that early intravenous amino acids are well tolerated and can be utilized as a substrate for protein synthesis during the first day of life [6]. The distribution of amino acids contributes to a more stable glucose homeostasis [4], and amino acids also act as precursors for the synthesis of various hormones, enzymes and neurotransmitters. Moreover, early intravenous lipids can usually be started during the first day of life as a concentrated substrate for energy. Administration of intravenous lipids also diminishes the risk of a deficiency of essential fatty acids. Total parenteral nutrition should be avoided in the immature infant and is given only in situations with intestinal malformations or severe necrotizing enterocolitis (NEC).

Parenteral nutrition can be administered as a solution containing glucose, amino acids, lipids, minerals, vitamins and trace elements. As an alternative,

196

the lipid solution including vitamins can be given separately. Most of the available components for parenteral solutions are not completely adequate for the special needs of ELBW infants, and there is a need for development in this area.

The ready-to-use solutions should, if not commercially available, be prepared under sterile conditions at the pharmacy.

Enteral Nutrition

Previously, there was a fear of causing NEC if enteral feeding was initiated early. However, it has been shown that enteral nutrition, preferably with breast milk, can be started a few hours after birth and the volumes gradually increased [5] with a low risk of developing NEC [7, 8]. After a few weeks the supplementary parenteral nutrition can usually be discontinued and the infant completely enterally fed. During the first days of life, banked milk (from another woman, preferably from another mother of a preterm infant) is given until the mother's own milk is available.

Tube feeding is mandatory until the infant can be fed by the nipple or bottle, usually at an age corresponding to 35–36 weeks of gestation. Whether the ELBW infant should be tube fed continuously or intermittently every 2nd or 3rd h is still a matter of controversy [8]. Also, there is no agreement on whether the tube should be placed by the orogastric or nasogastric route. In Sweden, most mothers manage to express their milk during the preterm period and breastfeed their infants at discharge from the hospital.

Superiority of Human Milk

During the last years, there is a growing body of evidence that human milk is superior to infant formula for all newborn infants including ELBW infants [9]. Human milk confers nutritional and non-nutritional advantages, and there is now a worldwide trend to using more human milk than infant formula in the feeding of preterm infants [10]. Outcome data support the improved neurological development when human milk is used [11], even if human milk intake has been limited to only a few weeks [12]. The risk of infection, retinopathy and NEC also seems to be lower if the infant is fed human milk as opposed to formula [7, 13]. Human milk is also better tolerated by the immature intestine than infant formula [3, 9].

If the mother's own milk is not available, banked human milk should be used [14]. Infant formula is used only in situations in which there is a complete lack of breast milk and, if used, only preterm formulas, not term formulas, should be given. To reduce the risk of transmission of viral and bacterial infections, banked milk is pasteurized before use (usually Holder pasteurization, 62.5°C for 30 min).

Preterm Milk

In the 1970s it was shown that the milk of mothers of preterm infants had higher concentrations of protein and fat, at least for the first weeks of lactation, but this difference may persist in some mothers for several months [15, 16].

Human Milk Macronutrient Variation

Unfortunately the misconception that human milk has a predictable and uniform composition is still widespread in many neonatal units throughout the world. However, several studies have underlined the enormous variation in the nutrient composition of human milk, particularly fat and also protein. There are variations between mothers, during the course of lactation, and during individual meals (fig. 1), and also as a consequence of the varying pumping techniques [17–20]. This has to be taken into account when using breast milk in the nutrition of ELBW infants.

Human Milk Analyses

To find a tool to determine the macronutrient content (protein, fat, carbohydrates and energy) of human milk from individual mothers, after evaluation of available chemical methods [21], we found that the most reliable method for analyzing the macronutrient content of milk is the infrared (IR) technique [18]. During the last 10–15 years, a system has been established in Sweden where most neonatal units use a centrally situated IR instrument for routine analyses [19, 22].

However, there is now a new and less expensive IR instrument available. It was originally developed for cow's milk, but modified and calibrated for human milk against reference methods for fat, protein, lactose and total solids (Rose-Gottlieb, Kjeldahl, Luff-Schorl and drying-oven, respectively) with an accuracy of $r \geq 0.98$ (Miris AB, Uppsala, Sweden) [23]. This equipment can be used bedside in the neonatal unit allowing analyses to be run on small amounts of milk (1 ml in duplicate or triplicate) at a low cost with the results available within 1 min for immediate use.

Analysis of the protein content in milk based on a calibrated Kjeldahl method probably slightly exaggerates the amounts of nutritionally available protein, but the method yields a reasonable appreciation of the need for fortification.

Perhaps equally important is how to get a representative human milk sample for analysis [24]. Fresh milk is usually not a problem, but when using the IR technique frozen-thawed milk can give unreliable results due

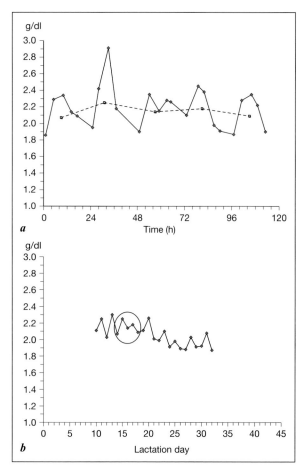

Fig. 1. **a** Day-to-day (—) and meal-to-meal (– – –) variation in milk protein content of a mother delivering a preterm infant. '0' indicates 6 a.m. on day 14. **b** Daily 24-hour protein collections. All spot samples were analyzed for 5 days (120 h) during lactation days 14–18 as indicated by the circle.

to the formation of complexes and may need homogenization before being analyzed.

The enormous meal-to-meal variation, mainly in fat and protein concentrations (fig. 1), makes it useless to analyze spot samples (milk from a single collection) [20, 22]. Instead, milk should be collected preferentially over 24 h, well mixed, and a representative sample taken for analysis [19]. Such 24-hour collections analyzed once or twice a week give sufficient information on the macronutrient content of the milk for reliable estimations of the actual macronutrient intakes [22].

Polberger

Techniques to reduce the variation in nutrient intake of ELBW infants are the following.
- Mother's own milk is given in chronological order, i.e. in the order it was pumped. As the protein content will slowly decrease during the course of lactation, the most immature infant will receive the earliest milk with a higher protein level.
- All milk is mixed in 24-hour collections before being given or frozen for later use. This will substantially reduce the day-to-day and meal-to-meal variation in nutrient content, which is likely to increase gut tolerance (fig. 1).

Fortification of Human Milk

The enteral nutrition of choice should always be breast milk [10]. However, the content of certain nutrients in the milk, such as protein, is not always sufficient to meet the extreme needs of ELBW infants [25, 26]. Therefore, there is usually a need to fortify the milk during the tube-feeding period.

There are various fortifiers available on the market, all of them (with one exception) of bovine origin. As there are no comparative studies, it is still unclear whether the source of energy should be carbohydrates or fat.

Various methods have been used to fortify milk for feeding of preterm infants.

Standardized Fortification
Standardized (blind) fortification, often started at 1 week of age, is widely used in the belief that all human milk has a uniform composition. The same amount of fortifier is added to the milk regardless of whether it is own or banked mature milk with quite different compositions. This method may cause under- or overnutrition and should be avoided [3, 19, 27, 28].

Semiquantitative Fortification
This seems to be a slightly better method, as the milk to be enriched is taken into account. For example, the preterm infant's mother's milk can be expected to have a higher protein content than the milk of a mother of a term infant after 3 months of lactation.

Individualized Fortification
The individualized feeding regimen is used in Lund, Sweden. This feeding system focuses firstly on protein intake, secondly on energy intake, and is used, at least in part, in most neonatal units throughout Sweden [22].

By analyzing the macronutrient content of the milk, the intake of the individual infant can be adjusted accordingly [19, 21]. Aiming initially at a daily protein intake of 3.5–4 g/kg in the ELBW infant or, later during the preterm period 3 g/kg, the milk can be individually fortified in relation to the gestational age of the infant. Short-term studies of the individualized feeding system indicate improved growth corresponding to the intrauterine growth rate [19, 28, 29].

Computerized Calculations

A computerized calculation system for nutrient intakes will increase the safety of the calculations and diminish the time required to evaluate the need for appropriate fortification. Such a system is used at our unit and is also available as part of various clinical information systems used in intensive care units.

Individualized Fortification (table 1)

Milk is fortified as deemed necessary (after calculating the protein intake starting at 10–14 days of age). There is no reason to start analyzing the nutrient content earlier due to the rapid changes in protein concentrations and the enhanced protein intake by the increased enteral volumes during the first weeks of life.

After fortifying the milk to achieve the desired protein intake, extra energy may be added if needed (usually using a liquid lipid preparation).

Even in situations of intestinal intolerance, try to avoid discarding the fortification completely. Instead try to diminish the amount of fortifier added to the milk.

Protein markers such as serum urea and transthyretin may be used to evaluate the metabolic capacity of the protein utilized [28, 30].

Growth

Growth corresponding to the intrauterine growth rate of a fetus of corresponding gestational age is the current goal in the nutrition of preterm infants [25, 26]. Not because growth itself is important but rather because poor growth is a marker of inadequate nutrition, which is associated with less favorable cognitive development [27].

Nutritional Status

To assess the nutritional status of the infant, the variables given in table 2, including protein markers, should be monitored continuously during the preterm period.

Table 1. Individualized nutrition of preterm infants: the Swedish model as performed in Lund, Sweden

---

- All preterm infants are fed human milk (mother's own milk is preferred), at least until 34 weeks of gestation
- The mother is encouraged to start pumping her milk (as soon as possible or at least within 24 h after birth) using an electric pump
- Banked milk (preferably preterm milk) is given during the first days of life, and later (rarely) if the mother's own milk is not available
- All banked milk is analyzed for macronutrient content (fat, protein, lactose and energy), and the most protein-rich milk is chosen when a new preterm infant is born
- Enteral feeding with banked milk is started within 2–4 h of life
- Parenteral nutrition with glucose and amino acids is started at birth, and lipids are initiated within the first 24 h of life. Supplementary parenteral nutrition is continued until enteral feeding constitutes 75–80% of the total volume intake
- The intake of human milk is gradually increased as tolerated (with corresponding decreased parenteral nutrition) until full amounts
- All mother's own milk (<32 weeks gestation) is analyzed for macronutrient content (24-hour collections, never spot samples) once (twice) a week, starting at 10–14 days of life
- Mother's own milk is used in chronological order to diminish the day-to-day variation in protein and particularly fat intake
- All mother's milk is mixed in 24-hour collections before being frozen or administered to reduce the meal-to-meal variation in protein and fat content
- Using a specific calculator, macronutrient intakes and the need for fortification are regularly calculated, at least after each milk analysis
- When the milk volumes can no longer be increased and there is a need of higher protein or energy intakes, fortification with a commercial fortifier is started, aiming at daily intakes of 3.5–4 g protein (the higher protein intake in the more immature infant) and 110–120 kcal/kg (or higher if there are lung problems)
- Growth is monitored (weight every 2nd day, length and head circumference weekly), and a computerized growth curve is used
- Protein status is assessed by analyses of serum urea and transthyretin once a week
- Fortification of the milk is continued throughout the tube-feeding period, usually until 35–36 weeks of gestation when breastfeeding is initiated
- Infant formula (preterm formula) is used when there is a lack of human milk, but never <32 weeks of gestation

---

Conclusion

A new approach to optimizing the early diet of preterm infants is presented. The nutrition of the growing number of surviving very preterm infants is extremely important in order to diminish neurological problems, especially in infants with less than 30 weeks of gestation. Human milk is more advantageous than infant formula for the feeding of these infants. However, human milk does not have a uniform composition. Due to the huge variation in the

Table 2. Nutritional status of the preterm infant

1.Growth
    Weight
    Crown–heel length
    Head circumference
2.Nutrient intakes
    Protein
    Energy
3.Metabolic markers
    Protein markers, e.g. serum urea and transthyretin
4.Clinical data
    Gastric residuals
    Abdominal distension
    Vomiting
    Apneas

---

content of various nutrients, particularly protein and fat, there is a need to analyze the macronutrient content of the individual mother's milk, allowing individualized fortification and nutrition including assessment of a protein marker. So far, macronutrients have been analyzed, but in the future certain minerals may also be evaluated and supplied individually.

Acknowledgement

The individualized feeding system described was funded in part by a grant from the Nils W. Svenningsen Foundation for Neonatal Research.

References

1 Wood NS, Costeloe K, Gibson AT, et al: The EPICure study: associations and antecedents of neurological and developmental disability at 30 months of age following extremely preterm birth. Arch Dis Child Fetal Neonatal Ed 2005;90:F134–F140.
2 Barker DJP: Fetal origins of coronary heart disease. Br Med J 1995;311:171–174.
3 Lucas A, Fewtrell M: Feeding low-birthweight infants; in Rennie JM (ed): Roberton's Textbook of Neonatology. Amsterdam, Elsevier, 2005, pp 314–324.
4 Ziegler EE, Thureen PJ, Carlson SJ: Aggressive nutrition of the very low birthweight infant. Clin Perinatol 2002;29:225–244.
5 Bellander M, Ley D, Polberger S, Hellström-Westas L: Tolerance to early human milk feeding is not compromised by indomethacin in preterm infants with persistent ductus arteriosus. Acta Paediatr 2003;92:1074–1078.
6 te Braake FWJ, van den Akker CHP, Riedijk MA, van Goudoever JB: Parenteral amino acid and energy administration to premature infants in early life. Semin Fetal Neonatal Med 2007;12:11–18.
7 Lucas A, Cole TJ: Breast milk and necrotising enterocolitis. Lancet 1990;336:1519–1523.
8 Newell SJ: Enteral feeding of the micropremie. Clin Perinatol 2000;27:221–234.
9 Heiman H, Schanler RJ: Enteral nutrition for premature infants: the role of human milk. Semin Fetal Neonatal Med 2007;12:26–34.

10 American Academy of Pediatrics Committee on Nutrition: Nutritional needs of low-birth-weight infants. Pediatrics 1985;75:976–986.

11 Vohr BR, Poindexter BB, Dusick AM, et al: Persistent beneficial effects of breast milk ingested in the neonatal intensive care unit on outcomes of extremely low birth weight infants at 30 months of age. Pediatrics 2007;120:e953–e959.

12 Isaacs EB, Gadian DG, Sabatini S, et al: The effect of early human diet on caudate volumes and IQ. Pediatr Res 2008;63:308–314.

13 Boyd CA, Quigley MA, Brocklehurst P: Donor breast milk versus infant formula for preterm infants: systematic review and meta-analysis. Arch Dis Child Fetal Neonatal Ed 2007;92:F169–F175.

14 Williams AF, Kingdon CC, Weaver G: Banking for the future: investing in human milk. Arch Dis Child Fetal Neonatal Ed 2007;92:F158–F159.

15 Atkinson SA, Bryan MH, Anderson GH: Human milk. Difference in nitrogen concentration in milk from mothers of term and premature infants. J Pediatr 1978;93:67–69.

16 Butte NF, Garza C, Johnson CA, et al: Longitudinal changes in milk composition of mothers delivering preterm and term infants. Early Hum Dev 1984;9:153–162.

17 Hibberd CM, Brooke OG, Carter ND, et al: Variation in the composition of breast milk during the first 5 weeks of lactation: implications for the feeding of preterm infants. Arch Dis Child 1982;57:658–662.

18 Michaelsen KF, Skafte L, Badsberg JH, Jørgensen M: Variation in macronutrients in human bank milk: Influencing factors and implications for human milk banking. J Pediatr Gastroenterol Nutr 1990;11:229–239.

19 Polberger S, Räihä NCR, Juvonen P, et al: Individualized protein fortification of human milk for preterm infants: comparison of ultrafiltrated human milk protein and a bovine whey fortifier. J Pediatr Gastroenterol Nutr 1999;29:332–338.

20 Weber A, Loui A, Jochum F, et al: Breast milk from mothers of very low birthweight infants: variability in fat and protein content. Acta Paediatr 2001;90:772–775.

21 Polberger S, Lönnerdal B: Simple and rapid macronutrient analyses of human milk for individualized fortification: basis for improved nutritional management of very low birth weight infants? J Pediatr Gastroenterol Nutr 1993;17:283–290.

22 Omarsdottir S, Casper C, Åkerman A, et al: Breastmilk handling routines for preterm infants in Sweden: a national cross-sectional study. Breastfeed Med 2008;3:165–170.

23 Selander B, Polberger S: Improved individualized nutritional management of preterm infants using a bedside, low-volume human milk analyzer (poster). Pediatric Academic Society Annual Meeting, Toronto, May 2007.

24 Picciano MF: What constitutes a representative human milk sample? J Pediatr Gastroenterol Nutr 1984;3:280–283.

25 Gartner LM, Morton J, Lawrence RA, et al; American Academy of Pediatrics Section on Breastfeeding: Breastfeeding and the use of human milk. Pediatrics 2005;115:496–506.

26 Nutrition and feeding of preterm infants. Committee on Nutrition of the Preterm Infant, European Society of Paediatric Gastroenterology and Nutrition. Acta Paediatr Scand Suppl 1987;336:2–14.

27 Ziegler EE: Breast-milk fortification. Acta Paediatr 2001;90:720–723.

28 Arslanoglu S, Moro GE, Ziegler EE: Adjustable fortification of human milk fed to preterm infants: does it make a difference? J Perinatol 2006;26:614–621.

29 de Halleux V, Close A, Stalport S, et al: Advantages of individualized fortification of human milk for preterm infants. Arch Pediatr 2007;14(suppl):S5–S10.

30 Polberger SKT, Fex GA, Axelsson IE, Räihä NCR: Eleven plasma proteins as indicators of protein nutritional status in very low birth weight infants. Pediatrics 1990;86:916–921.

Discussion

Dr. Lafeber: It is very important that you have shown in this meeting that it is possible to use breast milk even for extremely small preterm infants. Nevertheless I would like to put your setting in Sweden in perspective to the rest of the world. I am from Amsterdam, the Netherlands, and we also have an affluent society that is pre-pared to invest a lot of money in extremely preterm infants of 24–25 weeks gestational age. However, if you are going to promote the use of breast milk I would put more emphasis on somewhat older preterm infants. The reason for this remark is the fact that we performed several studies measuring protein turnover using stable isotope ^{13}C-glycine in very low birthweight preterm infants with a birthweight of <1,000 g. We found that even using the maximum of fortification in breast milk, it was difficult to achieve a protein turnover of >2 g protein/kg per day. We published that about 3 years ago and using the special preterm formula we could indeed reach levels above that limit [1]. So especially in preterm infants with a gestational age of <27–28 weeks, it is important that you must be aware that we have to fortify human milk with extra protein. Another issue when giving breast milk to preterm infants is the fact that you also have to keep in mind the supplementation of calcium, phosphate, and vitamin D. I told you yesterday after the presentation of Dr. Kalhan that we performed a study comparing the feeding of preterm infants after discharge from the hospital with a spe-cial post-discharge formula or breast milk, and what we found at 6 months corrected age was that the most important issue in very preterm infants is to add extra protein and calories until the moment of term, and from then onwards only extra protein and a normal amount of calories were given, like that in a normal standard formula [2]. We did not fortify human milk after discharge from hospital and we observed a similar growth rate compared to infants fed post-discharge formula. The only difference that we found at 6 months was that the mineral content measured by DEXA scan was lower in breastfed infants, so we might also not be sufficient in supplying enough cal-cium and phosphate between term age and 6 months corrected age in preterm infants fed breast milk. On the other hand the body composition at 6 months of the breastfed preterm infants showed less fat at 6 months and there was less insulin insensitivity, so I really do believe in your concept that it is very important to give breast milk to preterm infants but be aware that it is not always possible to establish the Swedish system in other countries because it is a phenomenal cost to have pasteurization and completely individualized care. The level of hygiene you need in the neonatal unit is tremendous, and to date we have not been successful in establishing that situation in the Netherlands [3].

Dr. Polberger: First a comment about the fortifiers. Today we use multicomponent fortifiers but with the individual system we rarely need full fortification. We need a separate system where we can supply extra minerals, which we actually do. So from my point of view I would in the future prefer having different fortifiers consisting of protein, some sort of energy source, and a mineral preparation which would allow us to deliver a more individualized fortification system to these infants.

Dr. De Curtis: I agree that human milk is the best food for premature infants; how-ever, giving fresh breast milk to extremely low birthweight infants could lead to some neonatal infectious problems, such as cytomegalovirus infection. In your unit do you give the mothers' own fresh milk to all extremely low birthweight infants even if you ignore the mother's immunological status? What is the percentage of low birthweight infants breastfed at discharge in your unit? If these babies are extremely breast-fed, do you give any fortification at home to increase protein and mineral intake? Macronutrient analysis of human milk based on the infrared technique is expensive and time-consuming but it could be useful for scientific purposes. However, in clinical practice, as seen many years ago by Rigo et al. [4], the simple evaluation of growth or, if necessary, the evaluation of serum urea levels could be sufficient to estimate the adequacy of protein intake.

Dr. Polberger: For macronutrient analyses, we now have a new IR machine avail-able which costs less than USD 20,000, and that is good enough to buy it for separate neonatal units in Sweden. To reduce the risk of cytomegalovirus transmission from the mother's own milk, we give the milk in chronological order, and usually we freeze the milk for a few days before giving it to the baby during the preterm period. I am aware that Hamprecht et al. [5] have suggested that all milk, including mother's own milk, should be pasteurized before giving it to a baby to eradicate this risk, but so far this has not been accepted in Sweden. The final question was about breastfeeding after discharge. In our unit about 75–80% of the mothers are breastfeeding when they go home. Fortification at home is a difficult question. We usually do not fortify the milk after discharge, and at the moment we don't know the optimal method of feeding the baby after discharge. It is much easier during the preterm period when the baby is tube-fed and the milk is easily available for analyses and fortification, but it is much harder to do that when the baby is on full breastfeeding at home. We discussed this with Dr. Lafeber the other day and there are some studies going on, among them a multicenter study in Denmark, which hopefully will give us some answers. They are actually fortifying the milk when breastfeeding by giving the baby some extra fortified milk.

Dr. Bohles: This is possibly a very provocative question. In utero the child is basically alimented intravenously, even the liver is bypassed. So why are we so reluctant in parenteral nutrition with respect to the very immature child? We are relying much more on immature digestion processes and basically we don't really know what is finally reaching the metabolism of the child. Why don't we further develop the intravenous route?

Dr. Polberger: That is an interesting question and there has been a lot of discussion about this. The trend at the moment is to try to reduce parenteral nutrition and start enteral nutrition as soon as possible. There are a lot of negative side effects using parenteral nutrition, for instance infections and thrombosis in the vessels being used. The risk of necrotizing enterocolitis (NEC) can actually be reduced by using human milk. So from the theoretical point of view it would be interesting to continue placental function with cord circulation but I don't think that is realistic. Most neonatal units today are using parenteral nutrition as a supplement and an important part of the nutrition, starting at birth or very early, but then trying to proceed to enteral nutrition and withhold parenteral nutrition. Infection is a serious problem in these infants.

Anonymous: We know that once you feed very low birthweight babies very early with high calories they develop NEC. In your study how many babies with NEC did you encounter?

Dr. Polberger: We see only 1 or 2 NEC cases a year. I don't have the exact figures but we actually see more NEC in full-term sick babies than in preterm infants. We attribute the low figures to the use of human milk and enteral feeding.

Dr. Bhattacharya: You talked about bronchopulmonary dysplasia (BPD) and high caloric intake. Do all the chronic lung disease (CLD) babies have the same benefit if they are given high calories? The second question is about protein markers, urea and transthyretin. Do you do that mainly after parenteral nutrition or before or during the course of enteral nutrition, and what about infrared counting of macronutrients?

Dr. Polberger: In babies with BPD and CLD we evaluate their growth, and as some of these infants need extra energy, we usually use a commercial fortifier to supply the amount of protein needed and, if necessary, add extra fat in a liquid preparation.

Dr. Bhattacharya: Does this improve the outcome of BPD and CLD?

Dr. Polberger: It happens that we discharge babies who are still on oxygen, usually using an oxygen concentrator for a few weeks, but that only happens a few times a year. This problem has diminished over the years with more efficient ventilation modes and is not really a big issue in our unit, fortunately. We use protein markers on a routine basis and try to analyze them once a week during the preterm period. We start with human milk analysis mainly using the protein content of the milk and then we supply the extra fortifier needed. If in that situation we have low serum urea or transthyretin we add more protein.

Dr. Vaidya: So far we have been following the ESPGHAN committee recommendations for feeding our preterm infants, and we also use the same guidelines for the SGA infants. Before the metabolic syndrome, these guidelines were highly recommended in these babies. In light of the recent information, do you think these recommendations will undergo a change? With the aggressive nutrition of low birthweight babies, how is this going to affect the metabolic syndrome in the days to come? When these low birthweight and SGA infants go home, should we routinely start screening them for metabolic syndrome and at what age we should start?

Dr. Polberger: The metabolic syndrome may of course be a problem, but these infants are vulnerable from the cognitive point of view. During the preterm period, Lucas [6] has suggested that we have to think mainly about neurodevelopment. The protein intake cannot be decreased during these vulnerable weeks for that reason. But I am sure we have not seen the end of that discussion, and we really don't know the implications of the metabolic syndrome discussion for these tiny infants. So at the moment we try to feed them efficiently based on human milk. And your final question, we are following these infants for 5–6 years. We have no specific screening program for the metabolic syndrome, but that is an interesting question.

Dr. Haschke: First a comment on the device which measures protein, fat, and carbohydrates in human milk. It is definitely available in India and used by dairy companies to standardize cow's milk quality. My question is, in Sweden can you achieve intrauterine growth rates in low birthweight infants who are fed fortified breast milk or specialized formulas?

Dr. Polberger: As you know, all these infants are actually being discharged with some degree of malnutrition. At term they weigh almost 1 kg less than expected as compared to the in utero situation. So with our current methods we don't manage very well. We always use mother's own milk and we fortify it accordingly, and that is the best we can do right now. But there is a period, especially if you have a very sick preterm infant, when no catch-up growth occurs until sometimes 3–4 weeks of age. At the moment we have to accept that the baby is not always reaching the intrauterine growth rate. That can only be seen in the most healthy preterm infants.

Dr. Haschke: But to clarify this, in no case do you reach a so-called catch-up growth with your measures?

Dr. Polberger: We do it now and then. Usually we see catch-up growth later on. There has actually been a Swedish study where you can see catch-up growth still occurring at 11 years of age in previously preterm infants.

References

1 de Boo HA, Cranendonk A, Kulik W, et al: Whole body protein turnover and urea production of preterm small for gestational age infants fed fortified human milk or preterm formula. J Pediatr Gastroenterol Nutr 2005;41:81–87.
2 Amesz E, Schaafsma A, Lafeber HN: Similar growth but altered body composition in preterm infants fed enriched 'postdischarge' formula without extra calories, standard formula or human milk, from term until 6 months corrected age. J Pediatr Gastroenterol Nutr 2009, in press.
3 Lafeber HN, Westerbeek EA, van den Berg A, et al: Nutritional factors influencing infections in preterm infants. J Nutr 2008;138:1813S–1817S.

4 Rigo J, Salle BL, Putet G, Senterre J: Nutritional evaluation of various protein hydrolysate formulae in term infants during the first month of life. Acta Paediatr Suppl 1994;402:100–104.
5 Hamprecht K, Maschmann J, Müller D, et al: Cytomegalovirus (CMV) inactivation in breast milk: reassessment of pasteurization and freeze-thawing. Pediatr Res 2004;56:529–535.
6 Lucas A: Programming by early nutrition: an experimental approach. J Nutr 1998;128(suppl):401S–406S.

Kalhan SC, Prentice AM, Yajnik CS (eds): Emerging Societies – Coexistence of Childhood Malnutrition and Obesity.
Nestlé Nutr Inst Workshop Ser Pediatr Program, vol 63, pp 209–225,
Nestec Ltd., Vevey/S. Karger AG, Basel, © 2009.

Prevention of Low Birthweight

Dewan S. Alam

Public Health Sciences Division, International Centre for Diarrhoeal Disease Research, Bangladesh, Dhaka, Bangladesh

Abstract

Globally an estimated 20 million infants are born with low birthweight (LBW), of those over 18 million are born in developing countries. These LBW infants are at a disproportionately higher risk of mortality, morbidity, poor growth, impaired psychomotor and cognitive development as immediate outcomes, and are also disadvantaged as adults due to their greater susceptibility to type 2 diabetes, hypertension and coronary heart disease. Maternal malnutrition prior to and during pregnancy manifested by low bodyweight, short stature, inadequate energy intake during pregnancy and coexisting micronutrient deficiency are considered major determinants in developing countries where the burden is too high. LBW is a multifactorial outcome and its prevention requires a lifecycle approach and interventions must be continued for several generations. So far, most interventions are targeted during pregnancy primarily due to the increased nutritional demand and aggravations of already existing inadequacy in most women. Several individually successful interventions during pregnancy include balanced protein energy supplementation, several single micronutrients or more recently a mix of multiple micronutrients. Nutrition education has been successful in increasing the dietary intake of pregnant women but has had no effect on LBW. The challenge is to identify a community-specific intervention package. Current evidence supports intervention during pregnancy with increased dietary intakes including promotions of foods rich in micronutrients and micronutrient supplementation, preferably with a multiple micronutrient mix. Simultaneously a culturally appropriate educational component is required to address misconceptions about diet during pregnancy and childbirth including support for healthy pregnancy with promotion of antenatal and perinatal care services. While further research is needed to identify more efficacious interventions, an urgent public health priority would be to select and implement an optimal mix of interventions to avert the immediate adverse consequences of LBW and to prevent the impending epidemic of type 2 diabetes, hypertension and coronary heart disease which are negatively associated with LBW.

Introduction

Globally an estimated 20 million or 15.5% of babies are born with low birth-weight (LBW) defined as less than 2,500 g at birth with wide variations over different geographic locations [1]. However, over 90% of all LBW infants are born in developing countries and nearly a half of the total global burden of LBW infants is distributed in South Central Asian countries. LBW infants represent a heterogeneous group of infants which may result from suboptimal fetal growth relative to gestational age, called intrauterine growth retardation (IUGR) or small-for-gestational age (SGA), or too early delivery, called pre-term delivery (<37 week of gestation). In general, IUGR is the predominant type of LBW in populations in poorer settings where the prevalence of LBW is high, whereas preterm delivery predominates in settings where the prevalence of LBW is low as in developed countries [2]. The distinction between these two entities has important programmatic implications as the determinants are often different and so are the interventions.

LBW has enormous consequences for health and survival. Infants born with LBW are at an increased risk of mortality, morbidity, poor growth, impaired cognitive function, decreased motor and psychomotor development [3–7]. The mortality gradient increases several fold as birthweight decreases [8]. LBW also greatly increases the risk of infant death due to other causes, such as acute lower respiratory infection, pneumonia and diarrhea [9, 10]. Although very high birthweight also increases the risk of mortality and morbidity, such incidences in developing countries are low. Infants born LBW due to IUGR remain shorter and lighter as adults [11] and may also suffer immune incompetence as older children and as young adults compared to normal birthweight infants [12, 13].

The long-term negative consequences of LBW are associated with the risk of type 2 diabetes, hypertension, and cardiovascular diseases in later life [14–16]. The elevated risk of these disease outcomes is not just limited to LBW but ranges across the distribution of birthweights [17–19]. LBW has huge economic costs which are related to excess mortality, morbidity and productivity loss due to the disproportionately higher rate of stunting and cognitive deficits among those who born LBW [20].

Extensive review of studies from developed and developing countries identified determinants of LBW and population-attributable risk associated with each major determinant [21]. Subsequent studies also reported similar determinants [22–24]. In developing countries maternal nutritional factors that include low pre-pregnancy weight, short stature, low energy intake during pregnancy, or low gestational weight gain are the major determinants [21]. Teenage pregnancy and morbidity are also important risk factors for LBW. Cigarette smoking and alcohol consumption are important determinants but they are more important in developed countries. In some settings HIV status and malaria are also important determinants, particularly in African countries where HIV and malaria coexist with maternal malnutrition [25–27]. Micronutrients play an important role in the growth and development of the fetus. In communities where LBW exists as a significant public health problem, widespread maternal malnutrition [28, 29] coexists with multiple micronutrient (MMN) deficiencies [30, 31]. This chapter briefly discusses some interventions deemed to be successful and which can be considered in the prevention of LBW, mainly in developing countries where the burden is too high.

Interventions for Prevention of LBW

Success of public health interventions for the prevention of LBW depends on how well population-specific quantitatively important determinants are identified and targeted. Interventions with a life-cycle approach and targeting several generations are needed to alleviate this intergenerational effect. However, most of the interventions for LBW are targeted during pregnancy because the vulnerability of already existing dietary inadequacy is further aggravated during pregnancy. Major successful interventions which look at LBW as an outcome and have great relevance in developing countries include balanced protein energy supplementation, micronutrient supplementation (single or combination), and nutrition education.

Food Supplementation and LBW

Dietary deprivation during pregnancy has a negative effect on fetal growth. Studies on the Dutch Famine of 1944–1945 showed that, during the third trimester, pregnant women who were exposed to a severe energy-restricted diet delivered lighter babies than unexposed women [32]. This natural experiment provides strong justification for food supplementation during pregnancy in populations at risk of dietary inadequacy. A Cochrane Systematic Review of food supplementation trials during pregnancy concluded that only a balanced protein energy supplementation modestly increases birthweight and reduces the incidence of LBW [33]. The latest review of balanced protein energy supplementation trials included 6 trials which reported SGA as outcome and met the methodological criteria for the review (table 1). The trails represented populations from both developing (Taiwan, The Gambia, India and Columbia) and developed countries (Wales and USA). Although all the trials included were not similar in terms of timing and duration of supplementation, composition of the supplemental food, total energy content and allocation procedure, the homogeneity of effect with a lower relative risk for SGA was reported. All the trials, except the Gambian, obtained unity in the confidence interval for the relative risk due to the lack of adequate power. However, the pooled estimate showed a significant reduction (32%) in SGA in the intervention group. SGA infants

212

Table 1. Prenatal balanced protein energy supplementation and incidence of small-for-gestational age infants

Study	Population	Intervention	Treatment n/N[1]	Control n/N	Relative Risk (95% CI)
Blackwell 1973	Taiwan	Supplemented: 40 g protein and 800 kcal/d plus vitamins and minerals Controls: vitamins and minerals	6/94	10/88	0.56 (0.21, 1.48)
Cessay 1997	The Gambia	Supplemented: 1,017 kcal energy, 22 g protein, 56 g fat, 47 mg calcium and 1.8 mg iron daily Control villages: no supplement	69/620	94/553	0.65 (0.49, 0.87)
Elwood 1981	Wales	Supplemented: fat-free milk Controls: no supplement	27/591	27/562	0.88 (0.52, 1.50)
Girija 1984	India	Supplemented: 417 kcal energy and 30 g protein Controls: usual diet	0/10	5/10	0.09 (0.01, 1.45)
Mora 1978	Columbia	Supplemented: 865 kcal and 38.4 g protein Controls: usual diet	12/177	14/162	0.78 (0.37, 1.65)
Rush 1980	USA	Supplemented: 322 kcal energy and 6 g protein and vitamins/minerals Controls: vitamins/minerals only	30/265	43/264	0.70 (0.45, 1.07)
Total			1,757	1,639	0.68 (0.56, 0.84)

[1] n = Number of SGA infants; N = total number in the treatment/control.
Reproduced with permission from Kramer and Kakuma [33].

are the major contributor to the LBW burden in developing countries. Apart from the lower incidence of LBW (39% reduction), the Gambian study [34] reported several other beneficial outcomes including increased gestational weight gain, fetal growth, and a reduction in stillbirth and neonatal death. Birthweight benefit was greater in the hungry season than in the wet season (more food available), and supplementation benefited malnourished women more than well-nourished women.

A few supplementation trials not included in the Cochrane Review also reported LBW as an outcome. In Guatemala pregnant women were given either a high or a low calorie supplement. Those who received the high calorie supplement delivered heavier babies and had a lower rate of LBW infants [35]. Energy supplementation during pregnancy in Indonesia with high or low (465 or 52 kcal/day) energy found increased birthweight and a lower incidence of LBW in both groups [36]. A dose-response relationship between energy consumption and birthweight was also reported. The risk of LBW was modified by maternal pre-pregnancy weight, with those weighing more than 41 kg having less risk than those weighing less.

In a recent randomized food and micronutrient trial in Bangladesh in which pregnant women were either assigned to early (1st trimester) or usual (2nd trimester) food supplementation, and further randomly assigned to one of three micronutrient supplements (30 or 60 mg iron plus 400 folic acid or the UNICEF-recommended 15 micronutrient mix) during pregnancy. The results showed no significant difference in birthweight or the incidence of LBW between the food or micronutrient groups. No interaction between food and micronutrient supplementation on birthweight was reported [Arifeen and Persson, 2005, unpublished observation]. This study did not have a control group since all participants received both food and micronutrient supplements. However, the mean birthweight was higher and the incidence of LBW was lower relative to that reported earlier from the same population [37]. Other important food supplementation trials during pregnancy include high protein or isocaloric protein supplementation but none of those trials showed any beneficial effect on LBW. However, high protein supplementation in the relatively well-nourished population was reported to be harmful [38].

Despite strong theoretical plausibility that population groups at risk of dietary inadequacy should benefit from food supplementation during pregnancy, the effect on birthweight has been modest although the effect on LBW, particularly on SGA, has been stronger. Some inherent limitations of supplementation trials need to be carefully taken into consideration when interpreting the findings, including poor documentation of the adequacy of the usual diet and poor quantification of the real contribution of supplemental food to the pregnant woman's diet. Other issues also deserve attention in interpreting the findings including compliance, substitutions of usual diet, 'eating down' during pregnancy (fear of large baby), sharing with other family members, improper targeting, and above all choice of supplement and its cost. It is also critically important to evaluate whether supplementation resulted in net energy balance which is important for a positive birthweight outcome.

Micronutrient Intervention and LBW

Maternal micronutrient status during pregnancy plays an important role in fetal growth [39–42]. MMN deficiencies among women of childbearing age, particularly during pregnancy, are widespread in developing countries [30, 31, 43]. Anemia during early pregnancy is associated with poor fetal growth [44, 45]. Anemia mainly due to iron deficiency is highly prevalent in non-pregnant and pregnant women in developing countries [46–48]. In an Indian community two thirds of pregnant women were found to have zinc or iron deficiency and over half of the women had both zinc and iron deficiency coupled with inadequate intake of those nutrients [31]. This clustering of MMN deficiency and dietary inadequacy supports the contention that intervention with MMNs is more preferable to a single micronutrient. Often combined micronutrient intervention is more effective than when given individually. For example, intervention with both vitamin A and iron has been shown to be more effective in reducing anemia and improving vitamin A status than iron or vitamin A supplementation alone [49]. In 1999 UNICEF/WHO/UNU recommended a multi-micronutrient mix in developing countries for supplementing pregnant women who are supposedly suffering from MMN deficiencies [50]. This multi-micronutrient mix has been promoted since then with the aim of reducing the incidence of LBW as one of the major outcomes [51].

A recent systematic review of the literature on the effect of micronutrients on fetal growth concluded that there was no significant effect of prenatal micronutrient supplementation on fetal growth [52]. However, the authors recognized the paucity of evidence from well-designed, adequately powered, randomized trials on the efficacy of a single micronutrient on birthweight or LBW as the outcome. Among single micronutrient supplementation trials only calcium and magnesium supplementation during pregnancy has been found to reduce LBW in selected population groups [52]. Iron supplementation with or without folic acid during pregnancy has been shown to improve iron status and reduce anemia, but no effect on birthweight or LBW has been reported [53]. One recent study in the United States reported that iron supplementation during pregnancy in iron-replete non-anemic women improved birthweight and reduced the incidence of LBW [54].

Results of MMN supplementation on birthweight and the incidence of LBW have been mixed. Some studies showed no additional benefits on birthweight or LBW over traditional iron folic acid supplementation and some reported the superior efficacy of MMN. However, more recent studies have consistently shown the superior efficacy of MMN supplementations over traditional iron folic acid in reducing the incidence of LBW (table 2).

Table 2. Effect of multiple micronutrient supplementation as compared to iron or iron plus folic acid supplementation during pregnancy on the incidence of low birthweight

Study	Population	Intervention	Relative risk (95% CI)
Christian et al. [55], 2003	Nepal	Vitamin A	1.00
		FA	1.00 (0.88–1.15)
		FA + I	0.84 (0.72–0.99)
		FA, I, Zn	0.96 (0.83–1.11)
		MMN	0.86 (0.74–0.99)
Ramakrishnan et al. [56], 2003	Mexico	I	1.00
		MMN	0.98 (0.55–1.74)
Friis et al. [57], 2004	Zimbabwe	I + FA	1.00
		MMN	0.84 (0.59–1.18)
Osrin et al. [58], 2005	Nepal	I + FA	1.00
		MMN	0.69 (0.52–0.93)
Zagré et al. [10], 2007	Niger	FA + I	8.4±8.9
		MMN	7.2±5.9
		Supplementation	6.7±10.4
		>150 days	3.8±6.1
		FA + I	
		MMN	
Gupta et al. [59], 2007	India	FA + I	1.00
		MMN (29 vitamins and minerals)	0.30 (0.13–0.71)
Shankar et al. [60], 2008	Indonesia	FA+I	1.00
		MMN	0.86 (0.73–1.01)

I = Iron; FA = folic acid; Zn = zinc; MMN = multiple micronutrients.

A randomized trial in Nepal showed no additional benefit from prenatal MMN when compared to traditional iron and folic acid supplementation, although both groups had a lower incidence of LBW (MMN vs. iron and folic acid: 14 vs. 16% reduction) as compared to a placebo group who received vitamin A only [55]. Similar results were reported from a semi-urban community in Mexico [56]. One study in Zimbabwe reported a statistically nonsignificant decrease in LBW associated with MMN supplementation [57]. However, a more recent report from Nepal showed that prenatal MMN supplementation was associated with a 25% lower incidence of LBW than traditional iron folic acid supplementation [58]. Noticeably, the positive effect of MMN shown in Nepal selectively worked on heavier (normal BMI) women and female infants, which underscores the importance of pre-pregnant nutrition of women. In a randomized trial in Niger reported a 14% fall in LBW associated with MMN supplementation when compared with iron and folic acid supplementation [10]. The effect of MMN was even stronger in women who had a longer

Alam

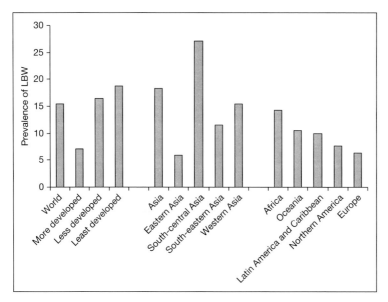

Fig. 1. Global and regional prevalence of low birthweight. Source: the United Nations Children's Fund and World Health Organization.

duration (150 days or longer) of supplementation. The effect on LBW was also stronger among women whose pre-pregnancy nutritional status was poorer. MMN supplementation in malnourished pregnant women in India has been shown to be associated with a 70% reduction in the LBW incidence as compared to iron folic acid supplementation [59]. In Indonesia MMN supplementation during pregnancy was reported to be associated with a 14% lower risk of delivering a LBW infant than for those who received iron and folic [60]. The effect was stronger for MMN in women who were anemic on enrollment. One earlier study in Tanzania showed that HIV-infected pregnant women who were supplemented with multivitamins had a 44% lower risk of delivering a LBW infant than those who received a placebo [61]. Dietary intervention with micronutrient-rich foods has also been shown to increase birthweight and reduce LBW in a poor Indian community [62].

Trials of prenatal MMN supplementations are not exactly comparable in supplement composition, timing of allocation, and total duration of supplementation; however, homogeneity of the effect on LBW findings is noticeable. From a programmatic point of view increasing micronutrient intake is a greater challenge than simply increasing the overall dietary intake. Most of the dietary intake of micronutrients depends on the contribution from animal sources, which is relatively low in the diet of pregnant women in developing countries [63].

Nutrition Education and LBW

Cultural rules relating to food proscription and prescription during pregnancy and lactation have been described in many populations, and approaches that have been used to successfully promote diet and nutritional status have some important common elements [64]. Apart from food availability, dietary intakes during pregnancy are guided by other cultural beliefs, food taboos and behavior, and relate to birth outcomes. Often nutrition knowledge of diet during pregnancy is guided by misconception and folk beliefs [65]. Women in developing countries even reduce food intake during pregnancy, commonly known as 'eating down', to avoid having a large baby [66].

Although it is expected that increased energy intake should have a positive effect on pregnancy weight gain and birthweight, review of nutrition education intervention trials concluded that educational intervention is successful in improving the dietary intake of pregnancy women, reducing the risk of fetal and neonatal death, but has no effect on LBW [33]. However, nutrition education has been shown to reduce the incidence of premature deliveries, one of the major causes of LBW [67]. Nutrition education may also potentiate the effect of other interventions in lowering the risk of LBW [68]. The efficacy of nutrition education in reducing LBW needs to be evaluated with respect to its content, cultural appropriateness and social acceptance, and above all its effect on dietary intake and net energy balance.

Intervention for LBW and 'Large Baby' Issue

Interventions for increasing birthweight have been criticized for increasing the risk of possible cephalopelvic disproportion and therefore obstructed labor [69] which is dangerous for women in developing countries where most deliveries take place at home and emergency obstetric care is rarely available. Increased birthweight is often accompanied by an increase in head circumference. However, data from different studies show that a very small increase (less than a third of a centimeter) in head circumference occurs due to supplementation, which is unlikely to cause such a problem [34]. Supplementation in a malnourished population is also of concern as it might contribute to increased adiposity in the offspring, a risk factor for insulin resistance [70, 71]. This issue of food supplementation on body composition needs further research in different settings.

Conclusions

This chapter focuses mainly on successful interventions that have potential in the prevention of LBW in developing countries. Interventions for LBW should be considered in a much broader perspective than just considering its immediate consequences. LBW is determined by multiple precipitating factors and lowering the incidence is obviously a formidable challenge particularly for resource-constrained developing countries. Improved dietary intake and micronutrient status before and during pregnancy are critically important in the prevention of LBW. Benefit from a single intervention seems to be small and unlikely to reduce the LBW burden effectively. This suggests that a population-specific optimal mix of interventions needs to be identified and implemented. However available evidence is sufficient to support a package of interventions that promotes increased dietary energy intake including micronutrients and culturally appropriate nutrition education that can remove misconceptions related to dietary intake during pregnancy and enhance mobilization of household resources to support healthy pregnancy. It is well documented that LBW is perpetuated through intergenerational effects, and therefore is strong justification for sustained effective interventions to improve maternal health and nutritional status for several generations. Thus household food security and intra-household food distribution issues with special emphasis on the diet of pregnant women require attention. Culturally appropriate nutrition education tools need to be developed, packaged and delivered to address the misconceptions related to diet, pregnancy and childbirth. While IUGR seem to respond well to intervention, preterm delivery is more complex and resilient to intervention and will require further research on the mechanistic aspects of this problem for identifying effective interventions. Prevention of LBW is an urgent public health priority not only for averting immediate adverse outcomes but also for preventing the impending global epidemic of diabetes, hypertension and cardiovascular diseases, which are negatively associated with size at b irth.

References

1 United Nations Children's Fund and World Health Organization: Low Birthweight: Country, Regional and Global Estimates. New York, UNICEF, 2004.
2 Villar J, Belizan JM: The relative contribution of prematurity and fetal growth retardation to low birth weight in developing and developed societies. Am J Obstet Gynecol 1982;143:793–798.
3 Arifeen SE, Black RE, Caulfield LE, et al: Infant growth patterns in the slums of Dhaka in relation to birth weight, intrauterine growth retardation, and prematurity. Am J Clin Nutr 2000;72:1010–1017.
4 McCormick MC: The contribution of low birth weight to infant mortality and childhood morbidity. N Engl J Med 1985;312:82–90.
5 Santos DN, Assis AM, Bastos AC, et al: Determinants of cognitive function in childhood: a cohort study in a middle income context. BMC Public Health 2008;8:202.
6 Silva A, Metha Z, O'Callaghan FJ: The relative effect of size at birth, postnatal growth and social factors on cognitive function in late childhood. Ann Epidemiol 2006;16:469–476.
7 Juneja M, Shankar A, Ramji S: Neurodevelopmental, functional and growth status of term low birth weight infants at eighteen months. Indian Pediatr 2005;42:1134–1140.
8 Ashworth A: Effects of intrauterine growth retardation on mortality and morbidity in infants and young children. Eur J Clin Nutr 1998;52(suppl 1):S34–S41.

9   Arifeen SE: Birth weight, intrauterine growth retardation and prematurity: a prospective study of infant growth and survival in the slums of Dhaka, Bangladesh; diss. Johns Hopkins University School of Hygiene and Public Health, Baltimore, 1997.
10 Zagré NM, Desplats G, Adou P, et al: Prenatal multiple micronutrient supplementation has greater impact on birthweight than supplementation with iron and folic acid: a cluster-randomized, double-blind, controlled programmatic study in rural Niger. Food Nutr Bull 2007;28:317–327.
11 Martorell R, Ramakrishnan U, Schroeder DG, et al: Intrauterine growth retardation, body size, body composition and physical performance in adolescence. Eur J Clin Nutr 1998;52(suppl 1):S43–S52.
12 Moore SE, Cole TJ, Collinson AC, et al: Prenatal or early postnatal events predict infectious deaths in young adulthood in rural Africa. Int J Epidemiol 1999;28:1088–1095.
13 Raqib R, Alam DS, Sarker P, et al: Low birth weight is associated with altered immune function in rural Bangladeshi children: a birth cohort study. Am J Clin Nutr 2007;85:845–852.
14 Barker DJ: The fetal origins of diseases of old age. Eur J Clin Nutr 1992;46(suppl 3):S3–S9.
15 Bavdekar A, Yajnik CS, Fall CHD, et al: Insulin resistance syndrome in 8-year-old Indian children: small at birth, big at 8 years, or both? Diabetes 1999;48:2422–2429.
16 Barros FC, Victora CG: Increased blood pressure in adolescents who were small for gestational age at birth: a cohort study in Brazil. Int J Epidemiol 1999;28:676–681.
17 Hales CN, Barker DJ, Clark PM, et al: Fetal and infant growth and impaired glucose tolerance at age 64. BMJ 1991;303:1019–1022.
18 Stein CE, Fall CHD, Osmond C, et al: Fetal growth and coronary heart disease in South India. Lancet 1996;348:1269–1273.
19 Rich-Edwards JW, Colditz GA, Stampfer MJ, et al: Birthweight and the risk for type 2 diabetes mellitus in adult women. Ann Intern Med 1999;130:278–284.
20 Alderman H, Berhman JR: Reducing the incidence of low birth weight in low-income countries has substantial economic benefits. World Bank Research Observer 2006;21:25–48.
21 Kramer MS: Intrauterine growth and gestational duration determinants. Pediatrics 1987;80:502–511.
22 Hirve SS, Ganatra BR: Determinants of low birth weight: a community based prospective cohort study. Indian Pediatr 1994;31:1221–1225.
23 Amin N, Abel R, Sampathkumar V: Maternal risk factors associated with low birth weight. Indian J Pediatr 1993;60:269–274.
24 Stevens-Simon C, McAnarney ER: Adolescent maternal weight gain and low birth weight: a multifactorial model. Am J Clin Nutr 1988;47:948–953.
25 Taha TT, Gray RH, Mohammedani AA: Malaria and low birth weight in central Sudan. Am J Epidemiol 1993;138:318–325.
26 Iroha EO, Ezeaka VC, Akinsulie AO, et al: Maternal HIV infection and intrauterine growth: a prospective study in Lagos, Nigeria. West Afr J Med 2007;26:121–125.
27 Brocklehurst P, French R: The association between maternal HIV infection and perinatal outcome: a systematic review of the literature and meta-analysis. Br J Obstet Gynaecol 1998;105:836–848.
28 Pryer JA, Rogers S: Epidemiology of undernutrition in adults in Dhaka slum households, Bangladesh. Eur J Clin Nutr 2006;60:815–822.
29 Ortolano SE, Mahmud Z, Iqbal Kabir AF, Levinson FJ: Effect of targeted food supplementation and services in the Bangladesh Integrated Nutrition Project on women and their pregnancy outcomes. J Health Popul Nutr 2003;21:83–89.
30 Ahmed F, Khan MR, Jackson AA: Concomitant supplemental vitamin A enhances the response to weekly supplemental iron and folic acid in anemic teenagers in urban Bangladesh. Am J Clin Nutr 2001;74:108–115.
31 Pathak P, Kapil U, Kapoor SK, et al: Prevalence of multiple micronutrient deficiencies amongst pregnant women in a rural area of Haryana. Indian J Pediatr 2004;71:1007–1014.
32 Stein AD, Lumey LH: The relationship between maternal and offspring birth weights after maternal prenatal famine exposure: the Dutch Famine Birth Cohort Study. Hum Biol 2000;72:641–654.
33 Kramer MS, Kakuma R: Energy and protein intake in pregnancy. Cochrane Database Syst Rev 2003;4:CD000032.

34 Ceesay SM, Prentice AM, Cole TJ, et al: Effects on birth weight and perinatal mortality of maternal dietary supplements in rural Gambia: 5 year randomised controlled trial. BMJ 1997;315:786–790.
35 Lechtig A, Martorell R, Delgado H, et al: Food supplementation during pregnancy, maternal anthropometry and birth weight in a Guatemalan rural population. J Trop Pediatr Environ Child Health 1978;24:217–222.
36 Kardjati S, Kusin JA, de With C: Energy supplementation in the last trimester of pregnancy in East Java: I. Effect on birthweight. Br J Obstet Gynaecol 1988;95:783–794.
37 Alam DS, van Raaij JMA, Hautvast GAJ, et al: Energy stress during pregnancy and lactation: consequences for maternal nutrition in rural Bangladesh. Eur J Clin Nutr 2003;57:151–157.
38 Rush D, Stein Z, Susser M: A randomized controlled trial of prenatal nutritional supplementation in New York City. Pediatrics 1980;65:683–697.
39 Masters ET, Jedrychowski W, Schleicher RL, et al: Relation between prenatal lipid-soluble micronutrient status, environmental pollutant exposure, and birth outcomes. Am J Clin Nutr 2007;86:1139–1145.
40 Muthayya S, Kurpad AV, Duggan CP, et al: Low maternal vitamin B_{12} status is associated with intrauterine growth retardation in urban South Indians. Eur J Clin Nutr 2006;60:791–801.
41 Neggers Y, Goldenberg RL: Some thoughts on body mass index, micronutrient intakes and pregnancy outcome. J Nutr 2003;133(suppl 2):1737S–1740S.
42 Gambling L, Danzeisen R, Fosset C, et al: Iron and copper interactions in development and the effect on pregnancy outcome. J Nutr 2003;133:1554S–1556S.
43 Khor GL: Update on the prevalence of malnutrition among children in Asia. Nepal Med Coll J 2003;5:113–122.
44 Xiong X, Buekens P, Fraser WD, Guo Z: Anemia during pregnancy in a Chinese population. Int J Gynaecol Obstet 2003;83:159–164.
45 Brabin BJ, Ginny M, Sapau J, et al: Consequences of maternal anaemia on outcome of pregnancy in a malaria endemic area in Papua New Guinea. Ann Trop Med Parasitol 1990;84:11–24.
46 Islam MZ, Lamberg-Allardt C, Bhuyan MA, Salamatullah Q: Iron status of premenopausal women in two regions of Bangladesh: prevalence of deficiency in high and low socio-economic groups. Eur J Clin Nutr 2001;55:598–604.
47 Ahmed F: Anaemia in Bangladesh: a review of prevalence and aetiology. Public Health Nutr 2000;3:385–393.
48 Hyder SM, Persson LA, Chowdhury M, et al: Anaemia and iron deficiency during pregnancy in rural Bangladesh. Public Health Nutr 2004;7:1065–1070.
49 Ahmed F, Khan MR, Jackson AA: Concomitant supplemental vitamin A enhances the response to weekly supplemental iron and folic acid in anemic teenagers in urban Bangladesh. Am J Clin Nutr 2001;74:108–115.
50 UNICEF/WHO/UNU: Composition of a Multi-Micronutrient Supplement to be Used in Pilot Programmes among Pregnant Women in Developing Countries. New York, UN Children's Fund, 1999.
51 Shrimpton R, Shrimpton R, Schultink W: Can supplements help meet the micronutrient needs of the developing world? Proc Nutr Soc 2002;61:223–229.
52 Fall CH, Yajnik CS, Rao S, et al: Micronutrients and fetal growth. J Nutr 2003;133(suppl 2):1747S–1756S.
53 Pena-Rosas JP, Viteri FE: Effects of routine oral iron supplementation with or without folic acid for women during pregnancy. Cochrane Database Syst Rev 2006;3:CD004736.
54 Cogswell ME, Parvanta I, Ickes L, et al: Iron supplementation during pregnancy, anemia, and birth weight: a randomized controlled trial. Am J Clin Nutr 2003;78:773–781.
55 Christian P, Khatry SK, Katz J, et al: Effects of alternative maternal micronutrient supplements on low birth weight in rural Nepal: double blind randomised community trial. BMJ 2003;326:571.
56 Ramakrishnan U, Gonzalez-Cossio T, Neufeld LM, et al: Multiple micronutrient supplementation during pregnancy does not lead to greater infant birth size than does iron-only supplementation: a randomized controlled trial in a semirural community in Mexico. Am J Clin Nutr 2003;77:720–725.

57 Friis H, Gomo E, Nyazema N, et al: Effect of multimicronutrient supplementation on gestational length and birth size: a randomized, placebo-controlled, double-blind effectiveness trial in Zimbabwe. Am J Clin Nutr 2004;80:178–184.
58 Osrin D, Vaidya A, Shrestha Y, et al: Effects of antenatal multiple micronutrient supplementation on birthweight and gestational duration in Nepal: double-blind, randomised controlled trial. Lancet 2005;365:955–962.
59 Gupta P, Ray M, Dua T, et al: Multimicronutrient supplementation for undernourished pregnant women and the birth size of their offspring: a double-blind, randomized, placebo-controlled trial. Arch Pediatr Adolesc Med 2007;161:58–64.
60 Shankar AH, Jahari AB, Sebayang SK, et al: Effect of maternal multiple micronutrient supplementation on fetal loss and infant death in Indonesia: a double-blind cluster-randomised trial. Lancet 2008;371:215–227.
61 Fawzi WW, Msamanga GI, Spiegelman D, et al: Randomised trial of effects of vitamin supplements on pregnancy outcomes and T cell counts in HIV-1-infected women in Tanzania. Lancet 1998;351:1477–1482.
62 Rao S, Yajnik CS, Kanade A, et al: Intake of micronutrient-rich foods in rural Indian mothers is associated with the size of their babies at birth: Pune Maternal Nutrition Study. J Nutr 2001;131:1217–1224.
63 Pathak P, Kapil U, Kapoor SK, et al: Prevalence of multiple micronutrient deficiencies amongst pregnant women in a rural area of Haryana. Indian J Pediatr 2004;71:1007–1014.
64 Gittelsohn J, Vastine AE: Sociocultural and household factors impacting on the selection, allocation and consumption of animal source foods: current knowledge and application. J Nutr 2003;133(suppl 2):4036S–4041S.
65 Everette M: Gestational weight and dietary intake during pregnancy: perspectives of African American women. Matern Child Health J 2008;12:718–724.
66 Hutter I: Reduction of food intake during pregnancy in rural south India. Trop Med Int Health 1996;1:399–405.
67 Villar J, Merialdi M, Gulmezoglu AM, et al: Nutritional interventions during pregnancy for the prevention or treatment of maternal morbidity and preterm delivery: an overview of randomized controlled trials. J Nutr 2003;133(suppl 2):1606S–1625S.
68 Taren DL, Graven SN: The association of prenatal nutrition and educational services with low birth weight rates in a Florida program. Public Health Rep 1991;106:426–436.
69 Garner P, Kramer MS, Chalmers I: Might efforts to increase birthweight in undernourished women do more harm than good? Lancet 1992;340:1021–1023.
70 Yajnik CS: Early life origins of insulin resistance and type 2 diabetes in India and other Asian countries. J Nutr 2004;134:205–210.
71 Yajnik CS, Fall CH, Coyaji KJ, et al: Neonatal anthropometry: the thin-fat Indian baby. The Pune Maternal Nutrition Study. Int J Obes Relat Metab Disord 2003;27:173–180.

Discussion

Dr. Kalhan: I have two questions. The outcome measures we are looking at, birthweight, head circumference, for example, are complex functions of a very large number of factors which may be related to a single micronutrient or to an array of micronutrients. Therefore are we realistic when we say that supplementing with zinc alone will solve the problem of head circumference, for example? I always have problems with these data that supplementation assumes that the society has a state of insufficiency. My second question is, when the meta-analyses were done, were these studies assuming that there is a state of insufficiency or do they correct for the state of sufficiency versus insufficiency? Assuming that the mother has an adequate caloric intake, the question that arises is whether supplementing another 300 kcal of energy is going to resolve the problem? My intuitive feeling is that if I give 300 kcal in a Western society, that is already eating plenty, it is probably not going to have any effect.

Dr. Alam: May I answer your second question first? The literature on food supple-mentation does not contain any information on the adequacy of a woman's usual diet, and therefore whether a 300-kcal/day supplementation would be sufficient to resolve the problem is hard to say. It has been observed that high protein supplementation in healthy women can even have a negative effect on birthweight. Of course while doing meta-analyses the authors set some criteria and they cannot go back. If the informa-tion regarding adequacy is not provided by the authors of the individual publications, then it is impossible to find, and most of the publications lack that information. But from the food balance, food distribution or food consumption data, population groups in which the low birthweight (LBW) burden is high have diets which are inadequate in both macro- and micronutrients. Regarding your first question whether a single micro-nutrient or single supplement could be effective in reducing the incidence of LBW: as you rightly mentioned it is a very complex issue. Evidence in the literature shows that an inadequacy of certain micronutrients coexists or is associated with a high preva-lence of LBW and supplementation of women during pregnancy is often targeted to deal with micronutrient deficiency. LBW is a multifactorial outcome and just a single or multiple micronutrient intervention is not the full solution to the problem; probably a comprehensive package of interventions is required to reduce the burden.

Dr. Sesikaran: With iron and folic acid supplementation, most of the studies have shown benefit, haven't they?

Dr. Alam: Prenatal iron and folic acid supplementation has so far not been shown to influence birthweight and LBW, although they have other maternal benefits like improved iron status in iron-deficient women and a reduced incidence of anemia. However, one very recent study in the United States reported that iron supplementa-tion in iron-replete non-anemic women improved birthweight and reduced the inci-dence of LBW [1].

Dr. De Curtis: I would like to know if in the studies in developing countries were carried out using regional neonatal growth charts or charts from developed countries? In Italy, for example, we have seen that there is a difference in birthweights between Italian newborns and those of families coming from developing countries. Moreover we have seen that in the last decades there has been a change in the percentage of SGA infants. I would like to underline that IUGR and SGA are not the same thing. An SGA newborn is an infant with a birthweight below the 10th percentile, while an IUGR baby is an infant who presents growth restriction during pregnancy which is detect-able only with prenatal ultrasound. Therefore, I think that in developing countries it is perhaps better and easier to speak only of SGA.

Dr. Alam: I accept your comment. We reviewed studies which looked at LBW as the outcome. We didn't take into account whether the LBW infants were SGA or appropriately grown. A normal birthweight infant may also be SGA. Use of a regional growth chart is a debated issue.

Dr. Rahman: You have shown us the positive effect of using these micronutrients in combination during pregnancy to prevent LBW. Would you like to tell us which period of gestation is best to give those micronutrients, what amount should be given, and for how long?

Dr. Alam: It is quite difficult to comment on the appropriate timing, choice of com-bination of micronutrients, dose, and duration to have maximum benefits. Kramer's [2] meta-analysis showed that maternal nutrition before entering pregnancy is a major determinant of LBW. So in my view, a lifecycle approach is more important than tar-geting a narrow window during pregnancy with any combination of supplementation. The current pregnancy should not be neglected because a better outcome is needed to ensure a heavier and healthier baby, and this should continue to ensure healthier babies in the next generation. The target of supplementation should not be making babies too big but ensuring optimal growth and development.

Dr. Agarwal: We published two national studies, one in the *Indian Journal of Medical Research* [3] and one in *Indian Pediatrics* [4]. There are two programs in India, one of which is integrated in the child development services. Two centers were chosen, in Hyderabad and Varanasi, to evaluate the impact of supplementation to pregnant women, and the final observations were analyzed on more than 6,000 deliveries in Varanasi. The women selected were deprived and of lower socioeconomic status. Food supplementation showed two things: women gain a mean of 100 g weight and the birthweight gain was about 65 g. This worked very well. The second program is a controlled national anemia program. We also evaluated this program which was run at 5–6 centers in the country to see what the impact was. Iron folate supplementation worked, birthweight increased, maternal iron stores increased as assessed by ferritin, and C-reactive protein was reduced. We came to the conclusion that instead of 60 mg we should raise the supplement to 100 mg. So the Indian national iron prophylaxis tablet contains 100 mg iron and 400 µg folate. All this work has been reported in the *Indian Journal of Pediatrics* and the *Indian Journal of Medical Research*. In 2003 and 2004 I surveyed maternal nutrition and anemia in 7 states of this country. To summarize in Himachal Pradesh the results were tremendously good, and what I learned from there is that a doctor will examine a pregnant women 3 times during pregnancy and delivery will be conducted by the doctor. Maternal mortality is lowest in Himachal Pradesh, there is no severe anemia, the anemia prevalence is low, and the LBW incidence in the Indian subcontinent is lowest in Himachal Pradesh. So the achievement is that during antenatal care, we only gave folate iron and it worked. A little more can be found on the internet about studies in the poor countries like ours.

Dr. Alam: Thank you for sharing this information. I used mostly a high-quality review level and some literature that was not included in those reviews. We should carefully look into these Indian experiences and evaluate the findings.

Dr. Christian: The meta-analysis that you showed on balanced protein energy supplementation, you said that it did not include the Gambia CC trial but in fact it does, the trial by Ceesay et al. [5], and it was highly weighted. Can you talk a little bit about the MINIMat trial from Bangladesh, and the lack of impact of food supplementation that you saw in that study? Given the high rates of LBW in that population and we know those women also had low BMIs and stunting, etc., why did you not see any benefit of food supplementation?

Dr. Alam: I accept your first comment, but the meta-analysis did not include the West Kiang trial which is what I meant. I will try to answer to your second question about the MINIMat [6] as I am also a part of the investigating team. Unfortunately we haven't been able to publish the work yet. As you know, it was not intended as a supplementation trial because the government program was distributing food, the equivalent of 600 kcal made of rice powder, pulse powder and a little bit of molasses mixed together. It was distributed through community nutrition centers to malnourished pregnant women (BMI <18.5). What the ICDDLB study did was to modify the government program a little bit. Some publications have shown that normally malnourished women cannot respond quickly to supplementation because they have a lot of deficit to replete, and maternal–fetal transfer only occurs when the maternal need has been satisfied. Pregnant women were identified by pregnancy testing in the community (<8 weeks gestation) and were invited to the clinic where pregnancy was further confirmed by ultrasound. Then they were randomly allocated to food supplementation early (1st trimester) or usual (2nd trimester), and further randomly assigned to iron (60 or 30 mg) and folic acid (400 mg) or the UNICEF recommended multiple micronutrients mix [7]. As all women received both food and micronutrient supplements, we did not have a true control group. In fact, there is evidence that women who attended the supplementation center shared this with their young children who loved the food more than the mothers actually did. We did not find any difference in energy intake as measured by repeated 24-hour dietary recall between supplemented and non-supplemented subjects. So it means that even though they attended the clinic or received the supplement, it did not affect the amount of energy in the total diet of the women; so it is obvious that the effect might not be there. On the other hand, we looked at the correlation between energy intake and birthweight where we found a positive correlation; it could be interpreted that the increased energy intake had a positive effect, although supplementation failed to show that. With respect to the multiple micronutrient and iron issue: as you did the first analysis from Nepal you know the results better than I, and we did not expect very much difference from that. Neither food supplementation nor micronutrient supplementation was associated with birthweight or the incidence of LBW.

Dr. Ganapathy: Just on iron and zinc, the micronutrient issue. There is an interaction between zinc and copper and zinc and iron. I think we should know about this as zinc can give rise to hypochromic microcytic anemia by blocking copper, and zinc can also prevent the absorption of iron. So it requires a very optimal ratio of iron to zinc if you want both of them to get into your system.

Dr. Kikafunda: You correctly said that the birthweight should, if possible, be kept around the median. That is good. However, although the lower limit of 2,500 g is strictly observed, I believe we should also set an upper limit and observe it. I fear that tomorrow somebody is going to come up with the theory that these bigger babies will have problems in the future. Especially in urban areas, the rate of cesarean births has greatly increased in recent times. I am not saying that cesarean births are the result of large babies, but I am sure that it is one of the factors.

Dr. Alam: Thank you very much for raising this issue that we should also look at the right side of the distribution; having too many big babies can cause not only perinatal problems, but may also cause some adverse health outcomes. Barker [8] and subsequent studies [9] have shown that there is a linear trend of a decreased risk of diabetes, cardiovascular disease and other health outcomes. But recent publications on diabetes show that there is a relationship between birthweight and type 2 diabetes, but the safer range is between 3,000 and 4,000 g [10], and an increased risk is associated with birthweight beyond that limit. So too a large baby is obviously an issue.

Dr. Prentice: I wonder if I could make a little comment here; I think there is a great deal of misunderstanding. Dr. Alam has just described the shape of the curve for birthweight and diabetes. If we look at the shape of the curve for birthweight versus neonatal mortality, which obviously would include a lot of those obstetric difficulties, then in fact if we set for any individual community at unity for a birthweight of 3,000–3,500 g then the odds of neonatal mortality continue to *decrease* as birthweight increases. As you go to 3,500–4,000 g it goes down to about 0.6; from 4,000 to 4,500 g it goes down to about 0.5, and you have to go up to very high birthweights before you start to see an increase in those neonatal mortality rates. Furthermore as Dr. Alam pointed out, the trials so far have shown no significant effect overall in the Cochrane analysis of increased head circumference. Perhaps head circumference is not the key measure, you may need to measure the chest circumference as well, but even in our trial where we have shown a significant increase, the increase was 0.3 cm, i.e. a diameter increase of 1 mm which I find difficult to imagine that that is going to increase any problems of CPD. And finally the thing we should concentrate on is that with any intervention trial we are trying not to *promote* abnormal growth, we are trying to *prevent* LBW.

Dr. Polberger: I have a question about chorioamnionitis or placental inflammation which seems to be an emerging cause of LBW and preterm birth. Is this a worldwide problem?

Dr. Alam: Chorioamnionitis or placental insufficiency may cause preterm delivery, which has not been well investigated.

Dr. Polberger: I mean chorioamnionitis or inflammation.

Dr. Alam: Yes, it is a cause of prematurity. There are a lot of publications showing that bacterial vaginosis or even asymptomatic urinary tract infection can increase the risk of preterm delivery. But treatment of these conditions does not have any effect on preterm delivery. Also in the MINIMat trial in Bangladesh, a randomized trial with metronidazole for those who had asymptomatic bacterial vaginosis and those who were symptomatic or syndromically classified as having bacterial vaginosis did not make any difference in preterm delivery.

Dr. Sesikaran: I think many of these studies have not taken the placental factors which could influence LBW into consideration. We have done a study where we compared the medical termination of pregnancy in terms of mothers who are underweight compared with mothers who are normal weight, and we looked at the placenta. A lot of factors seem to play a role in causing placental insufficiency: villous density, the number of blood vessels per villi, and the number of syncytial strokes, and several factors take place in underweight mothers in trying to improve the placental circulation to the baby. So in many supplementation studies we are probably not succeeding. No one has really looked and seen whether there are any other factors which could interfere with the full benefit of the supplementation, but rather blamed the supplementation that it did not work. So your point is very well taken and it needs to be looked into as far as placental function is concerned.

References

1 Cogswell ME, Parvanta I, Ickes L, et al: Iron supplementation during pregnancy, anemia, and birth weight: a randomized controlled trial. Am J Clin Nutr 2003;78:773–781.
2 Kramer MS: Intrauterine growth and gestational duration determinants. Pediatrics 1987;80:502–511.
3 Agarwal KN, Agarwak DK, Sharma A, et al: Prevalence of anaemia in pregnant and lactating women. Indian J Med Res 2006;124:173–184.
4 Srivastava M, Agarwal DK, Agarwal A, et al: Nutritional status of rural non-pregnant non-lactating women in reproductive age. Indian Pediatr 1998;35:975–983.
5 Ceesay SM, Prentice AM, Cole TJ, et al: Effects on birth weight and perinatal mortality of maternal dietary supplements in rural Gambia: 5 year randomised controlled trial. BMJ 1997;315:786–790.
6 Tofail F, Persson LA, El Arifeen S, et al: Effects of prenatal food and micronutrient supplementation on infant development: a randomized trial from the Maternal and Infant Nutrition Interventions, Matlab (MINIMat) study. Am J Clin Nutr 2008;87:704–711.
7 UNICEF/WHO/UNU: Composition of a Multi-Micronutrient Supplement to Be Used in Pilot Programmes among Pregnant Women in Developing Countries. New York, UN Children's Fund, 1999.
8 Barker DJ: The fetal origins of diseases of old age. Eur J Clin Nutr 1992;46(suppl 3):S3–S9.
9 Rich-Edwards JW, Colditz GA, Stampfer MJ, et al: Birthweight and the risk for type 2 diabetes mellitus in adult women. Ann Intern Med 1999;130:278–284.
10 Harder T, Rodekamp E, Schellong K, et al: Birth weight and subsequent risk of type 2 diabetes: a meta-analysis. Am J Epidemiol 2007;165:849–857.

Kalhan SC, Prentice AM, Yajnik CS (eds): Emerging Societies – Coexistence of Childhood Malnutrition and Obesity.
Nestlé Nutr Inst Workshop Ser Pediatr Program, vol 63, pp 227–257,
Nestec Ltd., Vevey/S. Karger AG, Basel, © 2009.

Community-Based Approaches to Address Childhood Undernutrition and Obesity in Developing Countries

Prakash Shetty

Institute for Human Nutrition, University of Southampton Medical School, Southampton, UK

Abstract

Community-based approaches have been the mainstay of interventions to address the problem of child malnutrition in developing societies. Many programs have been in operation in several countries for decades and originated largely as social welfare, food security and poverty eradication programs. Increasingly conceptual frameworks to guide this activity have been developed as our understanding of the complex nature of the determinants of undernutrition improves. Alongside this evolution, is the accumulation of evidence on the types of interventions in the community that are effective, practical and sustainable. The changing environment is probably determining the altering scenario of child nutrition in developing societies, with rapid developmental transition and urbanization being responsible for the emerging problems of obesity and other metabolic disorders that are largely the result of the now well-recognized linkages between child undernutrition and early onset adult chronic diseases. This dramatic change is contributing to the double burden of malnutrition in developing countries. Community interventions hence need to be integrated and joined up to reduce both aspects of malnutrition in societies. The evidence that community-based nutrition interventions can have a positive impact on pregnancy outcomes and child undernutrition needs to be evaluated to enable programs to prioritize and incorporate the interventions that work in the community. Programs that are operational and successful also need to be evaluated and disseminated in order to enable countries to generate their own programs tailored to tackling the changing nutritional problems of the children in their society.

Introduction

Three conceptual frameworks developed by international agencies have underpinned community-based approaches to improve child health and nutrition in developing countries. These include the 'life cycle approach to undernutrition' presented by a commission set up by the UN's Standing Committee on Nutrition [1] which underlines the importance of maternal and child nutrition as being essential for growth and healthy physical and mental development of children into adulthood and healthy old age, and to reduce the risk of premature morbidity and mortality due to adult-onset diseases. Secondly, the widely used 'food-care-health conceptual framework' developed by UNICEF [2] which explains the causes of malnutrition in society and their interactions at three levels: immediate (inadequate diet and infectious disease); underlying (household food insecurity, inadequate maternal and child care and poor health services in an unhealthy environment), and basic (i.e. structural factors including social, economic and political) – a framework that has considerable influence on approaches to remedial action and more recently has accorded recognition to the established links between child undernutrition and adult disease within this conceptual framework [3]. The 'triple A process', a framework again developed by UNICEF [2], is a cyclical and iterative participatory decision-making process wherein the problem of undernutrition is assessed, its causes analyzed, followed by a decision to implement an appropriate mix of actions.

Paradoxically community-based programs initiated by governments, aid agencies and NGOs have long preceded the evolution of these conceptual frameworks although they now influence and contribute significantly to the development and implementation of community-based interventions and programs in much of the developing world. Many of the earlier community intervention programs which preceded the evolution of those concepts were based on either the simple conviction that poor maternal and child nutrition is the result of inadequate intake of food thus resulting in programs that provide additional food supplements or are aimed more broadly at poverty reduction to alleviate food insecurity. The recognition of the high prevalence of nutritional deficiency diseases like anemia in pregnant women and children led to the development of community programs to supplement nutrients like iron and other micronutrients or reduce losses due to infections (malaria, worms, etc.) using treatment (e.g. deworming) or chemoprophylaxis. These interventions were expected to improve maternal nutrition during pregnancy and reduce maternal mortality, which in turn would have a beneficial impact on birth outcomes and child nutrition. Some of the community programs were national initiatives and were straightforward social welfare programs to improve overall nutrition or poverty reduction programs that were initiated for political reasons. In this chapter, the evidence from interventions through observational studies and well-designed trials will first be evaluated for their impact on reducing child undernutrition and obesity in developing country settings. A sample of the various national or regional level community-based programs aimed at reducing child undernutrition that have been operational for some time will be discussed and evaluated. This chapter will also make an effort to highlight those intervention strategies that work and are beneficial and hence need to be incorporated into national or regional level programs to address the problems of child nutrition in developing societies.

Do Community-Based Interventions Work? What Is the Evidence?

An attempt is made here to evaluate community-based intervention trials in pregnant women (antenatal, intrapartum and postnatal) and in infants and children, focusing mainly on developing countries. The objective is to identify key behaviors and interventions for which the weight of evidence is sufficient to recommend their inclusion in community- or population-based programs aimed at improving child nutrition and reducing the risk of later adult-onset diseases. With an understanding of the lifecycle approach, it is evident that poor maternal nutrition will result in poor birth outcomes such as low birthweight (LBW), which increases the risk of obesity and chronic disease in later adult life. LBW infants are at increased risk of illness and mortality. Weight at birth is a good predictor of size in later adult life, and intrauterine growth-retarded (IUGR) infants demonstrate poor catch-up growth, thus the incidence of LBW is reflected in an increased prevalence of underweight children. IUGR infants are also at greater risk of stunting during childhood and adolescence and, like other stunted children due to poor nutrition, end up as shorter adults [4]. It is also well documented that undernourished individuals show indications of an increased risk of obesity and metabolic abnormalities in childhood.

Maternal undernutrition manifested as small maternal size (short stature and underweight) at conception and low gestational weight gain are the principal attributable risk factors for IUGR and LBW [5], hence community interventions to improve birth outcomes will have to target pregnant women. Evidence for successful interventions that promote infant and child nutrition will also need to be evaluated in order to develop holistic community-based approaches to tackle child undernutrition and at the same time ward off the potential risk of childhood obesity and metabolic disorders. The evidence from well-designed intervention studies covering multifarious aspects will then have to be reviewed, analyzed and prioritized in order to facilitate their successful incorporation into community approaches and programs to further good nutrition in children and to prevent early adult-onset diseases. There have been several previous attempts to address the issues related to maternal nutrition, pregnancy outcomes and child malnutrition in the past [6–8].

Nutrition Interventions to Promote Maternal Nutrition and Health to Improve Birth Outcomes

Maternal undernutrition and its consequent impact on fetal and infant nutrition are major problems in developing countries. A high proportion of births in developing countries fall into the category of LBW which is a major underlying risk factor for an increase in morbidity and mortality during infancy and the increased risk of childhood malnutrition. A recent review evaluated the impact of nutrition interventions on pregnancy outcomes while highlighting the fact that few studies have addressed this problem in community settings in developing countries [9]. The Cochrane Library's pregnancy and childbirth database provides more evidence of the efficacy of interventions to improve maternal nutrition, health and pregnancy outcomes in addition to other summaries of reports in the literature [8, 10].

Prenatal Food Supplementation

In the Cochrane review [11], maternal food supplements that provided balanced protein and energy were the only interventions that improved pregnancy outcome measured as improved birthweight. Balanced protein-energy supplements provided <25% of the total energy content as protein. This review concluded that antenatal interventions with balanced protein-energy supplements significantly improved fetal growth, and reduced the risk of fetal and neonatal deaths. Fourteen trials were subjected to analysis and the intervention was associated with modest increases in maternal weight gain during pregnancy (+21 g), a small but significant increase in birthweight (+32 g), a smaller nonsignificant increase in birth length and head circumference as well as a tendency to a reduction in the prevalence of small-for-gestational age (SGA) babies (–32%) [12]. The interventions had a more substantial effect on reducing IUGR (OR 0.68; 95% CI 0.57–0.80) and a significant reduction in preterm births (OR 0.83; 95% CI = 0.65–1.06) [13]. Table 1 summarizes the significant features of many of these intervention trials, which were largely conducted in developing countries and in some cases in poor inner-city communities in industrialized countries.

It is important to note that the findings of the Cochrane review were largely biased by one recent large trial conducted in The Gambia [14]; excluding this study drastically alters the conclusions of this meta-analysis, leaving no demonstrable impact of antenatal interventions with food supplements. However, this trial provides a valuable example of an effective antenatal maternal intervention and has generated a resurgence of interest in this area of community interventions. This intervention trial showed remarkable increases in pregnancy outcomes: increase in birthweight (+136 g), decrease in LBW (–39%), increase in head circumference (+3.1 mm) with no changes in length or gestational age. Seasonal changes were also evident with even better outcomes when the intervention was in the hungry season. In addition

Table 1. Interventions with protein-energy supplementation on low birthweight

Setting and sample	Intervention	Outcome	Other effects	Reference; type of trial
The Gambia, rural; live births: 1,010 (I), 1,037 (C)	High protein energy biscuit supplement to pregnant women	Significant increase in birthweight (+136 g) and decrease (39%) in LBW	Decrease in incidence of stillbirths and reduced mortality first 7days	74; RCT
Indonesia, rural; n = 542 pregnant women	Assigned to low and high energy supplementation groups	Significant difference in birthweight (+463 g) and at 12 months of age (+421 g)		64; QET
Indonesia, rural; n = 741 pregnant women	Assigned to high energy and low energy groups	No significant effect of either supplement on birthweight or LBW rates when compared to baseline, i.e. no supplementation	No difference in maternal weight gain compared to non-compliers	65; DB-RPCT
Guatemala, rural; n = 169 mothers followed through 2 consecutive pregnancies	Two supplements (high protein energy gruel vs. no protein low calorie drink) offered during pregnancy and lactation	Linear trend for increased birthweight from highest (gruel) to lowest (drink) supplements		66; QET
Thailand, rural; n = 43 women in 3rd trimester	3 groups; control plus 2 different levels of supplementation	Significant increase in birthweight of supplemented groups: 3,089 g and 3,104 g (I) compared to 2,853 g (C)	Placental weight significantly higher in supplemented groups	67; RCT
India, urban, hospital setting; n = 20 pregnant women	3rd trimester supplementation	No significant difference in birthweights and birth lengths	No difference in maternal weight gain; significantly improved Hb levels in supplemented group	68; RCT

Table 1. (continued)

Setting and sample	Intervention	Outcome	Other effects	Reference; type of trial
The Gambia, rural; n = 1,229 pregnant women	Supplementation with peanut-based biscuits and vitamin-fortified tea from 16th week	Increase in birthweight of supplemented group (+101 g); benefit only during wet season 67.5% decrease in annual LBW; greatest effect in wet season (83.3% decrease)	Increased head circumference in infants of supplemented group	69; QET
Taiwan, rural; n = 212 women, supplemented from birth of first infant to birth of second infant	Supplements: high protein high calorie randomized with no protein low calories	Increase in birthweight of second infant (+161.4 g) in high protein-high calorie supplement LBW 2.8% compared to 6.8% but not statistically significant	No effect of supplements on prematurity rates	70; DB-RCT
Colombia, urban; n = 456 pregnant women in 3rd trimester	Supplements of dry milk, bread, and vegetable oil to families of intervention group	Significant increase in birthweight (+95 g) of males in intervened group No effect on LBW rates	Maternal weight gain significantly higher in supplemented group who had male infants	71; QET
Guatemala, rural; n = 405 chronically undernourished pregnant women	Two supplements (high calorie protein gruel and no protein low calorie drink) offered during pregnancy	No correlation between caloric supplementation and birthweights. Incidence of LBW halved in high calorie protein-supplemented group		72; QET

India, rural; n = 126 pregnant women from 20 weeks gestation	3 groups: group 1 iron-folate; group 2 high protein calories + iron-folate; group 3 control	Increase in birthweight: group 1 (= 270 g); group 2 (+810 g) compared to control group	Significant maternal weight gain (+1 kg) in group 2	74; RCT

RCT = Randomized control trial; QET = quasi experimental trial; DB-RCT = double-blind randomized control trial; DB RPCT = double-blind randomized placebo-controlled trial; I= intervention; C = control.

the antenatal food supplements were associated with a significant reduction in stillbirths and mortality of the newborn in the first 7 days.

As opposed to the interventions with balanced protein-energy supplementation, the benefits of protein supplements during pregnancy have been shown to be negligible following meta-analysis of the available evidence [11]. In studies conducted on Asian women in the UK [15] and Chilean women [16], where the habitual energy intake was iso-calorically replaced with protein, there was no effect on pregnancy outcome; if any a trend to a reduction in birthweights was observed. Even higher intakes of protein (>25% of energy) in relatively well-nourished women failed to show any benefit on pregnancy outcomes and birthweight [17].

One could safely conclude that supplementation during pregnancy with balanced protein and energy was the only intervention that improved birthweight, while high levels of protein alone cannot be recommended as an antenatal intervention. Most of the evidence comes from efficacy trials conducted under intense supervision with the weight of evidence in the meta-analysis being driven by the single large trial from The Gambia. Additional field evaluation is clearly required using available home diets or through dietary diversification strategies, and only by targeted supplementation in at-risk populations.

Prenatal Micronutrient Supplementation

Prenatal micronutrient supplementation was not considered an important intervention strategy for improving birth outcomes until the 1990s despite the concern with the high prevalence of iron deficiency among women of reproductive age in developing countries. Some of the earlier intervention studies aiming to increase energy and protein often provided some micronutrients with the food supplements. Since then evidence has been accumulating that the mineral and vitamin status of the mother can have a major impact on birth outcomes. Table 2 summarizes data from several intervention trials of micronutrient supplements either singly or as multiple micronutrients provided during pregnancy.

Iron Supplementation. There seems to be a U-shaped relationship between maternal anemia and birthweight because both low and high hemoglobin values are associated with increased risk of LBW [18, 19]. In developing countries, maternal iron deficiency is positively associated with LBW [20]. Meta-analysis of iron supplementation trials in the Cochrane collaboration [21] showed no detectable effect on birth outcome despite a significant reduction in maternal anemia. Community-based iron supplementation trials in developing countries have also failed to demonstrate any improvement in birthweights apart from a study in India [22], demonstrating a reduction in LBW rates with iron and folate supplementation from before 20 weeks of gestation, and another from rural Nepal where iron-folate supplementation slightly reduced the prevalence of LBW [23]. Oral iron supplementation may improve maternal anemia but has no clear impact on birth outcomes – a

Table 2. Community intervention trials with micronutrients on low birthweights

Setting and sample	Intervention	Outcome	Other effects	Reference; type of trial
Antenatal iron supplementation				
Niger, peri-urban; n = 197 women	100 mg/day elemental iron (I); placebo (C)	Supplemented group associated with increase in birth length but not birthweight	Significant effect on decreasing maternal anemia; drastic reduction in neonatal death	74; DB-RCT
The Gambia, rural; n = 550 multigravida women	60 mg/day elemental iron (I); placebo(C); all women received 5 mg folic acid weekly	Supplement had no significant effect on birthweights or LBW rates. Those who took supplement for >80 days delivered significantly heavier (+9.2 g) babies	Significant increase in Hb and plasma iron levels	75; DB-RCT
Sri Lanka, rural; n = 195 pregnant women	Fortified food supplement provided along with iron (60 mg) + folate (0.25 mg) per day	No effect on birthweight	Iron supplements improved maternal Hb status	76; PCS
India, rural; n = 418 women 16–24 weeks gestation	Supplement of iron (60 mg) + folate (500 mg) daily for 100 days	Significantly heavier babies – 2.88 kg (I) vs. 2.59 kg (C); 46% decrease in LBW. Birthweight higher in those supplemented before 20 weeks gestation	Iron+folate-supplemented group had increased Hb and serum ferritin levels	22; RCT
Antenatal folate supplementation				
South Africa, tertiary hospital; n = 354 women	3 groups: iron (200 mg/day); 5 mg folic acid+iron daily; 50 mg vitamin B12+folate+iron	Folic acid+iron-supplement group had a much lower number of infants weighing <2,270 g		24; RCT

235

Table 2. (continued)

Antenatal zinc supplementation

Setting and sample	Intervention	Outcome	Other effects	Reference; type of trial
Chile, urban slum; n = 804 pregnant adolescents, <20 weeks gestation	Zinc (20 mg/day) supplements until delivery (I) compared with placebo (C)	No effect on mean birthweights. Proportion of LBW significantly lower in supplemented group. Multiple regressions show significant effect of maternal nutritional status and supplements on birthweight		77; RCT
Indonesia, rural; n = 229 women between 10 and 20 weeks gestation	All 4 groups received iron + folate: group 1 + b-carotene; group 2 + zinc (30 mg/day); group 3 + b-carotene and zinc; group 4 only iron+folate (C)	Male infants born to mothers with all 4 nutrients were significantly heavier than the other 2 groups or controls		78; RCT
Peru, urban shanty town; n = 242 pregnant women 10–16 weeks gestation	Women receiving iron+folate were randomized to (25 mg zinc/day (I) or placebo (C)	No effect on birthweights	Positive effect of zinc on fetal femur diaphysis growth	79; RCT
Bangladesh, urban slum; n = 559 pregnant women; 12–16 weeks gestation	Randomized to 30 mg zinc/day (I) or placebo (C)	No significant effect on birthweight, length, head or chest cirumference. No difference in LBW rates (RR1.12)	Supplement had no effect on maternal weight gain	80; RCT
Peru, urban, hospital setting; n = 1,295 women, 10–24 weeks gestation	Randomized to iron, 30 mg zinc/day (I) or placebo (C)			81; RCT

Setting	Intervention	Outcomes	Additional outcomes	Reference
India, urban, hospital setting; n = 168 pregnant women	Intervention group (I) received zinc supplements (45 mg/day) compared to controls with no supplements (C)	Significant increase in birthweights of zinc supplemented group. Supplemented for 6–9 months (3.45 kg) compared to 1–3 months (2.98 kg) and controls (2.65 kg). gestational age higher with increased duration of supplementation		82; RCT
Antenatal iodine supplementation				
Zaire, rural; n = 109 pregnant women	28 weeks gestation at antenatal clinic either injection iodized oil (I) or iodine-free vitamins (C)	Birthweight increased (+109 g) in iodized oil group	Reduced infant mortality rate and improved maternal and infant thyroid hormone status in intervention group	83; PCS
Antenatal vitamin A supplementation				
Malawi, urban, hospital setting; n = 697 HIV-infected women; 18–28 weeks gestation until delivery	Randomized to receive daily iron+folate (C) or iron+folate+ vitamin A (3 mg retinol equivalent) (I)	Birthweights 2,895 g (I) vs. 2,805 g (C). Significantly lower proportion of LBW 14% (I) vs. 21.1% (C)	Significantly lower levels of anemic infants in vitamin A group (23.4%) compared to control group (40.6%) at 6 weeks postpartum	84; RCT
Antenatal multiple micronutrient supplementation				
Nepal, rural; n = 1,200 pregnant women	Individually randomized to either folate+iron (C) or MV supplements (I) during 2nd and 3rd trimesters	Birthweights 2,733 g (C) vs. 2,810 g (I) Difference 77 g (CI 24–130) 25% reduction in LBW in I group		85; DB-RCT
Nepal, rural; n = 4,926 pregnant women, 4,130 live births	Cluster/sectors randomized into 5 groups: folic acid; folic acid+iron; folic acid+iron+zinc;	Folic acid+iron increased birthweight (+37 g) and reduced LBW (−16%; RR = 0.84). MV supplements		23; DB-CRT

Table 2. (continued)

Setting and sample	Intervention	Outcome	Other effects	Reference; type of trial
Mexico, rural; n = 873 pregnant women before 13 weeks gestation	multivitamins; vitamins alone as control	increased birthweight (+64 g) and reduced LBW (−14%; RR = 0.86) Mean birthweight and birth length did not differ significantly between the 2 groups		86; RCT
	Randomized to receive supplements 6 days/week at home and antenatal care. Either iron (60 mg) alone or iron + 1–1.5 times RDA of several multivitamins			
Tanzania, urban; n = 1,075 HIV-infected women	Randomized to 4 groups: group 1 vitamin A daily; group 2 MV without vitamin A; group 3 MV with vitamin A; group 4 placebo controls	Vitamin A alone had no effect on LBW (OR = 1.14), or SGA (OR = 0.83). Risk of LBW and SGA significantly reduced in both MV groups 2 and 3. LBW decreased by 44% (OR = 0.56); SGA risk reduced by 43% (OR = 0.57)	Risk of preterm birth was significantly reduced in both MV groups 2 and 3. 40% decrease in fetal deaths in MV-supplemented groups	87; DB-RCT
Chile, urban; n = 709 pregnant women attending 9 prenatal clinics	Given either powdered milk with high milk fat or multiple micronutrient-fortified powdered milk. Non-consumers of any supplement were controls	Mean birthweights higher (+73 g) in the fortified powdered milk group than in other powdered milk supplement groups and even higher compared to controls (+335 g)	Significantly better maternal weight gain and iron status in the fortified milk group	16; PCS

South Africa, rural; n = 171 nutritionally deficient pregnant women >20 weeks gestation	Randomized to 4 groups: group 1, micronutrient fortified high bulk supplement (high I niacin +iron); group 2, micronutrient-fortified low bulk supplement (high in vitamin A, calcium, thiamine, riboflavin); group 3, zinc supplement; group 4, placebo controls	Mean birthweight higher in group 2 (low bulk) compared to group 1 (high bulk) by 9.5% and higher by 6.5% compared to placebo group	88; RCT

RCT= Randomized control trial; QET = quasi experimental trial; DB-RCT= double-blind randomized control trial; DB-CRT = double-blind cluster randomized trial; PCS = prospective cohort study; DB-RPCT = double-blind randomized placebo-controlled trial; I = intervention; C = control; RR = relative risk; OR = odds ratio; MV = multivitamins/multiple micronutrients; LBW = low birthweight; SJA = small-for-gestational age.

conclusion that is drawn largely on a paucity of robust trials of iron supplementation in community settings in developing countries.

Folate Supplementation. A study in South Africa in a tertiary hospital setting is the only one to show a significant decrease in the incidence of LBW births [24]. Along with iron supplements, folic acid has a demonstrable impact on improving maternal hemoglobin levels. The evidence is very strong that peri-conceptual folate supplementation reduces neural tube defects. However the impact on other beneficial birth outcomes resulting from folate supplementation during pregnancy is doubtful.

Zinc Supplementation. The potential for zinc supplementation to improve birthweight is largely based on a review of 17 studies which indicated an association between maternal indicators of zinc status and birthweight of the offspring [25]. An in-depth review of zinc supplementation trials showed that birthweight increased in 4 of 10 trials [26], although the Cochrane review on maternal zinc supplementation revealed no differences in birth outcome [27]. Evidence from other community-based studies summarized in table 2 suggest that overall zinc supplementation failed to show any impact on birthweight. Interestingly, two of the studies did show a reduction in the incidence of infectious disease morbidity among LBW infants [28] and mortality among SGA infants [29] born to zinc-supplemented mothers. This obviously has enormous implications in reducing childhood malnutrition, particularly given that LBW infants are at increased risk.

Neither iodine nor vitamin A supplementation trials have demonstrated any benefit on birth outcomes, although there is little doubt that iodine supplementation, even in mid-pregnancy, reduces deaths in infancy and early childhood while vitamin A supplementation reduces maternal mortality [8].

Multiple Micronutrient Supplementations. The benefits of multiple micronutrient supplements during pregnancy may be potentially high given the increased demand on nutrients for fetal growth. However, community-based intervention trials have not provided clear-cut evidence from studies in developing countries as either data are limited or the programs under evaluation are so varied. In addition many of the trials are complicated by the provision of additional energy or protein or food supplements alongside the micronutrient supplements. A recent Cochrane review [30] has shown that multiple micronutrient supplementation during pregnancy resulted in a decrease in LBW (RR 0.83; 95% CI 0.76–0.91) and SGA infants (RR 0.92; 95% CI 0.86–0.99). There is also evidence emerging that multiple supplements are not that superior to iron-folate supplements alone [23] and a meta-analysis comparing multiple micronutrients with folic acid and iron alone reports a small increase in birthweight (pooled effect of 21.2 g) [30]. Iron-folate supplementation alone also reduced LBW (RR 0.94; 95% CI 0.8–1.06) and SGA (RR 1.04; 95% CI 0.93–1.17). A recent report highlights the fact that the effects of antenatal multiple micronutrient supplementations on the fetus persist into childhood with increases in both bodyweight and body size [31].

Prevention of Maternal Infections

Maternal infections have an adverse impact on birth outcomes. The infections include malaria which greatly increases the risks of maternal anemia, preterm birth, LBW and neonatal mortality. The estimated population-attributable risk of LBW among primigravidae with malaria is 10–40% [32]. Hookworm infections and the associated maternal anemia are another problem and so is maternal sexually transmitted diseases like HIV, syphilis and gonorrhea.

Malaria chemoprophylaxis of mothers has been the main option in malaria endemic areas, although its efficacy is uncertain compared to intermittent presumptive treatment. A review of 15 trials by the Cochrane collaboration has shown that infants born to mothers on malaria chemoprophylaxis were heavier, especially so if they were born to primigravida [33]. In rural Uganda primigravidae on chloroquine had a significantly lower LBW rate (2% in treated vs. 9% in placebo group; p = 0.009) [34]. Other studies in Africa also support the findings of a benefit related to improved birthweights associated with malaria chemoprophylaxis during pregnancy. The increase in birthweight observed in almost all studies provides strong evidence for the beneficial effect of malaria chemoprophylaxis on birthweight in endemic areas. Compared to chemoprophylaxis, the use of insecticide-treated bed nets as a preventive measure had little impact on birthweights although they were effective in reducing mortality and morbidity from malaria [8].

Deworming is an accepted strategy to tackle helminthic infections like hookworm, which affect maternal health. The summary of evidence based on several small trials does favor deworming as being effective in reducing maternal anemia, improving maternal hemoglobin status and having some benefit in improving birthweights [8]. Maternal treatment of urinary tract infections and sexually transmitted diseases with antibiotics has also been shown to have benefits with regard to improving birth outcomes [8].

Other Interventions to Promote Maternal Health

Maternal Cessation of Smoking. Data on the effect of the cessation of smoking during pregnancy on birth outcomes are largely from industrialized countries and they seem to present mixed results on birth outcomes such as preterm birth or LBW rates. The important issue from a developing country perspective, i.e. the impact of the maternal environmental exposure to smoke and the beneficial effects of its reduction, has not been systematically examined in developing countries.

Interventions to Improve Diets and Weight Gain among Adolescent Mothers. Pregnant adolescents are at increased risk of inadequate gestational weight gain and micronutrient malnutrition due to inadequate intakes in their diets to support healthy fetal growth and promote good birth outcomes. Reviews of community interventions in developed societies show a predominance of medical models providing prenatal care with little emphasis on

241

nutrition education to alter the prenatal dietary behaviors of adolescents [35]. Positive effects on birth outcomes were evident when the approaches were driven by multidisciplinary teams supporting the nutritional and psychosocial needs of pregnant teenagers while individualized education and counseling encouraged optimal dietary intakes and appropriate gestational weight gain.

Interventions to Promote Initiation and Sustenance of Breastfeeding

Early initiation of breastfeeding is not a serious problem in developing countries as the initiation of breastfeeding is almost universal in the countries studied. However initiation rates remain low in many high income countries, particularly among the low income groups in their populations. A Cochrane collaboration report showed that the evaluation of all forms of breastfeeding education were effective in increasing breastfeeding initiation rates among low income groups in the USA [36].

Community-based intervention strategies to promote exclusive breast-feeding of infants up to 6 months of age and to sustain continued breast-feeding up to 12 months of age have also been evaluated. A Cochrane review that analyzed 34 trials of 29,385 mother–infant pairs in 14 countries provided evidence that any form of extra support increased the duration of both partial and exclusive breastfeeding up to 6 months [37]. All forms of extra support affected the duration of exclusive breastfeeding significantly. A review of specific breastfeeding promotion showed that both individual counseling (OR 1.93, 95% CI 1.18–3.15, $p < 0.0001$) and group counseling (OR 5.19, 95% CI 1.90–14.15, $p < 0.00001$) substantially increased exclusive breastfeeding at 6 months of age [13].

A Cochrane review of the potential benefits and drawbacks of exclusive breastfeeding for up to 6 months of age, based on trails and observational studies in both developed and developing country settings, showed no growth deficits in infant weight gain or increase in length [38]. The infants experienced less morbidity due to gastrointestinal infection compared to partially breastfed infants. The review in addition provided evidence of lactational amenorrhea and postpartum weight loss in the mothers.

Nutrition Interventions to Promote Child Growth and Development and to Prevent Undernutrition

Behavior and Practices of Caregivers
Caregivers provide food, healthcare, psychosocial stimulation and the emotional support necessary for the healthy growth and development of children [39]. The practices and the ways in which they are performed are critical for survival, optimum growth and proper development of children and in

the prevention of under- or malnutrition. Caregivers require time, energy and money to provide this important contributor of child health. A WHO review [40] concluded that interventions that incorporate care components are effective and identified the following conditions to maximize impact: interventions targeted to early life – both prenatally and in infancy; targeting children in poor households, and employing several types of interventions with more than one delivery channel and a high level of parental involvement. The significance of care practices on the nutrition status of children was demonstrated by a study in Ghana showing a close association of better scores for care practices with lower levels of stunting and underweight in children [41].

Complementary Feeding

Complementary feeding is the provision of foods and liquids along with continued breastfeeding of infants. Since the nutrient intake of an infant deteriorates when complementary foods start to be substituted for breast milk, many of the interventions that are central to complementary feeding include interventions with micronutrients and nutrition education [13].

Interventions that improve the intake of complementary foods by infants 6–12 months of age in developing countries have been shown to have a positive impact on their growth and nutrition [42]. A review of all the studies conducted on complementary feeds in developing countries is summarized in a recent report [12] and is based on two other compilations of trials published since 1988 in infants between 6 and 12 months of age [43, 44]. The trials varied in terms of the age of infant at intervention, the composition of the complementary food, and the extent of breastfeeding. Of the 14 trials reviewed, 3 demonstrated an increase in weight and length, and 2 showed only an increase in weight [12]. Nutrition education to improve complementary feeding in food-secure populations produced an increase in height for age Z scores compared to control groups [13], whereas in food-insecure populations educational interventions were of benefit only when combined with food supplements.

Community-Based Supplementary Feeding

Supplementary feeding implies the provision of extra food to children over and above the normal ration of their home diets. This intervention merits careful evaluation since several community-based programs have a component of supplementary feeding to improve child health and nutrition and to promote optimum growth. A Cochrane review has addressed the evaluation of the effectiveness of supplementary feeding at the community level for promoting the physical growth of preschool children [45]. Four randomized control trials were reviewed but no firm conclusions could be drawn on the effectiveness of supplementary feeding in improving child nutrition. Universal and untargeted supplementary feeding programs seem to have contributed to the rise in overweight and obesity among children in Chile [46].

Micronutrient Supplementation on Growth and Risk of Infections

Micronutrient supplementation either singly or as micronutrient mixes have been used as intervention strategies to improve child nutrition as well as to reduce the infectious disease burden which in turn has an impact on child undernutrition. Micronutrients have also been added to interventions with complementary foods or during supplementary feeding interventions in the community. Iron supplementation resulted in weight gain in anemic children but had a variable impact on improving heights [47] while the risk of diarrheal disease increased, demonstrating that iron supplementation in children has adverse effects on infectious diseases and no major gains with regard to growth [48]. Zinc supplementation or fortification of foods, on the other hand, reduces morbidity and mortality due to diarrheal disease and respiratory illness [49]. A meta-analysis of 25 studies provided evidence of an overall small but significant impact on the height of children with zinc supplementation, but only in children who had evidence of stunting [50]. The impact of vitamin A supplementation of infants is expected to reduce morbidity (and mortality) but the overall findings are largely variable with several randomized control trials failing to show any benefit on the risk of infections and growth [12]. Multiple micronutrient supplements also provide variable impact – improvements have been noted in stunted children in Vietnam and Mexico with no impact on growth in Peru and Guatemala [12].

Prevention and Treatment of Infections

Many of the interventions with micronutrient supplements have relevance on the prevention of infections in childhood and hence reduce the risk of child undernutrition. Treatment of infections and infestations also has a positive impact on child growth and nutrition. Deworming and use of anti-helminthics is particularly effective in children. A systematic review of 25 studies has documented the impact of single and multiple doses of anti-helminthics on growth [51]. While a single dose was associated with an average 0.24 kg increase in weight and 0.14 cm increase in height, several doses over a year resulted in 0.10 kg increase in weight and 0.07 cm in height over that time. A recent Cochrane review provided data only on weight gain and showed a 0.34 kg gain (95% CI 0.05–0.64) from 9 trials with a single dose while several doses over a year had no impact [52].

Other Interventions to Promote Infant and Child Nutrition

Interventions that promote hand washing, water quality treatment, sanitation and health education also reduce the risk of diarrheal disease and thus have impacts on promoting child nutrition [13].

Interventions to Prevent Childhood Obesity

The Cochrane database provides one review on the impact of interventions for preventing obesity in children [53]. All the studies were conducted in industrialized societies and there are no studies reported in the literature on interventions to reduce childhood obesity in developing countries. The only studies from developing countries were two conducted in Cuba where the intervention was dietary restriction [54] and hence cannot be considered as a community-based intervention. The Cochrane collaboration reviewed 22 studies: 10 considered long-term, i.e. at least 12 months duration, and 12 short-term, i.e. 12 weeks up to 12 months. Nineteen of the intervention trials were school-based, one was a community-based intervention targeting low income families, and 2 were family-based interventions targeting non-obese children of obese/overweight parents. The interventions either focused on dietary change or were targeted to increase physical activity, and in some instances was a combination of both. As the interventions were heterogeneous in design and quality, target population and outcome measures, the review was unable to provide statistical analysis of the impact. The review concluded that the interventions employed to date have largely not had an impact on the weight status of children. A recent comprehensive multicenter, multifactorial behavioral change intervention carried out over 3 years has been unable to demonstrate any change in the weight status among American Indian children [55]. Despite the global epidemic of obesity, the prevalence of obesity in most developing countries is small and there is no evidence that well-designed intervention trials to deal with childhood obesity have been carried out or reported.

Summary of Community-Based Intervention Trials: What Works?

Strategies that aim to improve maternal nutrition and health are the most significant interventions that have the best possible pregnancy outcome. An adequate and diversified diet promotes weight gain in pregnancy and hence food supplements or balanced energy-protein supplementation may be used to target vulnerable groups such as undernourished low BMI pregnant women and adolescent mothers. Multi-vitamin supplements have been shown to be effective not only in improving maternal health and birth outcomes but also on subsequent infant growth and health. Promotion of exclusive breastfeeding in early infancy followed by optimum complementary feeding in the presence of good hygienic practices diminishes risk of infections, promotes infant growth and prevents child undernutrition. Table 3 summarizes the most important interventions for good pregnancy outcomes and infant and child nutrition that are supported by evidence from community-based intervention studies and trials.

Table 3. Summary of interventions that have a positive impact on pregnancy outcomes and infant and child nutrition

	Comments
Interventions with evidence of positive impact on good birth outcomes, e.g. LBW	
Maternal supplementation of balanced energy and protein supplements/food supplements	Issues to be addressed: Should target only low BMI mothers and adolescents? Second or third trimester? Continue during lactation? Benefit-cost ratio?
Supplementation with iron-folate or multiple micronutrients	Impact on maternal morbidity and mortality
Micronutrient fortification of food	Fortification strategies cheaper than supplementation
Dietary diversification strategies	Sustainable approach in the long-term
Non-nutritional interventions: increase age of marriage/ conception; reduce physical activity during pregnancy; malaria prophylaxis and deworming; cessation of smoking/reduce smoke exposure	
Interventions for better infant and child nutrition and growth	
Promotional strategies and support for breastfeeding	Exclusive breastfeeding recommended for first 6 months
Educational strategies and support for better and safe complementary feeding	Breastfeeding to be continued when complementary foods added
Ensure adequate micronutrient intakes during complementary feeding	Evidence of positive impact of zinc, vitamin A, iron. Multiple micronutrient supplements and fortified foods beneficial
Prevent infections: hygienic interventions, deworming	Hygienic interventions reduce gastrointestinal infections which predispose to malnutrition. Probiotics also reduce risk

Community-Based Intervention Programs: Country Experiences

Some of the important community programs [56] with nutritional objectives and goals are summarized here. These are large district-wide or national programs that cover large sections of the population in developing countries – many of them ongoing even now. Many were initiated either by national governments or by aid agencies and bilaterals with the collaboration and support of the state. Some of them have been evaluated and others have adopted and evolved as the evidence for what works emerges.

Kenya – Applied Nutrition Project (ANP)

Started in 1983, the ANP covers 3 food-insecure divisions in Kenya. Although the main goals of this community-based project are related to food production, it also has nutrition and health objectives since nutrition education, promotion of breastfeeding and better weaning foods as well as improving water and sanitation are also objectives. Initially largely external aid driven, its long existence has institutionalized several components of the program with incorporation into existing community structures.

Madagascar – Expanded School and Community Food and Nutrition Surveillance and Education Program (SEECALINE)

Started in 1993 and funded by the World Bank, SEECALINE has been expanded nationally since 1998 and has received support from the state. The program has a supplementary feeding component with specific nutrition objectives. Data on growth monitoring indicate considerable improvement in child nutrition with between 8 and 15% reductions in underweight in 5 provinces. It is, however, a top-down program with weak community participation.

Zimbabwe – Community Food and Nutrition Program (CFNP)

In existence since 1987, this national program evolved from an earlier supplementary feeding program. State funded, it has both food security and nutritional objectives and integrates both agricultural and nutritional activities in the community. Until the recent troubles in Zimbabwe, CFNP demonstrated a reduction in both underweight and stunting in children.

Brazil – Child Pastorate Program

This large program in all 27 states of the country has been in existence since 1982 and is run by the Catholic Church with funding from the Ministry of Health. In addition to poverty reduction, the program has specific objectives related to health and nutrition. The program has been very successful with significant impact on maternal and child health. The achievements include: a reduction in underweight pregnant mothers; reduction in LBW (from 14% in 1988 to 5% in 2001); reduction in child malnutrition (18% in 1988 to 4% in 2001), and a considerable reduction in maternal and child morbidity and mortality. It is a politically popular and visible community program with strong support nationally and an interesting mixture of partners – the church, state, and NGOs.

Mexico – Education, Health and Nutrition Program (PROGRESA)

Started in 1997, PROGRESA is a large nationally funded initiative with broad objectives aimed at poverty reduction. This complex multi-sectoral program provides educational grants and food and income supplements. The food supplements provided were fortified with micronutrients and given to both to children and pregnant women and showed that supplemented children had gains in stature and lower levels of undernutrition and better hemoglobin and vitamin A status. An evaluation report showed that children receiving PROGRESA supplements had improved growth and a reduced probability of stunting [57].

Chile – Supplementary Feeding Program (Programa Nacional Alimentacion Complementaria; PNAC)

This national program with universal coverage is financed by public and private sectors. PNAC targets all children below 6 years of age and pregnant women in Chile. Since 1983, it operates at two levels – one basic for all and the other enhanced targeting specific vulnerable groups. The program has demonstrated good nutritional outcomes and benefits, although more recently concern has been raised about the program contributing to the rise in overweight and obesity in Chilean children [46].

The Philippines – Program on Good Nutrition for Health (LAKASS)

LAKASS is a nationally funded program with aid from Japan, and has been operational since 1989. It has a high level and consistent support and claims significant improvements in the nutritional status of young children. The program includes growth monitoring, micronutrient supplementation and supplementary feeding and weaning food components as well as other broader community development projects. With the built-in community participation, this is a sustainable community program.

India – The Integrated Child Development Services Scheme (ICDS)

ICDS is the largest program for the promotion of maternal and child health and nutrition in India, and was launched in 1975 in pursuance of the National Policy for Children. It is a multi-sectoral program run by the national government with the cooperation of the provincial governments. The beneficiaries are preschool children and women of reproductive age including those pregnant and lactating. ICDS provides an integrated approach to converge all the basic services for improved childcare, early stimulation and learning, health and nutrition, and water and environmental sanitation. Independent evaluation has demonstrated an improvement in the nutrition of children under the scheme as compared to those with no access to the program [58, 59], while other evaluations of ICDS have found its impact on nutrition to be limited [12].

Tamil Nadu, India – Tamil Nadu Integrated Nutrition Project (TINP)

Initiated in 1980, TINP goes beyond supplementary feeding to focus on improving caring practices and has achieved significant success in reducing severe malnutrition among children in participating districts as compared to non-participating ones [60]. In 1991 the second TINP (TINP-II) was launched and aimed to move beyond the reduction of severe malnutrition and was aimed at reducing the high prevalence of moderate undernutrition in children. The completion report of TINP-II found that the project had been successful in reducing severe undernutrition and infant mortality rates, but was less successful in reducing moderate undernutrition or LBW prevalence [61].

Bangladesh – Bangladesh Integrated Nutrition Project (BINP)
BINP is a large national program which evolved from its forerunner – the TINP in India and is an example of the pursuance of the food-care-health conceptual framework. It has been operational since 1995 funded largely by the World Bank with the overall aim to reduce malnutrition until it ceases to be a public health problem. This is an example of collaboration between an aid agency and national government. Among the various components of this program, the community-based elements, which consume most of the budget, are largely nutritional interventions including growth monitoring and supplementary feeding. BINP claims to have made a significant positive impact on the nutritional status of children and on the incidence of LBW, although doubts have been raised about the impact of this huge intervention program [62, 63].

The community-based programs summarized above are not exhaustive, and several programs with some degree of success have not been covered and include countries like Sri Lanka, Pakistan, Indonesia, Thailand, Cambodia and Vietnam in Asia. The success, effectiveness and impact of large scale nutrition intervention programs depend on both contextual success factors, i.e. the macro-environment in which the program operates, and the program success factors, i.e. the components, features and structure of the program itself [12, 56]. In addition the sustainability of the program depends on political will, the availability of resources (both monetary and human), community participation and involvement, and the level of institutionalization of the program that takes place over time. Table 4 provides a summary analysis of some of these features carried out by the Food and Agriculture Organization on some of the community-based intervention programs summarized above.

Community-based approaches can work if established as broad-ranging, multi-sectoral and integrated food and nutrition programs, often as part of poverty reduction and social welfare initiatives in developing countries. Because maternal and child undernutrition is the result of many factors, multiple sectors and strategies will have to bear on the objective of eradicating this problem. With child undernutrition and obesity and adult disease linked, as evident in the life cycle approach, and the consequent double burden of malnutrition manifesting in developing societies, tackling this emerging problem of malnutrition is a priority. Hence community-based approaches have to ensure a minimum package which addresses the 'food-health-care' triad recognizing the documented synergies in these approaches [12]. Thailand is often cited as an sterling example to demonstrate the success of community-based approaches in dramatically reducing child undernutrition [1].

Table 4. Summary of Community based Intervention Programs with food and nutrition objectives

	Countries						
	Kenya	Madagascar	Zimbabwe	Brazil	Mexico	Philippines	Bangladesh
Duration of program, years[1]	18	8	14	19	4	12	6
Coverage[2]	S	L	L	L	L	L	L
Impact on nutritional status	Yes	Yes	Yes	Yes	Yes	Yes	Yes
Inter-sectoral collaboration[3]	3	1	4	1	2	4	1
Program approach[4]	2	1	3	2	1	3	2
Level of institutionalization[5]	3	2	4	4	2	4	3

Adapted from FAO [56].
[1] Duration at the time of the analysis of the country programs in 2002/2003.
[2] S = Limited coverage (e.g. one district); L = wide or national coverage.
[3] Inter-sectoral collaboration: 1 = weak; 2 = good at central level; 3 = good at local level; 4 = good at all levels.
[4] Program approach: 1 = top-down; 2 = both; 3 = largely community driven.
[5] Level of institutionalization: 1 = total reliance on external funding and technical input; 2 = mostly reliant from outside; 3 = mostly reliant from outside but some state contributions and local technical inputs; 4 = good government contribution with or without external resources and technical inputs; 5 = fully institutionalized and totally funded by state – no external inputs.

References

1 Commission on the Nutrition Challenges of the 21st Century: Ending Malnutrition by 2020: An Agenda for Change in the Millennium. Geneva, UN Standing Committee on Nutrition, 2000.
2 UNICEF: Strategy for Improved Nutrition of Children and Women in Developing Countries. New York, UNICEF, 1990.
3 Black RE, Allen LA, Bhutta ZA, et al: Maternal and child undernutrition: global and regional exposures and health consequences. Lancet 2008;371:243–260.
4 Martorell R, Ramakrishnan U, Schroeder DG, et al: Intrauterine growth retardation, body size, body composition and physical performance in adolescence. Eur J Clin Nutr 1998;52(suppl 1):S43–S53.
5 Kramer MS: Determinants of low birth weight: methodological assessment and meta-analysis. Bull World Health Organ 1987;65:663–737.
6 Raiten D, Mittal R (eds): Proceedings of the Indo-US workshop on nutrition and health of women, infants and children, Hyderabad, India. February 10–12, 2000. Nutr Rev 2002;60:S1–S138.
7 Bhutta ZA, Jackson A, Lumbiganon P (eds): Nutrition as a preventive strategy against adverse pregnancy outcomes. Proceedings of a consultative meeting. Oxford, United Kingdom. July 18–19, 2002. J Nutr 2003;133(suppl 2):1589S–1767S.
8 Bhutta ZA, Darmstadt GL, Hasan BS, Haws RA: Community-based interventions for improving perinatal and neonatal health outcomes in developing countries: a review of the evidence. Pediatrics 2005;115:519–617.
9 Merialdi M, Carroli G, Villar J, et al: Nutritional interventions during pregnancy for the prevention or treatment of impaired fetal growth: an overview of randomized controlled trials. J Nutr 2003;133(suppl 2):1626S–1631S.
10 De Onis M, Villar J, Gulmezoglu M: Nutritional interventions to prevent intrauterine growth retardation: evidence from randomised controlled trials. Eur J Clin Nutr 1998;52:S83–S93.
11 Kramer MS: Isocaloric balanced protein supplementation in pregnancy. Cochrane Database Syst Rev 1996;4:CD000118.
12 Allen L, Gillespie S: What Works? A Review of the Efficacy and Effectiveness of Nutrition Interventions. Manila, Asian Development Bank, 2001.
13 Bhutta ZA, Ahmed T, Black RE, et al: What works? Interventions for maternal and child undernutrition and survival. Lancet 2008;371:417–440.
14 Ceesay S, Prentice A, Cole T, et al: Effects on birth weight and perinatal mortality of maternal dietary supplements in rural Gambia: 5 year randomised controlled trial. BMJ 1997;315:786–790.
15 Viegas O, Scott P, Cole T, et al: Dietary protein energy supplementation of pregnant Asian mothers at Sorrento, Birmingham. I: Unselective during second and third trimesters. BMJ 1982;285:589–592.
16 Mardones-Santander F, Rosso P, Stekel A, et al: Effect of a milk-based food supplement on maternal nutritional status and fetal growth in underweight Chilean women. Am J Clin Nutr 1988;47:413–419.
17 Rush D: Effects of changes in protein and calorie intake during pregnancy on the growth of the human fetus; in Chalmers I, Enkin M, Keirse M (eds): Effective Care in Pregnancy and Childbirth. Oxford, Oxford University Press, 1989, pp 92–101.
18 Scholl T, Hediger M: Anemia and iron deficiency anemia: compilation of data on pregnancy outcome. Am J Clin Nutr 1994;59(suppl):492S–501S.
19 Steer P: Maternal hemoglobin concentration and birth weight. Am J Clin Nutr 2000;71(suppl):1285S–1287S.
20 Rasmussen K: Is there a causal relationship between iron deficiency and iron deficiency anemia and weight at birth, length of gestation and perinatal mortality. J Nutr 2001;131:590S–603S.
21 Pena-Rosas, Viteri FE: Effects of routine oral iron supplementation with or without folic acid for women during pregnancy. Cochrane Database Syst Rev 2006;3:CD004736.
22 Agarwal K, Agarwal D, Mishra KP: Impact of anaemia prophylaxis in pregnancy on maternal haemoglobin, serum ferritin and birth weight. Indian J Med Res 1991;94:277–280.
23 Christian P, Shrestha I, LeClerq C, et al: Supplementation with micronutrients in addition to iron and folic acid does not further improve the hematologic status of pregnant women in rural Nepal. J Nutr 2003;133:3492–3498.

Shetty

24 Baumslag N, Edelstein T, Metz J: Reduction of incidence of prematurity by folic acid supplementation in pregnancy. BMJ 1970;i:16–17.
25 Tamure T, Goldbrg R, Kohnston K, et al: Serum concentrations of zinc, folate, vitamins A and E, proteins and their relationships to pregnancy outcomes. Acta Obstet Gynaecol Scand 1997;165:63–70.
26 Ramakrishnan U, Manjrekar R, Rivers J, et al: Micronutrients and pregnancy outcome: a review of the literature. Nutr Res 1999;19:103–159.
27 Mahomed K: Zinc supplementation in pregnancy. Cochrane Database Syst Rev 2000;2:CD000230.
28 Osendarp S, van Raaij J, Darmstadt G, et al: Zinc supplementation during pregnancy and effects on growth and morbidity in low birth weight infants: a randomised, placebo-controlled trial. Lancet 2001;357:1080–1085.
29 Sazawal S, Black R, Menon V, et al: Zinc supplementation in infants born small for gestational age reduces mortality: a prospective, randomised control trial. Pediatrics 2001;108:1280–1286.
30 Haider BA, Bhutta ZA: Multiple-micronutrient supplementation for women during pregnancy. Cochrane Database Syst Rev 2006;4:CD004905.
31 Vaidya A, Saville N, Shrestha BP, et al: Effects of antenatal multiple micronutrient supplementation on children's weight and size at 2 years of age in Nepal: follow-up of a double-blind randomised controlled trial. Lancet 2008;371:492–499.
32 Brabin B: An assessment of low birth weight risk in primiparae as an indicator of malaria control in pregnancy. Int J Epidemiol 1991;20:276–283.
33 Garner P, Gulmezoglu A: Interventions to prevent malaria during pregnancy in endemic malarious areas: prevention vs treatment for malaria in pregnant women. Cochrane Database Syst Rev 2003;1:CD00169.
34 Ndyomugyenyi R, Magnussen P: Chloroquine prophylaxis, iron-folic acid supplementation or case management of malaria attacks in primigravidae in western Uganda: effects on maternal parasitemia and haemoglobin levels and on birth weight. Trans R Soc Trop Med Hyg 2000;94:413–418.
35 Nielsen JN, Gittelsohn J, Aniker J, O'Brien K: Interventions to improve diet and weight gain among pregnant adolescents and recommendations for future research. J Am Diet Assoc 2006;106:1825–1840.
36 Dyson L, McCormick F, Renfrew MJ: Interventions for promoting the initiation of breast-feeding. Cochrane Database Syst Rev 2005;2:CD001688.
37 Britton C, McCormick FM, Renfrew MJ: Support for breast-feeding mothers. Cochrane Database Syst Rev 2007;1:CD001141.
38 Kramer MS, Kakuma R: Optimal duration of exclusive breast feeding. Cochrane Database Syst Rev 2002;1:CD003517.
39 Engle, P, Bentley M, Pelto G: The role of care in nutrition programmes. Proc Nutr Soc 2000;59:25–35.
40 WHO: A Critical Link: Interventions for Physical Growth and Psychological Development: A Review. Geneva, World Health Organization, 1999.
41 Ruel MT, Levin C, Armar-Klemesu M, et al: Good Care Practices Can Mitigate the Negative Effects of Poverty and Low Maternal Schooling on Children's Nutritional Status: Evidence from Accra. Food Consumption and Nutrition Division Discussion, paper 62. Washington, International Food Policy Research Institute, 1999.
42 Caulfield LE, Huffman SL, Piwoz EG: Interventions to improve intake of complementary foods by infants 6 to 12 months of age in developing countries: impact on growth and on the prevalence of malnutrition and potential contribution to child survival. Food Nutr Bull1999;20:183–200.
43 Brown KH, Dewey KG, Allen LH: Complementary Feeding of Young Children in Developing Countries: A Review of Current Scientific Knowledge. Geneva, World Health Organization, 1998.
44 Dewey KG: Approaches for Improving Complementary Feeding of Infants and Young Children. Background paper for WHO/UNICEF Technical Consultation on Infant and Young Child Feeding. Geneva, World Health Organization, 2001.
45 Sguassero Y, de Onis M, Carroli G: Community based supplementary feeding for promoting the growth of young children in developing countries. Cochrane Database Syst Rev 2005;4:CD005039.

46 Uauy R, Kain J: The epidemiological transition: need to incorporate obesity prevention into nutrition programmes. Publ Health Nutr 2002;5:223–229.
47 Allen LH: Nutritional influences on linear growth: a general review. Eur J Clin Nutr 1994;48(suppl 1):S75–S89.
48 Iannotti LL, Tielsch JM, Black MM, Black RE: Iron supplementation in early childhood: health benefits and risks. Am J Clin Nutr 2006;84:1261–1276.
49 Aggarwal R, Sentz J, Miller MA: Role of zinc administration in prevention of childhood diarrhoea and respiratory illnesses: a meta analysis. Pediatrics 2007;119:1120–1130.
50 Brown KH, Peerson JM, Allen LH: Effect of zinc supplementation on children's growth: a meta-analysis of intervention trials. Bibl Nutr Diet 1997;54:76–83.
51 Dickson R, Awasthi S, Williamson P, et al: Effects of treatment for intestinal helminth infection on growth and cognitive performance in children: systematic review of randomised trials. BMJ 2000;320:1697–1701.
52 Taylor-Robinson DC, Jones AP, Garner P: De-worming drugs for treating soil transmitted intestinal worms in children: effects on growth and school performance. Cochrane Database Syst Rev 2007;4:CD000371.
53 Summerbell CD, Waters E, Edmunds LD, et al: Interventions for preventing obesity in children. Cochrane Database Syst Rev 2005;3:CD001871.
54 Gibson LJ, Peto J, Warren JM, et al: Lack of evidence on diets for obesity for children: a systematic review. Int J Epidemiol 2006;35:1544–1552.
55 Caballero B, Clay T, Davis SM, et al; Pathways Study Research Group: Pathways: a school-based, randomized controlled trial for the prevention of obesity in American Indian schoolchildren. Am J Clin Nutr 2003;78:1030–1038.
56 FAO: Community-Based Food and Nutrition Programmes – What Makes Them Successful: A Review and Analysis of Experience. Rome, Food & Agriculture Organization, 2003.
57 Behrman J, Hoddinott J: An evaluation of the impact of PROGRESA on pre-school child height. Discussion paper No. 104. Washington, International Food Policy Research Institute, 1999.
58 Balaji, LN Arya S: Study of physical and psycho-social development of pre-school children. J Trop Pediatr 1987;33:107–109.
59 Kapil U: Integrated child development services (ICDS) scheme: a program for holistic development of children in India. Indian J Pediatr 2002;69:597–601.
60 Shekar M: The Tamil Nadu Integrated Nutrition Project: a review of the project with special emphasis on the monitoring and information system. Cornell Food and Nutrition Policy Program. Working paper No. 14. Ithaca, Cornell University, 1991.
61 Gillespie SR, Measham A: Implementation completion report of the Second Tamil Nadu Integrated Nutrition Project. Washington, World Bank, 1998.
62 Hossain SM, Duffield A, Taylor A: An evaluation of the impact of a US$60 million nutrition programme in Bangladesh. Health Policy Plan 2005;20:35–40.
63 Begum HA, Mascie-Taylor C, Nahar S: The impact of food supplementation on infant weight gain in rural Bangladesh; an assessment of the Bangladesh Integrated Nutritional Program (BINP). Public Health Nutr 2007;10:49–54.
64 Kusin J, Kardjati S, Houtkooper J, Renqvist U: Energy supplementation during pregnancy and postnatal growth. Lancet 1992;340:623–626.
65 Kardjati S, Kusin J, DeWith C: Energy supplementation in the last trimester of pregnancy in East Java. I. Effect on birthweight. Br J Obstet Gynaecol 1988;95:783–794.
66 Villar J, Rivera J: Nutritional supplementation during two consecutive pregnancies and the interim lactation period: effect on birth weight. Pediatrics 1988;81:51–57.
67 Tontisirin K, Booranasubkajorn U, Hongsumarn A, Thewtong D: Formulation and evaluation of supplementary foods for Thai pregnant women. Am J Clin Nutr 1986;43:931–939.
68 Girija A, Geervani P, Rao N: Influence of dietary supplementation during pregnancy on lactation performance. J Trop Pediatr 1984;30:79–83.
69 Prentice A, Whitehead R, Watkinson M, et al: Prenatal dietary supplementation of African women and birth weight. Lancet 1983;8323:489–492.
70 McDonald E, Pollitt E, Mueller W, et al: The Bacon Chow study: maternal nutritional supplementation and birth weight of offspring. Am J Clin Nutr 1981;34:2133–2144.
71 Mora J, Clement J, Christiansen N, et al: Nutritional supplementation and the outcome of pregnancy. III. Perinatal and neonatal mortality. Nutr Rep Int 1978;18:167–175.

72 Lechtig A, Habicht J, Delgado H, et al: Effect of food supplementation during pregnancy on birthweight. Pediatrics 1975;56:508–520.

73 Qureshi S, Rao N, Madhavi V, et al: Effect of maternal nutrition supplementation on the birth weight of the newborn. Indian Pediatr 1973;10:541–544.

74 Preziosi P, Prual A, Galan P, et al: Effect of iron supplementation on the iron status of pregnant women: consequences for newborns. Am J Clin Nutr 1997;66:1178–1182.

75 Menendez C, Todd J, Alonso P, et al: Malaria chemoprophylaxis, infection of the placenta and birth weight in Gambian primigravidae. J Trop Med Hyg 1994;97:244–248.

76 Atukorala S, de Silva L, Dechering W, et al: Evaluation of effectiveness of iron-folate supplementation and antihelminthic therapy against anemia in pregnancy – a study in the plantation sector of Sri Lanka. Am J Clin Nutr 1994;60:286–292.

77 Castillo-Duran C, Marin V, Alcazar L, et al: Controlled trial of zinc supplementation in Chilean pregnant adolescents. Nutr Res 2001;21:715–724.

78 Dijkhuizen M, Wieringa F: Vitamin A, Iron and Zinc Deficiency in Indonesia; PhD diss. Wageningen, University of Wageningen, 2001.

79 Merialdi M: The Effect of Maternal Zinc Supplementation during Pregnancy on Fetal Growth and Neurobehaviour Development. Baltimore, Johns Hopkins University, 2001.

80 Osendarp S, van Raaij J, Arifeen S, et al: A randomised placcbo control trial of the effect of zinc supplementation during pregnancy on pregnancy outcome in Bangladeshi urban poor. Am J Clin Nutr 2000;71:114–119.

81 Caulfield L, Zavaleta N, Figueroa A, Leon Z: maternal zinc supplementation does not affect size at birth or pregnancy duration in Peru. J Nutr 1999;129:1563–1568.

82 Garg HK, Singhal KC, Arshad Z: A study of the effect of oral zinc supplementation during pregnancy on pregnancy outcome. Indian J Physiol Pharmacol 1993;37:276–284.

83 Thilly C, Delange F, Lagasse R, et al: Fetal hypothyroidism and maternal thyroid status in severe endemic goiter. J Clin Endocrinol Metab 1978;4:354–360.

84 Kumwenda N, Miotti P, Taha T, et al: Antenatal vitamin A supplementation increases birth weight and decreases anemia among infants born to immunodeficiency virus-infected women in Malawi. Clin Infect Dis 2002;35:618–624.

85 Osrin D, Vaidya A, Shrestha Y, et al: Effects of antenatal multiple micronutrient supplementation on birthweight and gestational duration in Nepal: double-blind, randomised controlled trial. Lancet 2005;365:955–962.

86 Ramakrishnan U, Gonzalez-Cossio T, Neufeld L, et al: Multiple micronutrient supplementation during pregnancy does not lead to greater infant birth size than does iron-only supplementation: a randomized controlled trial in a semirural community in Mexico. Am J Clin Nutr 2003;77:720–725.

87 Fawzi W, Msamaga G, Spiegelman D: Randomised trial of effects of vitamin supplements on pregnancy outcomes and T cell counts in HIV-1 infected women in Tanzania. Lancet 1998;351:1477–1482.

88 Ross S, Nel E, Naeye R: Differing effects of low and high bulk maternal dietary supplements during pregnancy. Early Hum Dev 1985;10:395–302.

Discussion

Dr. Mathur: In the theme of this conference, you showed the obesity interventions in one slide but the focus has been on changing undernutrition. The successes and failures of the programs which you mentioned were mainly on undernutrition. In these societies where undernutrition and overnutrition coexist, can we give this country or any country a single package of nutrition as a policy? While we are tackling undernutrition we are looking at overnutrition also. The policymakers are confused on what would be an appropriate nutritional package. Undernutrition strategies aim at providing something extra, whereas overnutrition policies are restrictive. As a human behavior it is easier to take than to give up, and that is the challenge for all nutrition intervention trials. I suggest we look at some of the behavioral aspects and the new social determinants of health in tackling nutrition problems in coexisting societies.

Dr. Shetty: I think that is a very apt comment. I must apologize because I knew I was the last speaker and the main focus of the symposium was childhood obesity and undernutrition. I have about 5 or 6 slides which deal with the whole issue of population-based approaches and I wanted to highlight how, if you take this population-based approach, you can actually use the success stories of Finland and Norway to show that if you make the sort of changes that are required you can address the problem of chronic diseases in the population. I don't think I have the time to do that here. There are several lessons to be learned. Dr. Popkin spoke first at this meeting and I last, but we both believe that there are major macroeconomic and structural drivers of the changes happening in developing societies, which are contributing to the problem of obesity in these countries. Norway and Finland are two good examples of how they actually went about implementing policies that reduce coronary heart disease in a reasonably short period of time [1].

Non-communicable diseases are preventable. There is good evidence that population-based prevention is cost-effective, and is an affordable option for major public health improvement with regard to both obesity and non-communicable diseases and can bring about major changes in disease burden in a relatively short time. We have to learn lessons from countries which have addressed this issue very seriously. Not all countries have done that. We have to have population-based approaches, we have to use the experience that they have used in changing their food and agricultural policies which have had an impact on the prevention of non-communicable diseases. Norway and Finland are very good examples. In the recent literature there are examples of economic and food policy analysis that implicate the US agricultural policies and farm subsidies from the 1950s in the epidemic of obesity [2, 3]. The European Union promotes the increased consumption of fruits and vegetables; on the other hand it actually subsidizes farmers who are unable to sell their fruits and vegetables by providing what is called 'withdrawal compensation' for the destruction rather than promotion of the consumption of fruits and vegetables by making them available cheaply, particularly to low income households [4]. That is a paradoxical policy and I highlight this only to emphasize that the health sector cannot achieve much unless it understands the whole situation at the national level and acts to influence and change opposing policies and deals with other economic interests to achieve it goals. There are several such examples from which we can learn, and we can learn from positive experiences, and also from negative experiences. The last point that I would like to address is that the health sector, i.e. the people concerned with obesity and non-communicable diseases or undernutrition, has very little power within the system of governments. If you look at the health minister's budget in most countries, it is a very small fraction compared to what is spent on everything else. And yet the health sector makes several demands and recommendations for a healthy diet and lifestyles which end up having little impact. We in the health sector have to realize that we have to work with other people in other sectors while understanding their points of view and help influence policies that will be beneficial from a health perspective. We need to temper our demands or do it in such a way that it does not antagonize the interests of other sectors and ensures that all sectors recognize that the health of the population is important because of the economic burden on the nation. The examples of Finland and Norway I provided earlier show how the involvement and close cooperation of other sectors are crucial to success. We also need to emphasize that when we make recommendations for dietary intakes or healthy body weights or BMIs, for example, with population-based approaches we are actually referring to the population mean or median, and our attempt is to shift the distribution so that the median shifts below the recommended level. If we progress towards shifting the distribution we will achieve a lot more in terms of public health benefit. If you shift the median of the distribution of the risk factor, the incidence or burden of the disease is lowered [5]. In summary, we need the sort of approaches which take into consideration the macro changes within the food system that occur with economic development and the political will to implement the necessary policies to favor healthy diets and lifestyles.

Dr. Popkin: I just want to add a couple of things to Dr. Mathur's comments because they are relevant. First, in many countries around the world, particularly in Latin America today, there are still pockets of undernutrition as you mentioned. In contrast, Mexico has effectively eliminated acute malnutrition except for tiny pockets. In Asia and Sub-Saharan Africa we have larger numbers of acutely malnourished children. India is not at the point of Mexico. In South Asia the difficulty is we know what we need to do for children to deal with underweight and so much of it relates to birthweight and weaning foods in that critical period from prenatal to infants. But the difficulty we are facing in many countries is how to shift the lower end of the BMI distribution without much more rapidly shifting the upper end rightwards. This is where the complexity lies at the national level. We haven't figured out how to do that and it is particularly worrisome for India because we are beginning to see IGT forming in rural areas, with low BMIs for women and men and so forth. So the question of what BMI we need to shift to, and given this very unique etiology, is a complex one. Then we come to all the classic strategies. We clearly know breastfeeding can work for everyone. Once we move beyond that we usually deal with energy density issues for infant feeding, and we typically even think about protein density for pregnancy. But the complexity here is that very quickly, depending where you are in the spectrum, it creates negative things. Now Dr. Shetty mentioned a very small, not so well-done study in Chile showing that in programs dealing with undernutrition, when undernutrition improved and the –1 z score was changed for targeting children and preschoolers for food programs, and the children became overweight from those programs. PROGRESA is a huge study affecting 20 million people in Mexico, which is a much bigger country than Chile with over 100 million people, and the same thing has happened. In fact we just changed the whole PROGRESA program to move from whole milk to skim milk and a number of other things to try to deal with some of the programs in that country. In India where there is still so much undernutrition in rural areas; could you imagine for example moving to skim milk, it would be wonderful if you could even get some milk into children and infants in the rural areas. This is really a unique circumstance in South Asia, but in general it is not so different from what we faced in China. I could show the same kind of evidence for China as for Mexico and Chile. So we really have an issue in Asia. Africa is very different because there you have got either HIV in South Africa, or CHD. We have got two worlds presenting some extremely complex public health challenges related to body image. How do we reduce adult obesity while not making people think that adult has HIV/AIDS.

Dr. Ganapathy: Our patients visit a doctor when their child is thin and frail, undernourished as they call it. There is no awareness of obesity. Obesity is still a cosmetic problem and a storage issue. I think there is a need for the awareness that adipose tissue is an important endocrine system, a source of inflammatory cytokines that can give rise to chronic disease. Health education definitely plays a role. In rapid urbanization, children skip breakfast and get packed lunches. With working parents, not even a single meal is shared by the family. Their sleep patterns are also messy; no proper sleep hygiene.

Dr. Sesikaran: When we were students in school in India, we used to have the National Cadet Corps which ensured regular physical activity of at least 1 h almost every alternate day. That has been stopped, and now in schools we are unable to bring in physical activity.

Dr. Sawaya: For the last 2 years at our centers, we have been treating both obese and malnourished children. Although the social problems might be slightly different talking about slum children, it is true that at least 40% of the families have 1 malnourished child and 1 obese adult in the same family. If you a good adequate diet is given, body mass, especially fat mass, decreases and lean mass increases, and there is also recovery from malnutrition. In our experience it is much more a social question, for example the way the mother cares for her child, if lunch and dinner are provided and the type of food eaten, thinking more of the environment in the context of the family. But in terms of nutrients and food, in our experience the treatment for obesity in children and the treatment for malnutrition are practically the same.

Dr. Subramanian: In one of your slides you showed that there seems to be no evidence about the role of iodine in birth outcome, but the later slide includes salt iodization as part of the package for improving maternal and child nutrition. Why is iodine not considered important for birth outcome?

Dr. Shetty: I just looked at the evidence in the Cochrane review showing that iodine supplementation alone has no impact on birthweight, on pregnancy outcome. Iodine cannot be ignored because we know that there are periods with iodine deficiency, and also that there are other ill effects of not having enough iodine. Therefore we want to ensure that there is enough iodine. But giving iodine alone has no impact, that is the paradox.

Dr. Subramanian: You mentioned the LAKASS program and made a good summary of all the strengths as well as some weaknesses of what make community-based programs successful. We want to call them area-based, starting from a good analysis of the situation in an area. The combination and presentation of the package of services need not be the same for different communities, even in the same country because of cultural and regional differences. What is really very important here is political commitment, good leadership. Especially in a country like ours where political exercise happens more often than we desire. When there is a change in local leadership, we have to make sure that the program is sustained. Political participation is very important; how the program is run. When there is a change in local leadership and the people who run the government, surveillance is necessary. Local government needs feedback on what is happening, so that they continue to support the local programs.

References

1 Shetty PS, Mc Pherson K (eds): Diet, Nutrition and Chronic Disease: Lessons from Contrasting Worlds. London, Wiley, 1997.
2 Institute for Agriculture and Trade Policy: The Farm Bill and Public Health: An Overview. Minneapolis, Institute for Agriculture and Trade Policy, 2007. http://www.healthobservatory. org/library.cfm?RefID=99606. Accessed October 2007.
3 Muller M, Schoonover H, Wallinga D: Considering the Contribution of US Food and Agriculture Policy to the Obesity Epidemic: Overview and Opportunities. Minneapolis, Institute for Agriculture and Trade Policy, 2007. http://wwwhealthobersvatory.org/library. cfm?RefID=99607. Accessed October 2007.
4 European Public Health Alliance: Public Health Aspects of EU Common Agricultural Policy. Brussels, European Public Health Alliance, 2006. http://www.epha.org/a/2359?var_ rechrche=CAP+vegetables. Accessed November 2007.
5 Rose G: The Strategy of Preventive Medicine. Oxford, Oxford University Press, 1992.

Kalhan SC, Prentice AM, Yajnik CS (eds): Emerging Societies – Coexistence of Childhood Malnutrition
and Obesity.
Nestlé Nutr Inst Workshop Ser Pediatr Program, vol 63, pp 259–268,
Nestec Ltd., Vevey/S. Karger AG, Basel, © 2009.

Concluding Remarks

I am going to summarize very briefly what I understood from the talks in the session which I shared with *Bhaskar Raju*. The first one was given by *Andrew Prentice*. It was a brilliant lecture, and he spoke of a number of things which I had always tried to understand, but I had never understood them before. Today I don't have much difficulty actually putting this together. His talk was the evolutionary origins of obesity and the contribution of rapid nutritional transition. He stressed that the rapid increase in obesity has only been over the last few decades. Then he raised the question, 'Are developing populations more susceptible? Do we have any indications in the evolutionary analysis?' He discussed the thrifty gene hypothesis which proposes that the thrifty genes deposit more fat during food availability. These are positively selected when food is not available because these people are able to use their energy stores. He then raised the issue that all populations have faced, famine which is episodic rather than a long-term supply problem. By definition everyone alive today must carry the thrifty genes. He challenged the original description that selection is related to viability and showed evidence that selection is more related to fertility. He quoted recent work from Cambridge on genetic syndromes of obesity. Almost all of them are related to the control of appetite in the hypothalamus, there is hardly any genetic syndrome related to an energy expenditure problem. We don't have any experimental support for the thrifty genes. The recently describe FTO gene polymorphism has been replicated in the majority of European populations, but not in Africans., In Indians it is strongly related to diabetes, but weakly or not related to obesity. So in Indians it remains a diabetes gene but not an obesity gene. I interpret this to indicate a basic difference in Indians and Europeans about how obesity is related to diabetes. I think the geneticists have provided us with an exciting marker whose epigenetic regulation may reveal fundamental processes in this pathway. Dr. Prentice also thought that with the genome-wide search clever statisticians are going to provide us with some answers very soon.

Concluding Remarks

Parul Christian spoke on the prenatal origins of undernutrition and made the important point that the high prevalence of childhood stunting and wasting occurs in parts of the world where low birthweight is common. She showed that low birthweight increases the risk of stunting by 2–5 times. She then highlighted that IUGR rather than prematurity contributes to subsequent stunting. She discussed factors which determine birthweight and IUGR. Intervention is possible for pre-gestational factors, e.g. maternal age, parity, inter-pregnancy interval, maternal size at the time of pregnancy and maternal education, and a number of gestational factors, such as weight gain, diet, physical activity, stress, toxins including tobacco. Clearly more research is needed and we had a lot of discussion on this. During the discussion I think we all agreed that rather than weight we need more refined measurements of size and body composition so that we can dissect these problems further. Animal models could be useful, and we discussed some of these models.

Marc-André Prost told us about postnatal origins and he showed us that, despite a lot of interest in obesity, nutritional deficiencies are still among the top 15 causes of mortality in the world. Nutritional problems lead to impaired physical growth, cognitive development, reduced economic productivity, and increased morbidity and mortality. He also discussed the UNICEF scheme of undernutrition. He showed a graph, which I found very interesting, that length faltering starts much earlier than weight faltering. He stressed 3 factors which affect postnatal nutrition and postnatal growth, i.e. inadequate nutrition, infections, and problems related to care. He pointed out that mothers' nutrition is important for the quality of the breast milk and that problems could arise by relatively early complementary feeding at the cost of breastfeeding. Iron and zinc are important for growth between 6 and 23 months of age. He finally stressed the issue of societal care and its components including the GDP of the country, safe water supply, sanitation and healthcare facilities.

Finally *Anne-Lydia Sawaya* made a brilliant presentation. She said that stunting in the slums of Brazil reflects both malnutrition and poverty which are inseparable, therefore any approach and intervention must tackle both. In her experience 70% of stunted children had low birthweight. She shared with us her experience with these children and stressed the team approach which makes a lot of difference to the results. The comprehensive approach includes dietary, educational, social support, and treatment of associated conditions. She also talked of her research on risks of stunting, which is associated with adiposity and metabolic risk factors. In her studies successful height recovery reverses the majority of these changes except blood pressure. Further intervention studies are needed in this population.

Chittaranjan S. Yajnik

We had a session on the mechanisms of metabolic damage or what we should be calling the mechanisms of injury. We started with an outstanding summary of genomic methylation and epigenetics from a geneticist perspective. It was important to learn that there is only a small group of genes that have been identified so far, so-called metastable epialleles which are sensitive to environmental influences, and they undergo molecular changes such as methylation, acetylation, and that these changes remain permanent and for a lifetime. There was an important lesson to be learned from that. The second lesson was that the lifestyle of one generation can significantly influence the health of the next generation. The best example is that the intrauterine environment can influence growth of the embryo at multiple developmental stages.

Then *Emma Whitelaw* left us with the challenge: what the true transgenerational genetic inheritance of these traits is, is the embryo affected by the maternal environment or nutrient environment or whatever the other components of the environment are. So far there is not a very good evidence to confirm the transgenerational inheritance of these traits in humans, and it will require a definitive confirmation with improved modern and newer technologies. I am not sure that we will find the answer because as we learned that the blastocyst goes through massive demethylation and all the methyls are lost, and the fertilized embryo becomes a pleuripotent stem cell from where all the tissue's specific genes are expressed, and for example the liver cells become the liver and the brain cells become the brain. Then the question arises: what are these inheritable traits that are affecting the genome, and why they are surviving through that demethylation stage? This question has not been answered and is a challenge for the future.

In my own talk I tried to convey that methionine along with folate are the key methyl donors for a large number of methyltransferase reactions, there are a lot of methylation processes occurring on throughout the organism/and that every cell expresses the methionine cycle. Because methionine metabolism requires several vitamins, B_{12}, folate, pyridoxine, etc., and cofactors, it is regulated by a number of hormones, nutrient and environment changes can easily influence methionine metabolism and therefore the methylation status of the developing organism, and possibly cause permanent effects and programming. The last part is a speculation which needs to be confirmed. There is experimental evidence showing that alteration in folate metabolism does cause some changes in the methylation status of the genome and this can be reversed by appropriate nutrient supplementation and interventions.

Then we heard from *Eric Ravussin,* and the highlight of his talk was the issue of calorie restriction. As we know from a lot of animal studies, calorie restriction has a favorable effect on a number of physiological, hormonal and biochemical parameters and biomarkers of longevity. The interest in the biomarkers of longevity has to do with the changes in mitochondrial biogenesis particularly in the skeletal muscle, the change in the core temperature and in overall energy metabolism. He discussed at length that, in the presence of increased mitochondrial biogenesis, the changes in energy metabolism were going somewhat in the opposite direction, which is a very interesting and challenging issue to address in the future.

Vidya Subramanian next convinced us that obesity induces a complex inflammatory state by both inter- as well as intracellular signaling pathways. There is infiltration of macrophages in the adipose tissue associated with systemic metabolic responses such as the development of insulin resistance in the skeletal muscle, in the liver, through various cytokines and other molecular mechanisms. There is a whole corollary to this phenomena and she showed us evidence to support these concepts.

Finally *Arthur McCullough* introduced us to the consequences of atopic fat in the liver and non-alcoholic fatty liver disease, a rapidly emerging disease worldwide. We recognize it in Western societies with a rapidly increasing obesity, insulin resistance and inflammation. Ultimately it leads to hepatocellular degeneration, cirrhosis and other consequences. He showed us a number of intervention strategies, described the molecular mechanisms of fibrosis. Thus far the success of many of these interventions has been low. This particular syndrome is not necessarily confined to Western societies, it is rapidly increasing in emerging societies too.

Satish C. Kalhan

It is the end of a long day and a very fruitful meeting, so I will try to be rapid. We started our meeting by setting the scene for the later discussions. *Barry Popkin* gave us a lot of information that actually we are very well aware of, and we are well aware of it mostly due to Barry's work and his writing about this and the infiltration into the mass media. Congratulations. He addressed the global juggernaut in terms of food policies, changes in the dietary supply, changes in transportation and all the issues that are associated with this enormous global transformation. This is the first time that any species has so radically changed its own environment in such a way as to profoundly change its pattern of lifestyle and ultimately its physiology. We want to use that to perhaps amend some of the changes that we can predict are going to occur in the emerging nations. We got a picture of that for China from *Shi-an Yin*, for India from *Srinath Reddy* and for Africa. What we saw was that although these regions are at very different stages of change, in fact if the underlying themes are examined there is a very strong unified story as to where we come from and where we are going. I guess the overall message is that because some continents, and I am thinking particularly of the US and then Europe, have gone there first, surely those of us who are later behind the malnutrition-demographic transition should be able to learn something from the mistakes that have gone before. Whether we are able to do that or not remains to be seen.

In summarizing Session 4, there is again an underlying theme to all of the talks. I think it is possible to take away from any one of these talks something that we in the audience can do about the problem because that is ultimately what we are here for: to try to design interventions, be they in our pediatric clinic, be they in our special care baby unit, or wherever we work whether that is perhaps as a director of an institute of medical research or someone working in the private sector. We want to do something about this problem.

Ranjan Yajnik in his usual manner displayed his innovative thinking in the way that his research here in India has really lead the field. Obviously we have to give *David Barker* a great deal of credit for this, but I think *Ranjan Yajnik* is the one who is pushing the boundaries now and I think it is an immense credit that it is happening here in India, and congratulations to you and all your colleagues. What he told us was that diabetes is going to show a 300% predicted increase and we will have 18 million diabetics in India by 2025. He told us very clearly that the preventative efforts are starting too late and they are far too costly; we already cannot afford them and if you project those numbers forward, then we definitely cannot afford to be treating these people who have already got all these obesity-related comorbidities. He also made the important point that it only postpones the problem anyway, and in fact a very interesting cost-effectiveness analysis was published a couple of months ago [1] showing that actually the aggregated costs of keeping people alive and treating their obesity and diabetes are in the end going to cost us more. The sad fact is that people who die are very cheap. Keeping people alive is going to cost a lot more if those people have the associated obesity and metabolic defects. It is not an argument that he actually used but I think it strengthens very strongly the argument that *Ranjan Yajnik* was making, that we have got to stop trying to look at these things in the post-reproduction phase because that brings no benefit to the offspring and therefore is really not investing in the future. We are just trying to put out fires as they exist at the moment. And so there is a very strong imperative to look at the life-course approach. That was the real essence of *Ranjan Yajnik's* message. The situation is still confusing, a lot of it is an unfinished agenda, we don't understand yet how best to tackle this, but work is in progress. Disharmonious growth was obviously a very important part of the problem, and we find ourselves in a sort of intellectual trap: if we can't affect growth at any stage of the lifecycle without having problems downstream, then how can we do anything, and that is something that *Ranjan Yajnik* has written and talked about. The core of his interest at the moment relates to B_{12} and folate and the intriguing imbalances between those and the fact that we really need to be very careful how we intervene, and there will be issues of course for discussions as to how extrapolatable that is.

Staffan Polberger gave us a micro example of interventions and what we could do. He described the necessity of dealing with very low birthweight babies and how in his particular special care baby unit they are trying to individualize that. Very impressive work within that setting, there were controversy and arguments later as to whether that is affordable even in a Swedish special care baby setting. But clearly it points the way forward and ultimately this kind of individualized approach to nutrition is going to be something that will be affordable in many populations. We can add to that the possibility that we will know every individual's genetic profile which will help form that argument also.

Dewan Alam gave us a wide ranging review of the factors that affect low birthweight, and the fact that some of these are modifiable, some of them are not. Most of his talk was really about supplementation. He warned us that there are many reasons why there may be limited effectiveness of supplementation, and then he gave us a summary of the effects of those supplements as we know them so far. He talked about balanced protein energy supplementation, really very modest effects. I totally accept the points that were made later about the fact that our Gambian trial really has major weighting in the Cochrane analysis and that if you take that out then there is a very minor effect altogether, and the cost-effectiveness of that is very dubious. Single micronutrient interventions showed surprisingly little evidence of positive effects. Many multiple micronutrient trials have been published recently. We are starting to get a much more informed evidence based on this, some of them showing benefits, some of them showing benefits over and above iron and folate, and some of them not. I guess if you came down and said what is interesting about the issue you would say actually it is difficult to shift birthweight by more than 50 g, and that is a very small effect on birthweight. So then we talk about increasing the left hand side of the birthweight distribution, and a lot of these programs are quite effective at reducing low birthweight, so that is good news.

Finally *Prakash Shetty* gave us a really comprehensive analysis of community-based intervention trials. There is evidence to suggest that interventions to improve maternal nutrition and health are the most successful, which comes back to *Ranjan Yajnik's* point about lifecycle approaches. Again if there is a theme coming out of this meeting, it is the huge importance of early intervention and lifecycle approaches. The nutrition transition definitely places new challenges and the need for a modification of programs. We have discussed the fact that we need to be looking at both ends of the spectrum of undernutrition and overnutrition. The new interventions need to be integrated and joined up. They must start very early in life and must concentrate on both ends of the burden. It is very important that evaluation is conducted. A lot of programs must be scaled up if they are available, and sustainability requires political will, resources in terms of both money and people, and community involvement. When invited to give us other additional slides, he made some very pertinent comments about not just the community-based interventions but what we should be aiming for at the national level, and gave us examples of where there has been success.

There are some final cross-cutting conclusions. It is critical to tackle the issues very early in the lifecycle. I think that has come out loud and clear from our meeting here. The evidence base on how to intervene is growing but there remain huge research questions. I know scientists are always saying we need more research money and there is more research to be done, and I genuinely think this is the case. In whom should we intervene, when, at what stages in the lifecycle should we intervene, and how do those interact with each other? How do we balance the short- and long-term benefits and risks? It seems that if we benefit one short-term endpoint, we may be harming a longer term end-point, so we have to learn a lot about that. How do we disentangle the very complex matrix of possibly conflicting effects of interventions? The material we heard from *Satish Kalhan* in terms of the complexities of the methionine cycle and a rather overlapping complexity from *Ranjan Yajnik* in terms of the folate-B_{12} angle, just give us a little glimpse at some of the enormous complexities of this. And finally, in the meantime how do we guide health professionals and governments; what as pediatricians can we do, and what do we tell our colleagues as a result of this meeting?

Andrew M. Prentice

Discussion

Dr. Prentice: I had a specific request from the audience for a final discussion: can we please talk about what messages we take back to our pediatric clinics and our colleagues? I think it would be especially useful if we could just spend a few minutes discussing that.

Anonymous: To me the topics that have been discussed during these 3 days have been very diverse. From the very depth of the presentations from the biomedical level to the community level, it is difficult to think who will take what kind of message home. Probably it depends on individual interests. As a pediatrician the message that I have taken from these presentations is that we should look into the totality of the matters, as far as the children are concerned, undernutrition is concerned, and obesity is concerned. Unless and until we take it as a total message, as a package and not in piecemeal fashion, and until we have sifted through the opportunities from the top to the bottom, it will be difficult to solve the problem.

Anonymous: The message that I as a pediatrician will take back would be first in all certainly prevent obesity in the child who was born low birthweight or SGA. We don't know what is catch-up growth is, but we certainly must not allow them to become obese at any time during their lifecycle. The second message would be that in all these babies, regardless the diets we give them or what growth monitoring we do, they must be monitored for the metabolic syndrome early in their lives because that will really show us what is harmful or beneficial to the baby.

Anonymous: From my understanding of all that we have discussed today, I think we are actually looking at supervisory nutrition for everyone, from childhood to adulthood, and even in the case of the obese child. During supervisory nutrition, when the child is catching up it gets to the point where you know that at this age there should be some control of the child's diet. With this supervisory nutrition you do not stop certain types of intervention and begin another type, and that is what I see in the issue of catch-up growth in the young child. Then for the general population at large, I think we need to begin to look at the situation of population intervention, whereby the government is responsible for making some policies as we heard yesterday; policies to ensure that globally nutrition is apt in our countries, support for the resources available in each nation as far as agricultural products are concerned, and in the light of research, I think preventive measures are something that a bigger authority ought to be looking at. I find it very sad that, within the same household, some people are undernourished and some people are overnourished. We have to ensure supervisory nutrition for all with education for the household, knowing what is needed for the household. That is one of the message I would like to take home as a community nutritionist. Individuals in the household should know what is right to eat; adequate nutrition is the key in every household. At the government level, the authorities have control over the resources of the country, and they are responsible for supporting food agriculture, the nutrition of the people, and also to make information available to the people. With regard to catch-up growth, the child must be observed so that it will not suffer all the disease outcomes in adulthood.

Dr. Singhal: Can I just go back to an important point for pediatricians, the monitoring of follow-up of SGA babies in terms of the metabolic syndrome. There was a consensus statement published last year on the management of the SGA baby which states that you should not be monitoring for the metabolic syndrome [2] because programming is based on populations an not on individuals. The positive predictive value of all programming factors is small for the individual. There is a difference between populations and individuals. Pediatricians are concerned with the individual for whom there is very little evidence of benefits of surveillance. Now regarding the question whether we promote growth fin SGA babies, I come back to the answer I gave early. It depends on the population you are interested in. The same consensus statement argues that in the West there is no indication for the promotion of catch-up growth in these babies [2].

Anonymous: I was actually very amazed by Finland where food habits changed and there was a major decrease in ischemic heart disease and diabetes by behavioral change. There the women definitely took the step. But what about the Third World; how do we communicate these things to our governments? It is difficult. I don't see epidemiologists trying to communicate this to the government. What they did in Finland is an excellent thing, simply taking skim milk instead of a lot of soft drinks. About the food habits, this is also a matter of mass media. Mass media can also help us to spread this message especially in underdeveloped countries where education is another problem.

Dr. Prentice: In relation to your question, I think this comes back to what Dr. Shetty was saying that money speaks and governments listen when it is going to hurt them, when it is going to hurt their pockets or going to hurt them being reelected. One of the problems is that it is mostly going to hurt the pockets of governments five governments ahead, so it is difficult to concentrate the mind of governments of today. In the UK our Prime Minister actually called in the head of National Westminster Bank to do a future analysis on this, and he made reports which really did paint a very gloomy picture of the future if we didn't do anything about it, and now I think the UK is really moving and trying to do things and certainly it is suddenly taking the issue seriously. So I think this comes back to the point Dr. Shetty was saying about the necessity of cost analysis.

Dr. Chittal: This has been a wonderful experience, like standing in front of the Mona Lisa painting or the Taj Mahal. I am admiring, I am appreciative, but I am also baffled and I don't know what I am admiring and I don't know what I am taking back home. I can't change government, I can't even change the government's opinion, but I need to take something home for my patients. I look after small IUGR preterm babies, I encourage them to put on weight, but yet I need to warn them somewhere. Dr. Singhal says there is no point monitoring individual babies for the risk of type 2 diabetes; I need some marker, I need to monitor that. Is HOMA the marker or is insulin resistance the marker? I need one biochemical marker with which I can predict that this baby is going the wrong way. If I take that home, then yes, I have learned something.

Dr. Prentice: Let's not lose sight of the certainties that we do have and one of those certainties was articulated in the very first point in this discussion which is, avoid obesity. Now how you measure that as a pediatrician is another issue, but I think let's hang on to at least some of the things that we do know and then we know other things which Dr. Sawaya has been articulating about balanced diet and common sense, not losing sight of common sense. It may sound boring when related to the complexities of the methionine cycle, but we must not lose sight of those things as well.

Dr. Pandit: The last two and a half days have been like a movie which played in the Western world, in the developed world, at the end of the 19th century and early 20th century, which exposed itself as diabetes and cardiovascular disease; in the mid 1950s, it kind of slowed down in the West. Now this same movie is being shown in the East, in the developing countries. Only the characters have changed, there is a new character called affluence, otherwise it is the same movie. The West had an infant mortality of 200 per 1,000 at the end of 19th century which was also here some years ago and that resulted in diabetes hybridization in the 1950s in the West, and today we are facing the same. So it is a movie replayed with a new character, affluence.

Dr. Prentice: It is a movie, and when they do screen tests in Hollywood they ask the audience to chose between different endings. What we have got to do is to try and chose a happy ending.

Dr. Pandit: There is no micro-message that comes from this. I think we should get sensitized to the fact that government programs are basically research to be conducted not on an individual child basis but looking at the associations, not a cause and effect relationship. What we have discussed for the last two and half days are association paradigms, they are not cause and effect. Pediatricians like us came here to look at cause and effect, and it is not possible in two and half days.

Dr. Kikafunda: My message is to Africa. As was reported on the first day, there are limited data on the problem of obesity and its consequences in most African countries, particularly Sub-Saharan Africa. When there are no data, you believe there is no problem. But the problem is huge. Every 5 years demographic and health surveys are carried out. On nutrition, they only report on stunting, underweight, wasting and micronutrient deficiencies. The columns for overweight and obesity are left blank! So let us get data, and then we can face the problem.

Dr. Prentice: Because I was presenting the last session, it is only by accident that I am standing up here. Dr. Kalhan and Dr. Yajnik, do you want to make any closing comments before we the conference is closed

Dr. Kalhan: My only comment is to look at the big picture. Biology has to move and we have to investigate all aspects of it. All these things that we have heard over the last two days, from basic sciences to genetics, to epidemiology, these are not mutually exclusive, they complement each other, we learn from these and create new paradigms and we tackle the problems.

Dr. Yajnik: I have to say that I enjoyed the last 3 days. Thanks to Nestlé for organizing this and thanks to everyone for your very active participation. I am taking home a number of new ideas to test in our studies. Thank you everybody.

Concluding Remarks

References

1 van Baal PH, Polder JJ, de Wit GA, et al: Lifetime medical costs of obesity: prevention no cure for increasing health expenditure. PLoS Med 2008;5:e29.
2 Clayton PE, Cianfarani S, Czernichow P, et al: Management of the child born small for gestational age through to adulthood: a consensus statement of the International Societies of Pediatric Endocrinology and the Growth Hormone Research Society. J Clin Endocrinol Metab 2007;92:804–810.

Subject Index